Atlas of Early Neoplasias of the Gastrointestinal Tract

Frieder Berr • Tsuneo Oyama
Thierry Ponchon • Naohisa Yahagi
Editors

Atlas of Early Neoplasias of the Gastrointestinal Tract

Endoscopic Diagnosis and Therapeutic Decisions

Second Edition

Springer

Editors
Frieder Berr
Department of Internal Medicine I
Paracelsus Medical University
Salzburg
Austria

Thierry Ponchon
Department of Digestive Diseases
Hôpital Eduard Herriot
Lyon
France

Tsuneo Oyama
Department of Endoscopy
Saku Central Hospital Advanced Care Center
Saku
Nagano
Japan

Naohisa Yahagi
Division of Research and Development
for Minimally Invasive Treatment
Cancer Center
Keio University School of Medicine
Shinjuku-ku
Tokyo
Japan

ISBN 978-3-030-01113-0 ISBN 978-3-030-01114-7 (eBook)
https://doi.org/10.1007/978-3-030-01114-7

Library of Congress Control Number: 2019930836

This Springer imprint is published by the registered company Springer Nature Switzerland AG
The registered company address is: Gewerbestrasse 11, 6330 Cham, Switzerland

This book is dedicated to all colleagues who strive for proficiency in image-enhanced endoscopic analysis of early gastrointestinal cancers. Accurate endoscopic staging of superficial neoplasias results in correct indications for appropriate resection technique and serves the best interest of the patients.

Salzburg, August 15, 2018 *The Editors*

Preface

"State-of-the-art endoscopic skills best serve the patient"

Since the first edition of this endoscopy atlas and compendium of indications, endoscopic en bloc resection based on ESD techniques has proven equally curative for the resection of early GI cancers as major resective surgery. And the techniques are now refined for ESD of early cancer as well as for endoscopic tunneling resection of symptomatic or pre-/malignant early intramural tumors. Consequently, some Western guidelines have adopted the principle of endoscopic en bloc resection of malignant appearing GI neoplasias, whereas others still adhere to piecemeal snaring techniques for early cancer in Barrett's esophagus or colorectum – assigning diagnostic competence exclusively afterward to the histopathologist.

In the last decade, a network of pioneering referral centers throughout Western countries has reported on implementation of ESD technique. And the endoscopic electrosurgical performance – as taken by high rates of en bloc resection and low rates of emergency surgery and mortality – are nearly approaching East Asian standards. However, the rates of curative resection by ESD still lag behind East Asian standards due mainly to poor prediction of submucosal invasion and less to inadequate delineation of lateral margins or multiple foci of early cancer.

The updated and slightly extended second edition of this atlas on early GI neoplasias *aims* to increase *detection* of pre-/malignant neoplasias in the earliest stage, predict the *tumor category* with high accuracy, and *make the indication* for the least invasive curative resection technique based on this diagnosis. An effort is needed to accomplish professionalism and best serve the patients. The learning curve to professional image-enhanced endoscopy and accurate endoscopic diagnosis of early GI cancers may take up to 2 years, until the technique becomes a rapid and accurate routine procedure. We publish this atlas and compendium for those who strive to accomplish state-of-the-art endoscopic diagnosis and treatment of early GI neoplasias.

Salzburg, Austria Frieder Berr
Saku, Nagano, Japan Tsuneo Oyama
Lyon, France Thierry Ponchon
Shinjuku-ku, Tokyo, Japan Naohisa Yahagi
August 20, 2018

Acknowledgments

The special thanks of the editors and authors go to all who have relentlessly contributed to the text and figures of the book, in particular Dr. Tobias Kiesslich of Salzburg and Dr. Akiko Takahashi of Nagano, as well as to the staff of Springer US, Clinical Medicine publishers, especially Mr. Andy Kwan and Mr. Richard Hruska, senior editor, Clinical Medicine.

Salzburg, August 15, 2018 The editors

Contents

Part I General Principles of Endoscopy for Early Gastrointestinal Neoplasias

1 Endoscopic Detection and Analysis of Mucosal Neoplastic Lesions: Enhanced Imaging and Tumor Morphology ... 3
Frieder Berr, Thierry Ponchon, and Toshio Uraoka

2 Histopathology of Early Mucosal Neoplasias: Morphologic Carcinogenesis in the GI Tract ... 25
Daniel Neureiter and Tobias Kiesslich

3 Principles of Endoscopic Resection: Diagnostic and Curative Resection of Mucosal Neoplasias ... 47
Tsuneo Oyama and Naohisa Yahagi

4 Subepithelial Gastrointestinal Tumors: Diagnosis and Indications for Resection ... 63
Frieder Berr, Jürgen Hochberger, and Tsuneo Oyama

5 High-Resolution Endoscopic Ultrasound: Clinical T-Staging of Superficial and Subepithelial Gastrointestinal Neoplasias ... 79
Hans Seifert, Daisuke Kikuchi, and Naohisa Yahagi

6 Endoscopic Screening and Surveillance: Indications and Standards ... 101
Thierry Ponchon, Frieder Berr, and Tsuneo Oyama

Part II Organ-Specific Endoscopic Analysis of Early Neoplasias

7 Squamous Cell-Lined Esophagus and Hypopharynx: Mucosal Neoplasias 121
Tsuneo Oyama

8 Columnar Epithelium-Lined (Barrett's) Esophagus: Mucosal Neoplasias 149
Pierre H. Deprez and Takashi Toyonaga

9 Stomach: Mucosal Neoplasias 175
Tsuneo Oyama

10 Duodenum and Small Bowel: Mucosal Neoplasias 223
Motohiko Kato, Naohisa Yahagi, and Thierry Ponchon

11 Colorectum: Mucosal Neoplasias 241
Andrej Wagner, Tadateru Maehata, Frieder Berr, and Naohisa Yahagi

12 Chronic Inflammatory Bowel Disease in Remission: Mucosal Neoplasias 291
Naohisa Yahagi, Tadateru Maehata, and Atsushi Nakayama

Appendix: Terminology 307

Index 311

Contributors

Frieder Berr Department of Internal Medicine I, Paracelsus Medical University, Salzburg, Austria

Pierre H. Deprez Department of Hepato-Gastroenterologie, Cliniques Universitaires Saint-Luc, Université Catholique de Louvain, Brussels, Belgium

Jürgen Hochberger Department of Gastroenterology, Vivantes Klinikum Berlin Friedrichshain, Berlin, Germany

Motohiko Kato Division of Research and Development for Minimally Invasive Treatment, Cancer Center, Keio University School of Medicine, Shinjuku-ku, Tokyo, Japan

Tobias Kiesslich Department of Internal Medicine I & Institute of Physiology and Pathophysiology, Paracelsus Medical University, Salzburg, Austria

Daisuke Kikuchi Department of Gastroenterology and Endoscopy Unit, Toranomon Hospital, Tokyo, Japan

Tadateru Maehata Division of Research and Development for Minimally Invasive Treatment, Cancer Center, Keio University School of Medicine, Shinjuku-ku, Tokyo, Japan

Atsushi Nakayama Division of Research and Development for Minimally Invasive Treatment, Cancer Center, Keio University School of Medicine, Shinjuku ku, Tokyo, Japan

Daniel Neureiter Institute of Pathology, Paracelsus Medical University, Salzburg, Austria

Tsuneo Oyama Department of Endoscopy, Saku Central Hospital Advanced Care Center, Saku, Nagano, Japan

Thierry Ponchon Department of Digestive Diseases, Hôpital Eduard Herriot, Lyon, France

Hans Seifert Department of Internal Medicine – Gastroenterology, University Hospital Oldenburg, Oldenburg, Germany

Takashi Toyonaga Department of Endoscopy, Kobe University Hospital, Kobe, Japan

Toshio Uraoka Department of Gastroenterology and Hepatology, Gunma University Hospital, Maebashi, Prefecture Gunma, Japan

Andrej Wagner Department of Internal Medicine I, University Hospital, Paracelsus Medical University, Salzburg, Austria

Naohisa Yahagi Division of Research and Development for Minimally Invasive Treatment, Cancer Center, Keio University School of Medicine, Shinjuku-ku, Tokyo, Japan

Part I
General Principles of Endoscopy for Early Gastrointestinal Neoplasias

Chapter 1
Endoscopic Detection and Analysis of Mucosal Neoplastic Lesions: Enhanced Imaging and Tumor Morphology

Frieder Berr, Thierry Ponchon, and Toshio Uraoka

1.1 Introduction

Worldwide, the gastrointestinal (GI) tract is the organ system with the highest cancer incidence (20.5% of all new cases) and annual mortality (22% = 1.81 Mio). Early endoscopic detection and resection has led to improved survival rates for colorectal and gastric cancer, especially for gastric cancer in Japan, where more than 70% are now detected as early gastric cancer [1, 2].

The majority of esophageal and gastric cancers and about 50% of colorectal cancers (CRC) develop from flat precursor lesions [3, 4]. However, small (5–10 mm) or minute (<5 mm) flat neoplasias are easily missed on standard upper or lower GI endoscopy. The miss rate of such lesions had been estimated to be up to 19% [5]. Detection of small early neoplasias requires familiarity with the endoscopic spectrum of neoplastic lesions on conventional white-light imaging (WLI)

F. Berr
Department of Internal Medicine I, Paracelsus Medical University, Salzburg, Austria
e-mail: frieder.berr@pmu.ac.at

T. Ponchon
Department of Digestive Diseases, Hôpital Eduard Herriot, Lyon, France
e-mail: thierry.ponchon@chu-lyon.fr

T. Uraoka (✉)
Department of Gastroenterology and Hepatology, Gunma University Hospital, Maebashi, Prefecture Gunma, Japan
e-mail: turaoka@a3.keio.jp

F. Berr et al. (eds.), *Atlas of Early Neoplasias of the Gastrointestinal Tract*,
https://doi.org/10.1007/978-3-030-01114-7_1

[3, 6], as well as image analysis with the proper use of magnifying and image-enhanced endoscopy (IEE) [7], such as chromoendoscopy (CE) and narrow-band imaging (NBI) techniques [8–12]. Endoscopic microsurface (S) and microvascular (V) architecture have been characterized in normal mucosa and neoplasias by surface microscopic morphometry in comparison with magnified IEE images [13–15].

1.2 Standard Endoscopy and Chromoendoscopy Techniques

Image quality depends on *resolution* and *contrast*. Contrast is the ratio of brightness (light density) between a pattern and its background. Resolution is determined by the pixel number of the image sensor chip (CCD = charge-coupled device) and the optical lens system, as well as the pixel capacity of the video processor and the display monitor; therefore, resolution is enhanced by high-definition endoscopy (HD > 850 000 pixel), thus improving the detection rate of flat neoplasias. Contrast is increased by surface staining (chromoendoscopy, CE, e.g., with indigo carmine) or narrow-band spectral image (NBI) endoscopy [8, 11]. Most video endoscopy systems use a bright xenon lamp as a white light source. But two different systems for color reproduction are in use: the color CCD system with tiny red-green-blue (RGB) color filters in each CCD pixel, used in Western countries (simultaneous RGB system); and the RGB sequential imaging system using a monochromatic (black and white) CCD and color transformation of the light pulses in the video processor (Fig. 1.1a, b), used in Japan, East Asia, and the UK. The color CCD system shows better motion imaging, and the RGB sequential system yields better resolution [11].

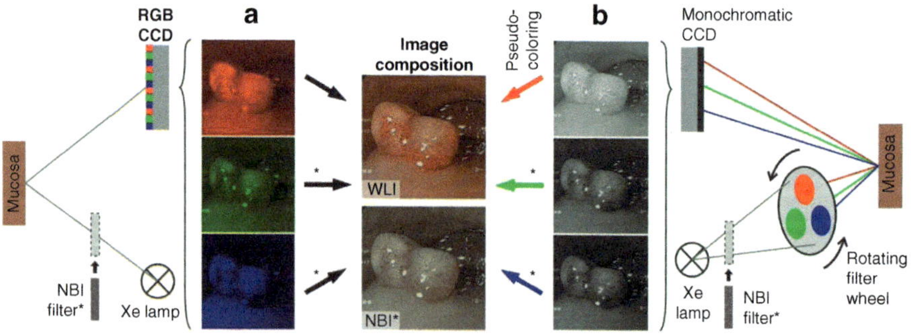

Fig. 1.1 (**a**) Schematic diagram of CCD-based simultaneous color imaging system (EVIS Excera III). *CCD* charge-coupled device. (**b**) Schematic diagram of red-green-blue (RGB) sequential imaging system (EVIS Lucera Spectrum)(Olympus Medical System Co., Tokyo, JP). Insertion of an NBI filter into the Xe-light path eliminates red light and illuminates mucosa with less intense, dual narrow-spectrum light of 415 nm and 540 nm – interacting with the two absorption maxima of hemoglobin. (Modified from Uedo et al. [11])

For *NBI observation* (Fig. 1.1a,b), a narrow band filter is switched into the light path. From the broadband white light of the xenon lamp, two bands with reduced light intensity are split, blue with wavelength of 415 nm and green with 540 nm, corresponding to the absorption peaks of hemoglobin. The light scattered in and reflected from the mucosa shows greenish blue color, and its absorption by hemoglobin in blood vessels shows the complimentary pseudocolor, i.e. brownish and dark cyan. The 415 nm blue light band highlights brownish-appearing capillaries in the lamina propria mucosae (LPM), and the more tissue-penetrating 540 nm green band shows cyan pseudocolored veins in the submucosa, together contrasting the superficial vascular (V) architecture [11, 15] (compare Fig. 1.4). On the other hand, Blue Light Imaging (BLI, Fujifilm Corp., Tokyo) generates similar light bands as NBI without a filter by using four LED (blue-violet, 415 nm / blue / green / red), and thus enhances magnifying surface (S) and vascular (V) imaging [8]. Based on the principles of NBI, alternative processing systems use computer-based filtering of reflected light for spectral light bands in the image processor, e.g., flexible spectral imaging color enhancement (FICE, Fujifilm Corp., Tokyo) or i-Scan tone enhancement (TE) mode (Pentax Medical Corp.,Tokyo) [10, 16].

1.3 Standard White Light Imaging (WLI) and Chromoendoscopy (CE)

Screening and surveillance use light-intense WLI endoscopy for *detection* of early neoplasias focusing on changes in *surface structure* (epithelial architecture) and/or *color* of the mucosa [17]. The more reddish color of neoplastic lesions is due to increased vascular density of the lamina propria mucosa (LPM), decreased glandular layer, or both alterations combined; a more pale color reflects increased gland density / neoplastic cell infitration, diminished vascularized connective tissue of the LPM, or both factors combined. Rarely, neoplasias display the same color as the mucosa. The *analysis* of suspicious lesions is facilitated by CE and HD endoscopy and often is feasible only with enhanced magnification imaging (60–120-fold) of microsurface (S) and microvascular (V) patterns in WLI and NBI or BLI technique [8, 18, 19].

Chromoendoscopy (CE) with acetic acid or indigo carmine enhances the surface structure, whereas Lugol (iodine) solution reacts with squamous epithelial cell membranes; methylene blue and crystal violet are internalized into columnar epithelial cells [3, 20]. Indications for and principles of CE are given in Table 1.1. For application of CE, wash the mucosa and lesion clean with water containing simethicone before absorptive stain – apply dye solution (e.g., 10 mL) for about 1 min, and wash again briefly before imaging. Esophageal squamous neoplasias show Lugol-*unstained* area on WLI, and appearance of slight pink coloring in unstained area after 1–2 min is highly specific for cancer (*pink coloring sign*) [21]. Neutralize the irritant action of Lugol solution immediately after iodine CE using sodium thiosulfate (5% aqueous sol., twice the volume of Lugol solution) [22]. Crystal violet staining is most accurate for irregular colonic microsurface (pit pattern type V; compare Chap. 11).

Table 1.1 Gastrointestinal chromoendoscopy and virtual chromoendoscopy (NBI or BLI)

A. Indications		
Location	**Neoplasia**	**Dye solution or VCE (NBI, BLI)**
Esophagus	Squamous cell cancer	Lugol[a] staining/NBI
	Barrett's HGIN, cancer	Acetic acid (AA)/indigo carmine (IC)/NBI
Stomach	Gastric adenoma, cancer	Indigo carmine (IC)/AIM[b]/NBI
Colon	Adenoma, HGIN, CRC	Indigo carmine (IC)/crystal violet/NBI
B. Application and principles of staining		
Principle	**Solution**	**Target structure/cells**
Reactive	Iodine-potassium iodide (0.75–1.0% aqu.) (Lugol solution)[a]	Squamous epithelial cell (SC) membranes; SC cancer: unstained area with clear demarcation line, "pink coloring sign" after 2 min
Contrasting	Indigo carmine (0.15% aqueous) AIM[b] (0.6% AA, 0.4% IC)	For macroscopic type and border of lesion AIM for identification of lesion border
Absorbed	Crystal violet (0.05% aqueous)[c]	Colonic epithelium

HGIN high-grade intraepithelial neoplasia, *VCE* virtual chromoendoscopy
[a]Avoid exposure of the larynx, iodine allergy, and hyperthyreosis! (comp. Chap. 7)
[b]AIM, freshly prepared mixture of 0.6% acetic acid and 0.4% indigo carmine [23]
[c]After spraying indigo carmine often combined (compare Chap. 11)

Note CE enhances surface pattern (S), NBI and BLI (or i-Scan TE mode) show microvascular architecture (V) and may indicate S structure of mucosal neoplasias, whereas CE better shows S structure and lateral margins of neoplasias.

1.4 Characteristics of Early Mucosal Neoplastic Lesions on WLI

Detection of a lesion depends on visible alterations in *surface structure* or *color* [6], whereas prediction of histopathological tumor (pT) category or invasiveness rests on *assessment* of three criteria – *macroscopic morphology*, *mucosal surface pattern* (S), and *microvascular pattern* (V) of the mucosa – and is performed with magnifying NBI or CE (see Sect. 1.5).

1.4.1 Macroscopic Classification (Paris-Japanese Classification)

The endoscopic classification developed in Japan [24] and promoted by international consensus in Paris is analogous for superficial neoplastic lesions of the esophagus, stomach, and colon [3, 20] (see Fig. 1.2a). Diagnostic failure mainly comes from mis-classification of type 0–IIa versus type 0–Is lesions, which is of minor importance for cancer miss rates, and from under-detection of type 0–IIc lesions, which is a major cause for missed cancer because even small 0–IIc neoplasias show a high rate of intramucosal cancer and progression to invasive cancer [3, 9].

Superficial protruding lesions (0–Ip, Isp, Is) are easily detectable. In the stomach, they comprise hyperplastic polyps (80–90%, multiple in chronic type B gastritis), adenoma (5–10%, with high risk of malignant foci), or differentiated adenocarcinoma (2–3%), inflammatory polyps (~2%, e.g. eosinophilic granuloma), rarely fundic gland polyps (e.g. in familial adenomatous polyposis), hamartomas (e.g. in juvenile polyposis or Peutz-Jeghers syndrome), or hereditary polyposes (e.g. Cowden syndrome, Cronkhite-Canada syndrome).

In the colon, most mucosal lesions are protruding; about two thirds are adenomas (some with high-grade intraepithelial neoplasia [HGIN] or early cancer), and one third are harmless hyperplastic polyps, which must not be confused with serrated adenoma. Submucosal tumors (lipoma, carcinoid [mainly in rectum], rare leiomyoma) are covered with normal or inflammatory mucosa; so are hamartomas (Peutz-Jeghers polyp and juvenile polyp) and inflammatory pseudopolyps.

Flat lesions, i.e. slightly elevated, completely flat, and slightly depressed lesions (IIa, IIb, IIc), are less striking on WLI and deserve continuous attention for changes in *color* and/or *surface structure* of the mucosa. In squamous and columnar epithelial esophagus and in the stomach, the majority of early cancers (75–80%) show flat

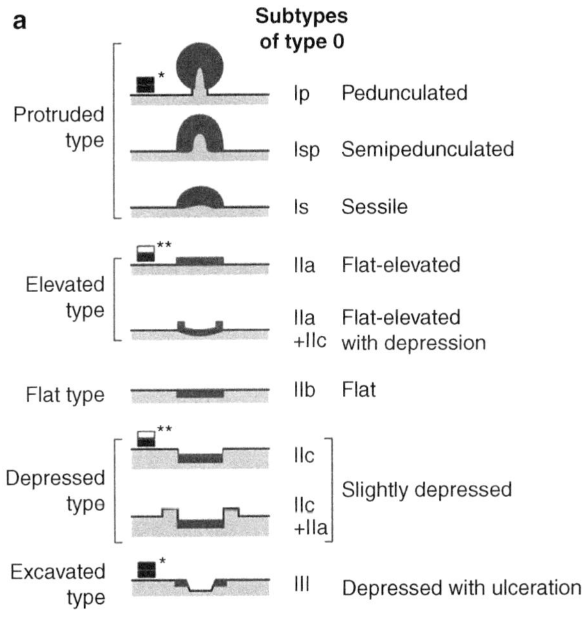

Fig. 1.2 (**a**) Endoscopic Paris classification of superficial neoplasias of the digestive tract (Modified acc. to [3, 20]): The macroscopic type is evident from the aspect of the lesion as compared with the size of a standard biopsy forceps (* closed cups of forceps = 2.5 mm; ** one jaw = 1.25 mm). Lesions are defined in relation to the adjacent surface as "protruding 0–I" (>2.5 mm↑ in columnar epithelium) and non-protruding, i.e., "flat-elevated = 0–IIa" (<2.5–0.5 mm↑), "flat = 0–IIb," and "depressed 0–IIc" (0.5–1.25 mm↓) or "excavated 0–III" (>1.25 mm↓). Composite lesions are described according to the combination of surface subtypes. In *esophageal* squamous epithelium, only *half* the sizes are used for the cutoff lines, e.g., ">1.25 mm↑ for 0–I," ">0.25 mm↑ for 0–IIa," ">0.25 mm↓ for 0–IIc," and ">0.5 mm↓ for 0–III." *, ** standard biopsy forceps (*gauge closed = 2.5 mm, **one jaw = 1.25 mm)

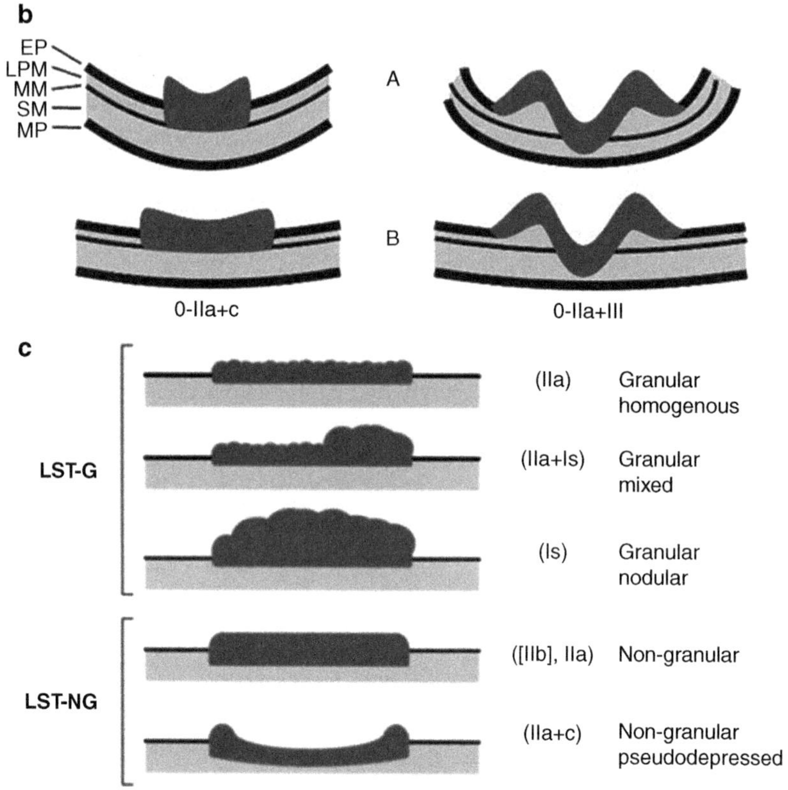

Fig. 1.2 (continued) (**b**) Desufflation (*A*)/insufflation (*B*) of a visceral organ provides information on depth of invasive growth. *Left*: Air-induced deformation of shape indicates infiltration of the muscularis mucosae (MM) layer. *Right*: Fixed shape of neoplasia indicates invasion of deep sm or MP layer. (**c**) Laterally spreading types of neoplasia (LSTs) [9]

lesions (IIa, IIb, IIc) [3]. Small early gastric cancers (EGC) typically display reddish type 0–IIc lesions when well differentiated, but small, pale type 0–IIb lesions, often with intact surface structure, when poorly differentiated. The latter are hard to detect and constitute about 15% of flat EGC in Japan and a higher fraction (up to 40%) in Western countries [25].

About 36% of *colonic neoplasias* present type 0–IIa flat lesions, and about 2% present type 0–IIc depressed lesions [9, 26]. As the tumor progresses in size and sm invasion, flat depressed neoplasia (0–IIc) may gain an elevated hyperplastic rim (types 0–IIc + 0–IIa) and become entirely elevated (types IIa + IIc) or ulcerated (0–III) in cases of deeply sm-invasive growth (Fig. 1.2a). Shape and deformation of a lesion during inflation/desufflation of the organ also provide information on invasive growth into the muscularis mucosae or deep sm/proper muscle layer (Fig. 1.2b).

Laterally spreading-type (LST) neoplasia (Fig. 1.2c) has been defined by Kudo et al. as a flat or elevated neoplastic lesion in the colorectum of more than 10 mm diameter [9]. These neoplasias (mostly adenomas) are barely distinguishable in color from the surrounding normal mucosa and can be quite flat or low elevated.

Chromoendoscopy with indigo carmine is advisable to demonstrate tumor extension. Uraoka et al. characterized the spectrum of LST, including nongranular-type LST with high probability of malignant foci (up to 50%) [27].

1.5 Magnifying and Image-Enhanced Endoscopy (IEE) for Analysis of Microarchitecture

1.5.1 Magnifying Endoscopy

Magnifying endoscopy with image enhancing endoscopy (IEE) techniques enables accurate diagnosis of early cancer lesions for appropriate curative resection technique [13, 28, 29]. High-definition (HD) endoscopes, even with the color CCD system, have a physical magnification up to 2 mm distance from the epithelial surface, yielding an optical magnification of 40-fold in dual-focus mode. With dual-focus endoscopes (e.g., GIF-H190Q or CF-H190Q for Exera III or GIF-HQ290 or CF-HQ290 for Lucera Spectrum, OLYMPUS), the user can switch between standard mode and near mode (40-fold) for close focus observation with depth of field (DoF) of 2–6 mm. In combination with the 1.5-times digital zoom, these endoscopes offer 60-fold magnification. The Multi Light™ system (ELUXEO, FUJIFILM) even allows switching from standard WLI or BLI to high-power magnifying (100×) WLI or BLI to obtain high-resolution IEE of micro-surface (S) and micro-vascular (V) structure. There are zoom endoscopes with adjustable image magnification up to 120-fold and depth of field (DoF) of 2–3 mm in both the sequential RGB and the simultaneous color CCD system. Moving the endoscope closer than 2 mm or further than 3 mm from the tissue causes the image to go out of focus. Therefore, a soft black hood as a distal attachment with depth equal to the DoFis essential on the zoom endoscope to keep the precise distance from the lens for clear, focused images (Fig. 1.3). To avoid contact bleeding,

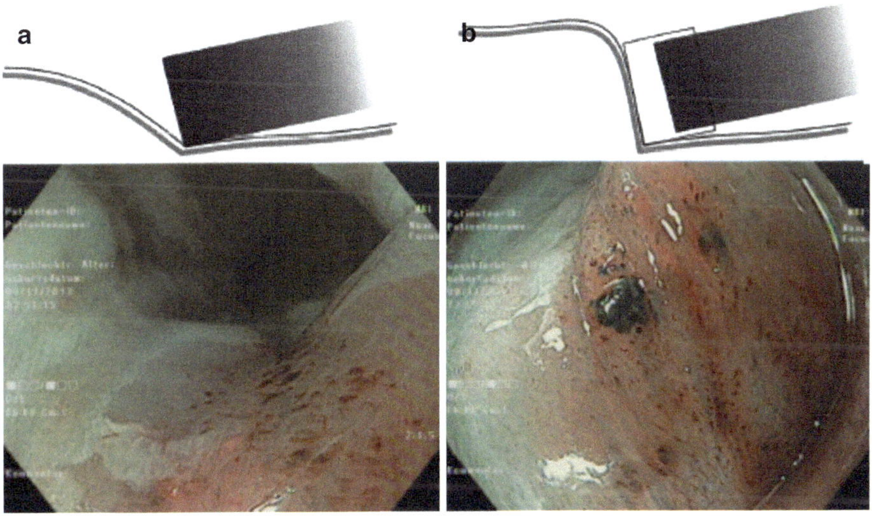

Fig. 1.3 M-NBI images of esophagus (**a**) without and (**b**) with distal attachment. (Modified from [11])

gently approximate the hood to the lesion and apply cautious suction/insufflation to optimize the focal distance. Observation under water with high magnification (60× – 120×) improves resolution and abolishes surface light reflection. In the stomach, there are two alternative techniques: (1) water filling of the stomach (e.g. with 500 mL water), or (2) water irrigation by injecting water from a syringe (20 or 50 mL) via a working channel into the distal hood when it is approximated to the target mucosa. The latter technique is also useful for acetic acid magnified CE of small lesions.

1.5.2 Image-Enhanced Endoscopy (IEE)

Narrow-band imaging (NBI), as well as *CE, augments the contrast* and enhances visibility of structures (IEE) while changing the image color [15, 30]. *NBI* based on hemoglobin absorbance images the microvessels in the superficial mucosal layer (lamina propria) and the submucosa [15, 29, 30] (Fig. 1.4), and sharpness of imaging depends on the index of hemoglobin color enhancement (IHb) [12]. The *structure enhancement function* improves image resolution on magnifying (M) observation in Olympus Lucera CV-260LS and Excera CV-190 *video processors*. There are two modalities (modes A and B) with eight levels each, and three of them can be preset. For the best structure enhancement settings see Table 1.2. The ELUXEO system (Fujifilm Corp., Tokyo) also has modes A and B with nine levels for BLI. The default setting for BLI is B4 for both standard and magnification.

The post-imaging digital filter technique (*i-Scan*, Pentax) needs tuning for enhancement of surface structure (SE mode) or of green-blue spectral bands for "tone enhancement" (TE) mode [16]. BLI, FICE, and *i-Scan* use principles established for NBI, and key findings reported for NBI also apply [8, 10, 16].

Key Points for Magnifying Endoscopy (60× – 130×):

- Proper structure enhancement settings of the video processor (Table 1.2)
- Soft distal hood (depth = DoF) to keep focal distance
- Water immersion (water filling or irrigation technique)
- Surface enhancement with acetic acid CE (Table 1.1, in irrigation technique).

Note Magnification (60-fold to 130-fold) combined with image-enhanced techniques (NBI, BLI, i-Scan, acetic acid, or crystal violet CE) yields maximum performance for diagnostic analysis of early neoplasias.

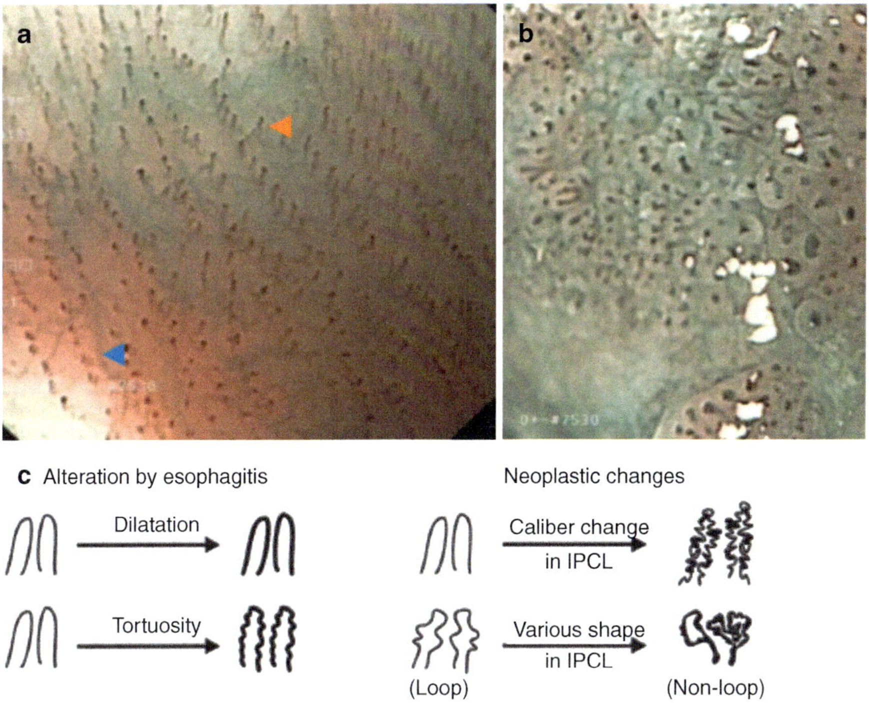

Fig. 1.4 Microvascular pattern (m-NBI, 60×) of squamous epithelial mucosa. (**a**) Normal esophagus. Faint submucosal collecting venules (cyan) ◀ and intrapapillary capillary loops (IPCL, light brown ◀) in LPM of squamous cell mucosa. (**b**) Neoplasia with HGIN. Disappearance of sm collecting venules, typical changes of IPCL (thickness, curling). (**c**) Basic alterations of schematic IPCL structure. (Modified from [11], permission granted by John Wiley & Sons Inc.)

Table 1.2 Structure enhancement settings (mode A vs. B, levels 1–8) [11, 12]

OLYMPUS	Excera III,CV-190	Lucera, CV-290
Standard WLI	A3 and A5	A5
M-WLI (>40-fold)	A8	A8 (or B8)
Standard NBI	B1 and B3	B1 and B3
M-NBI (>40-fold)	B8 (or A8)	B8

Color mode (level range 1–3): Level 1 for WLI, and for NBI level 1 and 3 in the GI tract

1.6 Capillary Structure of Squamous Mucosa and Neoplasias

Squamous epithelial esophagus displays rows of tiny reddish dots on WLI, which are identified on magnifying NBI as intrapapillary capillary loops (IPCL) in papillae of the mucosal LPM layer (Fig. 1.4a). Neoplasias in squamous epithelium induce angiogenesis and change vascular architecture of IPCL visible on IEE as alterations of IPCL morphology (Fig. 1.4b). Basic abnormal changes are in diameter ("caliber change" by 2×; "thick vessel" by 3×), irregularity in shape (non-loop due to fusion/destruction of papillae). This sequence of angiogenic alterations by early neoplasias (Fig. 1.4b, c) is well visible in squamous epithelial esophagus (*see* Table 7.2) and, in analogous fashion, is known in early cancer of columnar cell–lined mucosa (see below).

Key Points for Intrapapillary Capillary Loops (IPCL)

- Caliber change (thickness)
- Tortuosity
- Loop shape (loop / non-loop)

Note Squamous epithelial esophagus is best screened with both WLI (on scope insertion) and NBI observation (on scope withdrawal), whereas oropharynx and hypopharynx are screened with NBI on scope insertion, and during expiration for better overview (compare Sect. 6.4.2).

1.7 Analysis by IEE of Columnar Epithelial Mucosa and Neoplasias

Columnar epithelial mucosa extends between the squamocolumnar junctions at cardia and anal channel and presents different surface patterns depending on the type of mucosal glands. Single-layered columnar epithelium (in large intestine with mucin-rich goblet cells) covers the surface of mucosa and glands. Mucosa contains tubular glands with pitlike orifices in the colorectum and gastric fundus/corpus (fundic-type mucosa), displaying on IEE a pattern of *regular pits* in an even mucosal surface. In the antrum and pylorus, and in cardia and Barrett's esophagus, the mucosal surface forms villi or ridges surrounded by groove-like crypts; therefore, the surface pattern is *villous* (tubular) or *gyrus* (ridgelike). In small bowel, the mucosal surface is entirely villous (tubular).

On *NBI* of *columnar epithelial mucosa* (Barrett's esophagus, stomach, and intestine), the surface pattern of marginal crypt epithelium is superimposed onto the capillary pattern of the lamina propria, yielding complex surface (S) and vessel (V) patterns (Fig. 1.5). *Colonic mucosa* exhibits a regular surface pattern of pits on magnifying NBI and indigo carmine CE (explained in Fig. 1.5), which differs from adenoma.

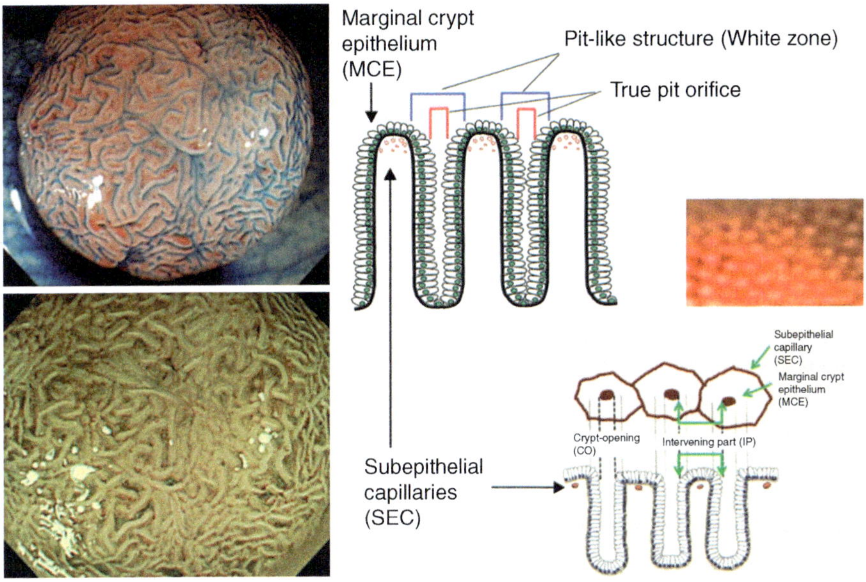

Fig. 1.5 Explanation of complex NBI patterns in columnar epithelial mucosa (*right side*; colon) and adenoma (*left side*). (Adapted from Tanaka et al. [32], permission granted by John Wiley & Sons Inc.). Magnifying colonoscopic images of normal mucosa (*right*) and tubulovillous adenoma (*left*, *top*: indigo carmine CE; *left*, *bottom*: NBI). The "white zone" (*WZ*) on the NBI image represents the perpendicularly illuminated layers of marginal crypt epithelium of glandular pits (the V pattern is extinct), which is the entire pitlike structure (*right panel*). An actual pit is hardly observed as a *dark dot* (mNBI 100×), because perpendicular illumination of the gland pit is rarely achieved. The vascular pattern (VP) of normal colonic mucosa is regular and brownish on NBI (*right upper panel*). Adenoma has a gyrous structure with ridges and groves (*left*)

1.7.1 Microarchitecture of Colonic Neoplasias

Adenomas in the gastrointestinal tract are defined on histology by cylinder epithelial cells with enhanced proliferation, *even* structure of pseudoglands, and *noninvasive* growth pattern (Fig. 1.6). These clonal epithelial neoplasms form different macroscopic types, e.g., flat types 0–IIb and 0–IIc or flat elevated types 0–IIa, which can also grow to sessile or polypoid adenoma or expansively spread out to larger, flat or flat-elevated, laterally spreading-type neoplasias (LST, in colon).

Note *Classic adenoma,* as compared with normal colonic mucosa on M-NBI (Fig. 1.6), is characterized by:

- *Regular surface pattern, SP* (evenly spaced WZ = MCE of pseudoglands)
- *Even but enhanced vascular pattern, VP* (reticular or spiral) around pseudoglands [15]
- *Clear margin* (without demarcation in surface relief)
- *Disappearance* of branched (dendritic) *sm vascular pattern*

Mucosal carcinoma arising in adenoma leads to irregular structures:

- *Irregular SP (uneven WZ, loss of structure* of crypt epithelium and pseudoglands)
- *Irregular VP* (sparse, curled vessel pattern due to destruction of pseudoglands)
- *Demarcation line* in surface *relief* (and *expansive nodule* or *encroachment*), if invasive into mucosal layer (Fig. 1.7a, c), or superficial submucosal (SM1) layer [19]

In general, the longer the adenomatous proliferation proceeds, i.e., with enlarging adenoma size, the greater the risk of malignant transformation. Even more so, the potential for cancerous transformation of colonic adenomas depends on histomorphologic type, increasing in the order of tubular, tubulovillous, villous, and serrated adenomas, and intraepithelial neoplasia (compare Fig. 2.2 and Table 2.1). Colorectal small depressed adenomas (types 0–IIc) tend to transform early to invasive adenocarcinoma that infiltrates the mucosa or sm layer. Some even arise as minute intraepithelial HGIN or carcinoma in situ [9].

These alterations of colonic mucosal surface and vessel structures induced by adenomatous and carcinomatous transformation have been characterized and classified as *pit patterns (PP)* by Kudo [9] and *capillary patterns (CP)* by Sano et al. [15] (Table 1.3; compare Fig. 11.2a–h). Combined analysis of vessel pattern

Table 1.3 Sano's capillary pattern types (CP) renamed as vessel types (V) in the Japan NBI Expert Team (JNET) classification using mNBI [19, 32]

Vessel type	V 1	V 2A	V 2B	V 3
CP type	CP I	CP II	CP IIIA	CP IIIB
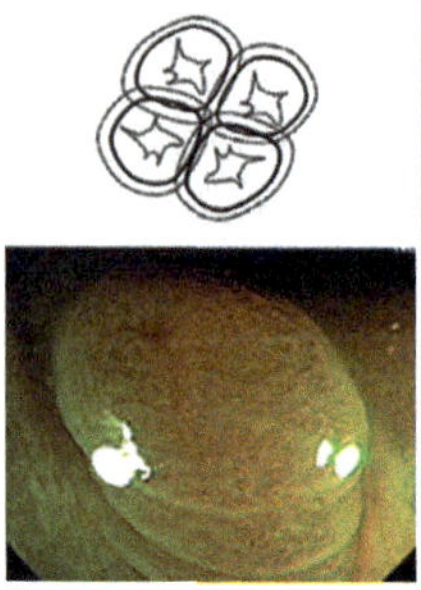		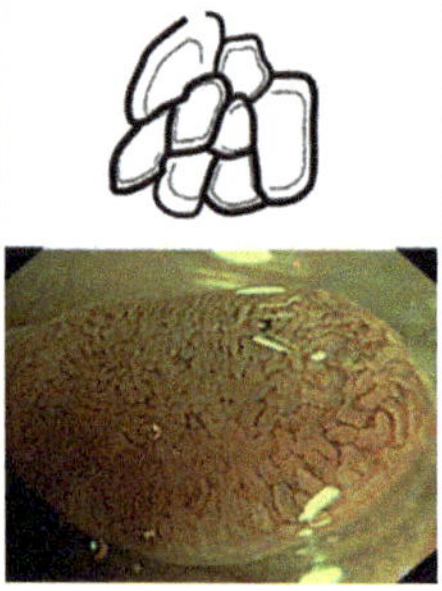	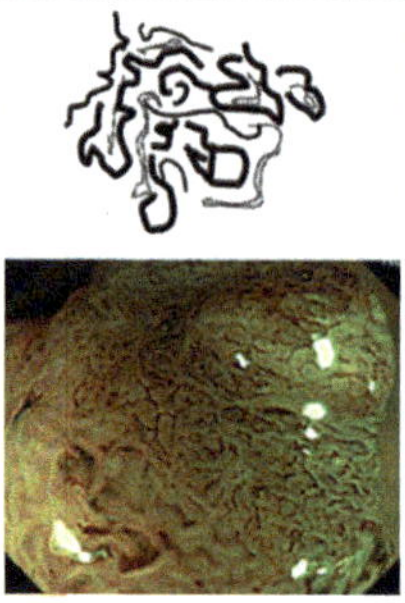	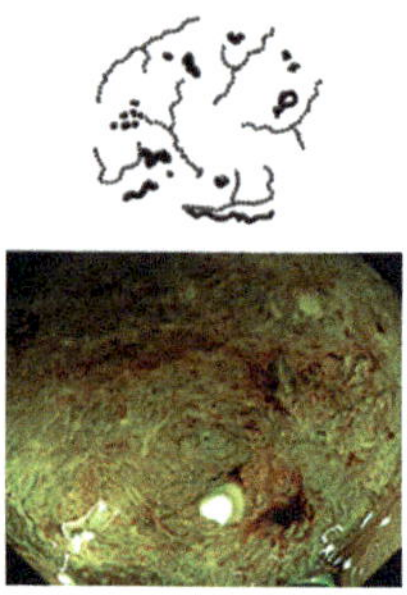
Meshed capillary vessels, invisible (−) or normal		Meshed capillary vessels, regular (+)	Meshed capillary vessels, characterized by branching, curtailed irregularity & blind endings	
		Capillary vessels surround mucosal glands	Lack of uniformity High density of capillary vessels	Nearly avascular, or loose capillary vessels
Hyperplastic polyp[a]		Adenoma, LGIN	Ca-m[b], sm–superficial[c]	Ca sm – deep[d]

Permission granted by the Japan Gastroenterological Endoscopy Society/Digestive Endoscopy, and John Wiley & Co.

[a]normal hyperplastic polyp or sessile serrated polyp [19]

[b]HGIN, intramucosal cancer Ca-m

[c]sm superficial invasion (<1000 μm)

[d]sm deep invasion (≥1000 μm)

(V = CP) and surface pattern (S = PP) of colonic mucosal neoplasias allows prediction of malignancy and submucosal invasion with high accuracy (>90%). (See Chap. 11 for details.)

An international panel has simplified these two classifications to the *Narrow-Band Imaging International Colorectal Endoscopic (NICE) classification*, applicable for *standard endoscopy* (indigo carmine CE and NBI) without magnification [32, 33]. The NICE classification has been evaluated, but only tentatively differentiates superficial from deep sm-invasive (≥sm2) cancer [33]. Based on magnifying NBI, the Japan NBI Expert Team (JNET) reached consensus on the *JNET classification* to better discriminate superficial from deep sm-invasive carcinoma [19] (Table 1.4).

Table 1.4 Relationship between Narrow-Band Imaging International Colorectal Endoscopic (NICE) classification[a], Sano's classification, and Japan NBI Expert Team (JNET) classification

NICE	Type 1	Type 2	Type 3
Color	Same or lighter than background	Brownish relative to background (verify color arises from vessels)	Brown to dark brown relative to background; sometimes patchy whiter areas
Vessels	None, or isolated lacy vessels might be present coursing across the lesion	Thick, brown vessels surrounding white structures[b]	Area(s) with markedly distorted or missing vessels
Surface pattern	Dark or white spots of uniform size or homogenous absence of pattern	Oval, tubular or branched white structures surrounded by brown vessels	Areas with distortion or absence of pattern
Most likely pathology	Hyperplastic	Adenoma, HGIN, intramucosal cancer[c]	Deeply submucosa invasive cancer
Sano's CP classification[d] [29]	Type I	Type II / Type IIIA	Type IIIB
JNET classification[e]	Type 1	Type 2A / Type 2B	Type 3

Modified from Tanaka et al. [32], Sano et al. [19]
[a]Can be applied using colonoscopes both with and without optical magnification
[b]These structures might be the pits and the epithelium of the crypt opening
[c]Type 2 consists of the Vienna classification types 3, 4, and superficial 5. In some countries (e.g., the USA), type 2 includes all adenomas with either low-grade or high-grade dysplasia. High-grade dysplasia in the USA includes adenomas with carcinoma in situ or intramucosal carcinoma. In Japan, intramucosal cancer might be termed *cancer* rather than high-grade dysplasia. Some lesions with superficially submucosal invasive cancer might also have type 2 appearance
[d]For description of Sano's types compare Table 1.3
[e]Types 1–3 of JNET classification correspond to types I to IIIB of Sano's CP classification

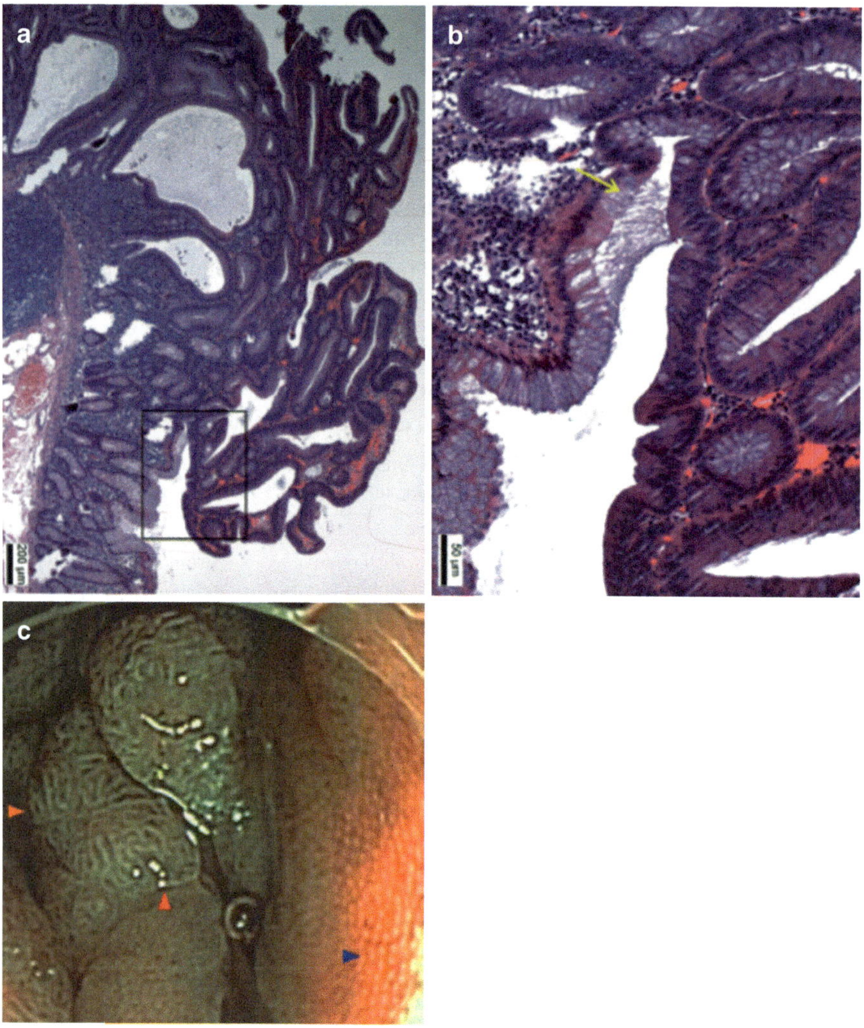

Fig. 1.6 (**a**) *Classic tubular adenoma* in the colon exhibits a noninvasive growth pattern of regular tubular glands. Coherent expansive growth of transformed epithelium creates pseudoglands with single-layered surface epithelium (*even WZ*) and may lead to protruding mucosal neoplasia 0–IIa or Isp (HE stain). (**b**) Magnified inset from **a**,: showing a sharp transition (*yellow arrow*) with even surface (*clear margin, even surface*) from colonic epithelium (*left side*) to adenomatous colonocytes (*right side*), which show an enhanced nucleus/cytoplasm ratio, loss of basal polar orientation, and clonal proliferation without goblet cells. (Courtesy Dr. Daniel Neureiter). (**c**) Magnifying NBI (60×) reveals normal colonic mucosa (*right side*, ▶) with round white dots representing marginal crypt epithelium (WZ) of tubular glands and a fine, brownish network of capillaries around glands in the mucosal layer. Top and left sides (▶) show protruding adenoma (0–Is) with a large tubular surface structure displaying even bands of WZ and ridgelike bands of brownish VP in LPM of adenomatous pseudogland tubule. The adenoma has a clear sharp margin (▲) to columnar mucosa

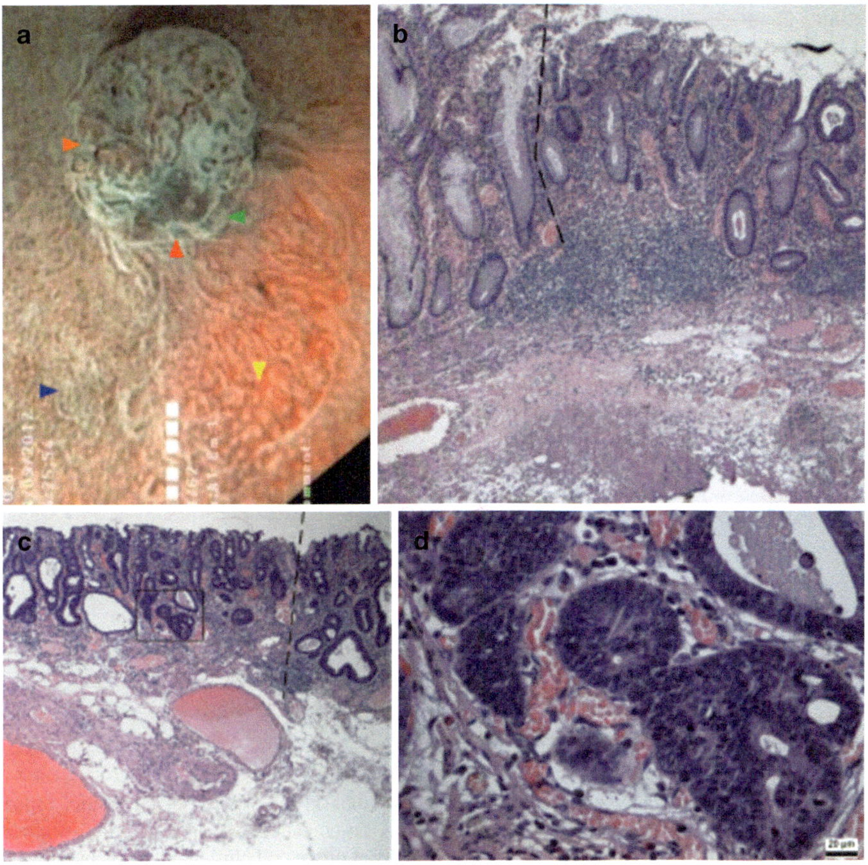

Fig. 1.7 (**a**) Colonic LST 0–IIb presenting ▶ meshed capillary pattern (CP II) and small nodule 0–IIa (▲ with demarcation line) displaying ▶ irregular dense CP (IIIA) and ◀ irregular sparse CP IIIB with thick vessels (magnifying NBI, 80×). ESD showed tubular adenoma with low-grade intraepithelial neoplasia (LGIN) in 0–IIb and adenocarcinoma pTis (LPM) in nodule IIa. *Vertical arrows* mark margins between hyperplastic and neoplastic mucosa (▼ in (**a**) represents *dotted line* in (**b**)) and between adenoma and intramucosal adenocarcinoma [G2, T1a LPM] (▲ in (**a**) marks *dotted line* in (**c**)). (**b**) Transition (*dotted line*) from hyperplastic mucosa with goblet cell–rich pits (*left*) to tubular adenoma with regular pseudoglands, lack of goblet cells, augmented capillaries in mucosa, LPM. (**c**) Transition (*dotted line*) from adenoma (*right*) to adenocarcinoma (*left*; *insert* = *d*) with irregular glands and thick microvessels. (**d**) Adenocarcinoma [G2, T1a LPM] (insert in **c**, 10× more magnified). (Courtesy Dr. Daniel Neureiter)

1.7.2 Microarchitecture of Gastric Mucosa and Neoplasia

Gastric mucosa exhibits columnar cell–lined epithelium with mucosal areas (*areae gastricae*) separated by fine grooves. The mucosa of the gastric fundus and corpus is lined with fundic-type glands presenting a regular pattern of round or oval pitlike gland openings surrounded by a brownish reticular network of microcapillaries on M-NBI (Fig. 1.8a, normal margin; Fig. 1.9). By contrast, the distal corpus and antropyloric region bear pyloric-type glands showing a villous surface and a regular open-loop pattern on M-NBI (Fig. 1.10a, normal margin). Normal *fundic*-type mucosa without gastritis displays a regular red pattern of starfish-like submucosal collecting venules (regular arrangement of collecting venules, *RAC*) on WLI, which vanishes in severe gastritis. Severe chronic *atrophic gastritis* – at increased risk for cancer – presents a prominent *submucosal* vascular pattern on WLI, and often intestinal metaplasia presenting mainly as whitish areas with uncertain margin and loss of sm vascular pattern on WLI, with light blue crests (*LBC* = brush border in cells) in the white zone of marginal epithelium on magnifying NBI [31]. (Compare Chap. 9.)

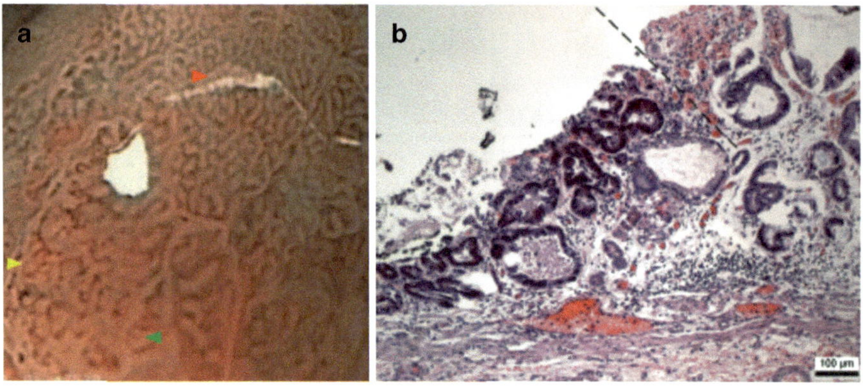

Fig. 1.8 Well-differentiated adenocarcinoma (WDAC, tub, G1, pT1a MM) 0–IIa, gastric corpus. (**a**) NBI (100-fold): ▶ fundic mucosa (top right side: oval pit pattern); ▶ clear margin (*demarcation line*) due to expansion of WDAC/MDAC as coherent tumor cell cluster; ◀ fine network with irregular microvascular pattern (VP). For respective VP, compare Fig. 1.9. (**b**) HE stain shows sharp margins (*dotted line*) to WDAC (*left side*). (Courtesy Dr. Daniel Neureiter)

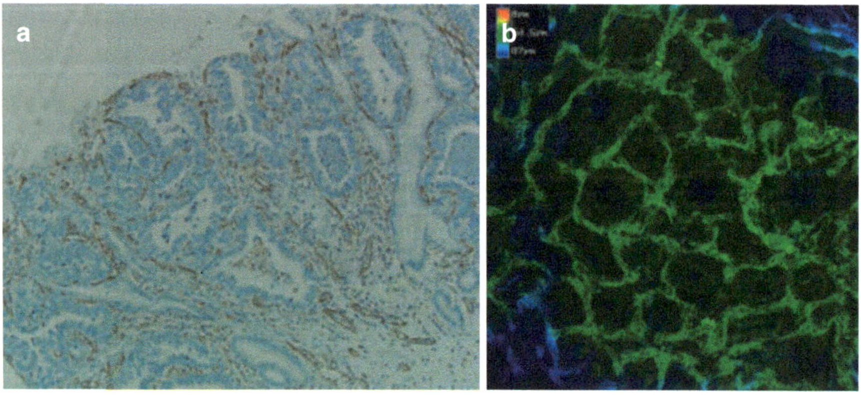

Fig. 1.9 (**a**) Histology of gastric WDAC demonstrates *coherent expansion* of mucosal cancer with relatively regular pseudogland and capillary structure (VP). (**b**) In analogy, intact VP of gastric WDAC, as revealed by laser scanning microscopy (LSM) of HE stain after CD31-immunohistological staining of capillary endothelia, displays a nearly regular network VP. (Permission of Thieme/Endoscopy [14])

Small early gastric cancer (<10 mm) (EGC) is easily missed when WLI does not focus on *discolored spots*, the hallmark for flat EGC, because only 15–20% are elevated lesions (0–IIa/Is, usually differentiated adenocarcinoma [AC]), but 80–85% are tiny flat (0-IIb) or depressed (0-IIc) lesions (Figs. 1.8 and 1.10). Up to 40% of small flat EGC is poorly differentiated diffuse-type AC (grading G3, PDAC) [25]. Unfortunately, most small PDAC is difficult to detect on WLI or even M-NBI, owing to pale or isochrome aspect. The histology explains why: The vascular pattern in the LPM often is sparse, and cancer cells diffusely spread in LPM and sm, hiding the vascular pattern (Figs. 1.10 and 1.11), and epithelium and gland openings may be preserved as normal on the luminal surface.

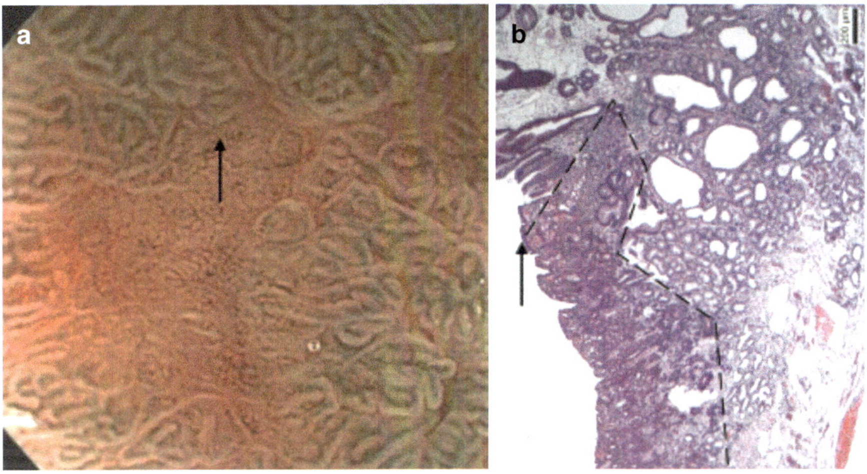

Fig. 1.10 (**a**) Poorly differentiated, diffuse-type early gastric cancer (PDAC). Absent microsurface structure, sparse VP with corkscrew-like irregular microvessels, with encroachment (*arrow*) (M-NBI), surrounded by pyloric-type mucosa with villous SP. (Permission of John Wiley and Sons/J Gastroenterol Hepatol [34]). (**b**) Histology of another PDAC (*left side of dotted line*) with surface encroachment (*arrow*) and undermining of mucosal margin, loss of surface gland structure, and LPM layer diffusely infiltrated by cancer cells. (Courtesy Dr. Daniel Neureiter)

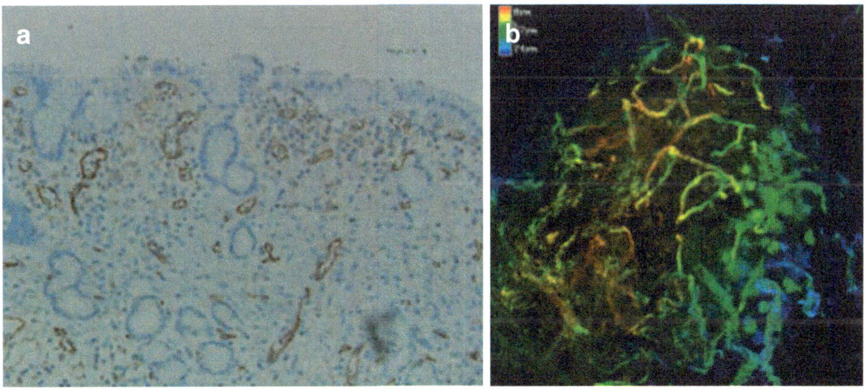

Fig. 1.11 Microarchitecture of small, depressed-type EGC of diffuse type with poorly differentiated grading (PDAC). (Permission of Thieme/Endoscopy [14]). (**a**) Histology of PDAC, HE stain, and CD31 immunostain of endothelium. (**b**) Laser surface microscopic reconstruction of VP in LPM layer of similar undifferentiated AC (PDAC) with a sparse, irregular capillary pattern and some corkscrew vessels

The vascular pattern (VP) shows a scanty and regular periglandular capillary network (mesh) in normal corpus/fundus mucosa with tubular glands, and spiral capillary patterns in normal antrum/pylorus mucosa covered with surface villi or ridges (Figs. 1.8 and 1.10). Early differentiated adenocarcinoma usually displays prominent irregular mesh VP and irregular surface pattern (SP) on magnifying NBI (Fig. 1.8). By contrast, in small 0–IIc lesions, a non-reticular, often sparse VP signals intramucosal poorly differentiated adenocarcinoma (PDAC, Fig. 1.10) or deep sm invasion of early well-differentiated AC (specificity 85%).

Correct mapping of *tumor extension* of EGC is necessary for endoscopic resection with free margins. Magnifying NBI helps to distinguish tumor margins from surrounding normal mucosa in cardia-type EGC, or more frequently from atrophic mucosa with intestinal metaplasia in chronic *Helicobacter pylori*–induced or autoimmune gastritis [18]. Surface enhancement using CE with acetic acid–indigo carmine mixture is very helpful for mapping of differentiated-type adenocarcinoma but tends to obscure pale-type 0–IIb small PDAC. (Compare Chap. 9)

Magnifying WLI followed by magnifying NBI endoscopy achieves >90% specificity and accuracy for endoscopic diagnosis of type 0–IIc small mucosal gastric adenocarcinoma and improves differential diagnosis for small flat or depressed lesions caused by chronic atrophic gastritis [18, 35]. The analysis of SP and VP in EGC is detailed in Chap. 9.

Note In stomach, assessment of SP and VP with M-NBI differentiates with high accuracy (>90%) [18, 35–37]:

- Non-neoplastic *versus* neoplastic mucosa
- Adenoma or differentiated mucosal adenocarcinoma (HGIN, T1 m/sm1) *versus* deeply sm-invasive carcinoma (≥sm2)

1.7.3 Microarchitecture of Columnar Mucosa-Lined Esophagus

Barrett's esophagus (BE) is an area of columnar epithelium-lined esophagus (*CLE*) extending for more than 1 cm oral to the gastroesophageal junction, which corresponds to the oral end of the gastric folds (Western definition) or the distal end of the longitudinal palisade vessel pattern (IPCL) in the esophagus (Japanese definition). According to the US definition, CLE with goblet cells on biopsy proves specialized intestinal metaplasia (SIM) which is required for diagnosis of BE in CLE. According to the Japan and British Gastroenterological Societies, BE is defined by CLE (without or with goblet cells). CLE increases the risk for adenocarcinoma of the esophagus or gastroesophageal junction to a similar extent in the absence or the presence of goblet cells [38–40]. In fact, even islets of columnar epithelial mucosa in an irregular Z-line (so-called *ultrashort BE*) may carry an increased risk of cancer, like non-goblet CLE [40] (Fig. 1.12).

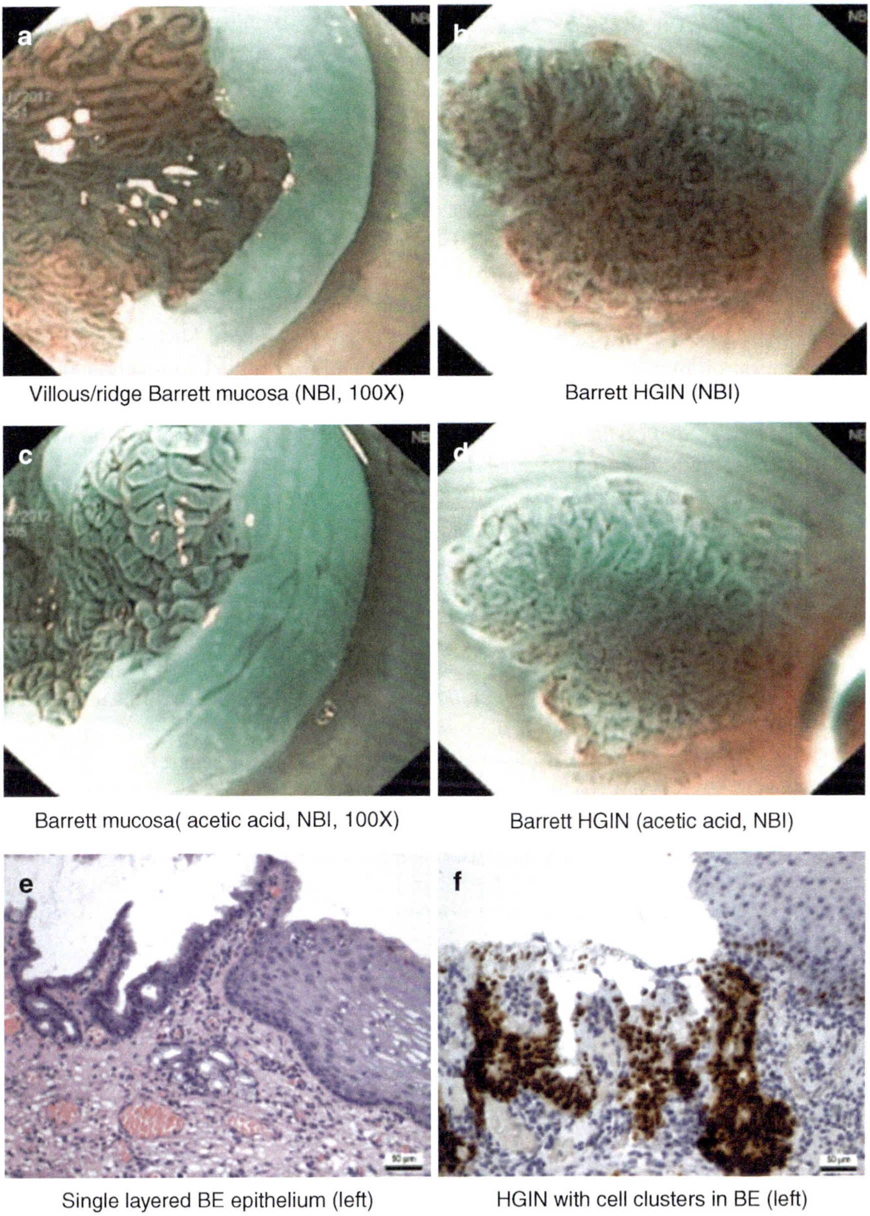

Fig. 1.12 Typical case of Barrett's mucosa with HGIN (Courtesy of Dr. H.P. Allgaier). *Left panels* (**a**, **c**, **e**): Linear WZ in villous/ridge-type Barrett's mucosa with (**a**) regular helix-like CP on M-NBI (100×); (**c**) even SP after 1.5% acetic acid; (**e**) margin of single-layered BE epithelium on the left side (HE stain, 100×). *Right panels* (**b**, **d**, **f**): HGIN in BE with irregular (**b**) CP, (**d**) SP, and (**f**) clusters of dysplastic cylinder cells. (**e**, **f**) HE stain after ESD, (**f**) with p53 immunohistochemistry. (Courtesy of Dr. Tsuneo Oyama, Nagano; and Dr. Daniel Neureiter, Salzburg)

Reports from Japan on the microsurface pattern (SP) and vascular pattern (VP) of Barrett's neoplasia are scarce because of its very low prevalence there, and the characterization of neoplastic alterations of surface structure lags behind that in colonic and gastric mucosa. At least four classifications of SP and VP of CLE mucosa are known [41–45], but none is universally accepted. In general, CLE shows five different regular patterns (round pits and tubular, linear, villous, or atrophic-absent surface patterns) (*See* Table 8.2). Linear/villous mucosal surface with "light blue crests" (LBC) on magnifying NBI is highly (~90%) sensitive and specific for specialized intestinal metaplasia (SIM) [31].

Early malignant neoplasias are mostly flat lesions (0–IIa–c, 85%) and hard to detect as minute (≤5 mm) or small lesions in Barrett's mucosa [46]. Basically, any slight alteration in reddish color or uneven surface relief on WLI must be analyzed with magnifying NBI endoscopy (>60×) and surface enhancement with acetic acid (*see* Fig. 1.12). *Neoplastic areas* (HGIN, early cancer), type 0–IIa–c, exhibit uneven surface relief and an irregular, speckled white zone of marginal epithelium, combined with irregularities in VP (irregular loop or spiral pattern) and clear margin of the suspicious area within surrounding BE mucosa [41, 43] The diagnosis of neoplasia should still be confirmed by targeted biopsy.

Note Irregular SP and VP in CLE distinguish with accuracy of 80–85% [41, 43, 45] between:

- Nonneoplastic CLE (−/+SIM) *versus* differentiated mucosal neoplasia (HGIN, T1 m, or sm1 adenocarcinoma)
- Deep submucosal invasion (≥sm2) of early cancer with severely irregular SP (destruction of gland structure) and CP (sparse and thick vessels)

Acknowledgments The contribution of cases or images by Dr. Hans-Peter Allgaier, Freiburg, Germany; Dr. Gerhard Kleber, Aalen, Germany; Dr. Tsuneo Oyama, Saku Central Hospital, Nagano, Japan; and Dr. Daniel Neureiter, University Institute of Pathology, Salzburg, Austria, is gratefully acknowledged.

References

1. Ferlay J, et al. Cancer incidence and mortality worldwide: sources, methods and major patterns in GLOBOCAN 2012. Int J Cancer. 2015;136:E359–86.
2. Inoue M, et al. Epidemiology of gastric cancer in Japan. Postgrad Med J. 2005;81:419–24.
3. The Paris endoscopic classification of superficial neoplastic lesions: esophagus, stomach, and colon: November 30 to December 1, 2002. Gastrointest Endosc. 2003;58:S3–43.
4. George SM, et al. Classification of advanced colorectal carcinomas by tumor edge morphology: evidence for different pathogenesis and significance of polypoid and nonpolypoid tumors. Cancer. 2000;89:1901–9.
5. Heresbach D, et al. Miss rate for colorectal neoplastic polyps: a prospective multicenter study of back-to-back video colonoscopies. Endoscopy. 2008;40:284–90.
6. Yao K, et al. Development of an e-learning system for teaching endoscopists how to diagnose early gastric cancer: basic principles for improving early detection. Gastric Cancer. 2017;20(Suppl 1):S28–38.

7. Kaltenbach T, et al. American Gastroenterological Association (AGA) Institute technology assessment on image-enhanced endoscopy. Gastroenterology. 2008;134:327–40.
8. Dohi O, et al. Diagnostic ability of magnifying endoscopy with blue laser imaging for early gastric cancer: a prospective study. Gastric Cancer. 2017;20:297–303.
9. Kudo S, et al. Colonoscopic diagnosis and management of nonpolypoid early colorectal cancer. World J Surg. 2000;24:1081–90.
10. Osawa H, et al. Present and future status of flexible spectral imaging color enhancement and blue laser imaging technology. Dig Endosc. 2014;26(Suppl 1):105–15.
11. Uedo N, et al. Role of narrow band imaging for diagnosis of early-stage esophagogastric cancer: current consensus of experienced endoscopists in Asia-Pacific region. Dig Endosc. 2011;23(Suppl 1):58–71.
12. Uraoka T, et al. Narrow-band imaging for improving colorectal adenoma detection: appropriate system function settings are required. Gut. 2009;58:604–5.
13. Kudo S, et al. Pit pattern in colorectal neoplasia: endoscopic magnifying view. Endoscopy. 2001;33:367–73.
14. Nakayoshi T, et al. Magnifying endoscopy combined with narrow band imaging system for early gastric cancer: correlation of vascular pattern with histopathology (including video). Endoscopy. 2004;36:1080–4.
15. Sano Y, et al. Magnifying observation of microvascular architecture of colorectal lesions using a narrow-band imaging system. Dig Endosc. 2006;18:s44–51.
16. Kodashima S, et al. Novel image-enhanced endoscopy with i-scan technology. World J Gastroenterol. 2010;16:1043–9.
17. Yao K, et al. Development of an e-learning system for teaching endoscopists how to diagnose early gastric cancer: basic principles for improving early detection. Gastric Cancer. 2017;20:28–38.
18. Muto M, et al. Magnifying endoscopy simple diagnostic algorithm for early gastric cancer (MESDA-G). Dig Endosc. 2016;28:379–93.
19. Sano Y, et al. Narrow-band imaging (NBI) magnifying endoscopic classification of colorectal tumors proposed by the Japan NBI Expert Team. Dig Endosc. 2016;28:526–33.
20. Update on the Paris classification of superficial neoplastic lesions in the digestive tract. Endoscopy. 2005;37:570–8.
21. Ishihara R, et al. Quantitative analysis of the color change after iodine staining for diagnosing esophageal high-grade intraepithelial neoplasia and invasive cancer. Gastrointest Endosc. 2009;69:213–8.
22. Kondo H, et al. Sodium thiosulfate solution spray for relief of irritation caused by Lugol's stain in chromoendoscopy. Gastrointest Endosc. 2001;53:199–202.
23. Kawahara Y, et al. Novel chromoendoscopic method using an acetic acid-indigocarmine mixture for diagnostic accuracy in delineating the margin of early gastric cancers. Dig Endosc. 2009;21:14–9.
24. Japanese Research Society for Gastric Cancer. Japanese classification of gastric carcinoma First English ed. Tokyo: Kanehara & Co., Ltd; 1995.
25. Everett SM, et al. Early gastric cancer in Europe. Gut. 1997;41:142–50.
26. Rembacken BJ, et al. Flat and depressed colonic neoplasms: a prospective study of 1000 colonoscopies in the UK. Lancet. 2000;355:1211–4.
27. Uraoka T, et al. Endoscopic indications for endoscopic mucosal resection of laterally spreading tumours in the colorectum. Gut. 2006;55:1592–7.
28. Yao K, et al. Novel magnified endoscopic findings of microvascular architecture in intramucosal gastric cancer. Gastrointest Endosc. 2002;56:279–84.
29. Yoshida T, et al. Narrow-band imaging system with magnifying endoscopy for superficial esophageal lesions. Gastrointest Endosc. 2004;59:288–95.
30. Gono K, et al. Appearance of enhanced tissue features in narrow-band endoscopic imaging. J Biomed Opt. 2004;9:568–77.
31. Toyoda H, et al. Detection of intestinal metaplasia in distal esophagus and esophagogastric junction by enhanced-magnification endoscopy. Gastrointest Endosc. 2004;59:15–21.

32. Tanaka S, et al. Aim to unify the narrow band imaging (NBI) magnifying classification for colorectal tumors: current status in Japan from a summary of the consensus symposium in the 79th Annual Meeting of the Japan Gastroenterological Endoscopy Society. Dig Endosc. 2011;23(Suppl 1):131–9.
33. Hayashi N, et al. Endoscopic prediction of deep submucosal invasive carcinoma: validation of the narrow-band imaging international colorectal endoscopic (NICE) classification. Gastrointest Endosc. 2013;78:625–32.
34. Okada K, et al. Diagnosis of undifferentiated type early gastric cancers by magnification endoscopy with narrow-band imaging. J Gastroenterol Hepatol. 2011;26:1262–9.
35. Ezoe Y, et al. Magnifying narrowband imaging is more accurate than conventional white-light imaging in diagnosis of gastric mucosal cancer. Gastroenterology. 2011;141:2017–25. e2013.
36. Abe S, et al. Depth-predicting score for differentiated early gastric cancer. Gastric Cancer. 2011;14:35–40.
37. Tanaka K, et al. Features of early gastric cancer and gastric adenoma by enhanced-magnification endoscopy. J Gastroenterol. 2006;41:332–8.
38. Gatenby PA, et al. Relevance of the detection of intestinal metaplasia in non-dysplastic columnar-lined oesophagus. Scand J Gastroenterol. 2008;43:524–30.
39. Kelty CJ, et al. Barrett's oesophagus: intestinal metaplasia is not essential for cancer risk. Scand J Gastroenterol. 2007;42:1271–4.
40. Riddell RH, et al. Definition of Barrett's esophagus: time for a rethink--is intestinal metaplasia dead? Am J Gastroenterol. 2009;104:2588–94.
41. Anagnostopoulos GK, et al. Novel endoscopic observation in Barrett's oesophagus using high resolution magnification endoscopy and narrow band imaging. Aliment Pharmacol Ther. 2007;26:501–7.
42. Goda K, et al. Usefulness of magnifying endoscopy with narrow band imaging for the detection of specialized intestinal metaplasia in columnar-lined esophagus and Barrett's adenocarcinoma. Gastrointest Endosc. 2007;65:36–46.
43. Kara MA, et al. Detection and classification of the mucosal and vascular patterns (mucosal morphology) in Barrett's esophagus by using narrow band imaging. Gastrointest Endosc. 2006;64:155–66.
44. Sharma P, et al. The utility of a novel narrow band imaging endoscopy system in patients with Barrett's esophagus. Gastrointest Endosc. 2006;64:167–75.
45. Sharma P, et al. Development and validation of a classification system to identify high-grade dysplasia and esophageal adenocarcinoma in Barrett's esophagus using narrow-band imaging. Gastroenterology. 2016;150:591–8.
46. Pech O, et al. Prospective evaluation of the macroscopic types and location of early Barrett's neoplasia in 380 lesions. Endoscopy. 2007;39:588–93.

Chapter 2
Histopathology of Early Mucosal Neoplasias: Morphologic Carcinogenesis in the GI Tract

Daniel Neureiter and Tobias Kiesslich

2.1 Introduction

The term *early cancer* suggests carcinoma curable with resection. This clinical concept was coined in Japan and over the years has been defined more and more by macroscopic and microscopic criteria throughout the gastrointestinal tract. It applies to mucosal differentiated cancers without (or with minor) submucosal invasion, with a low probability of lymph node metastasis and >90% rate of cure by surgical R0 resection [1–3].

In Japanese tradition, endoscopic features have been correlated with histopathological findings. Mucosal surface alterations of well-differentiated cancers and precursor lesions compared with non-neoplastic mucosa have been characterized by histology in parallel with stereomicroscopic observation and magnified image-enhanced endoscopy (M-IEE). Well-differentiated early mucosal neoplasias, e.g in colon, revealed distinct margins and typical alterations of epithelial surface and mucosal capillary structure [4, 5]. In addition, several morphological pathways of carcinogenesis exist in each organ [4, 6–9], so the endoscopist must be familiar with different early cancerous lesions and their precursors.

Western and Japanese classifications differed in the criteria for intraepithelial high-grade dysplasia vs. mucosal cancer [10, 11]. This difference has been largely resolved by the consensus Vienna Classification of gastrointestinal epithelial neoplasias [12], extended in Paris by the macroscopic and microscopic International

D. Neureiter (✉)
Institute of Pathology, Paracelsus Medical University, Salzburg, Austria
e-mail: d.neureiter@salk.at

T. Kiesslich
Department of Internal Medicine I & Institute of Physiology and Pathophysiology, Paracelsus Medical University, Salzburg, Austria

F. Berr et al. (eds.), *Atlas of Early Neoplasias of the Gastrointestinal Tract*,
https://doi.org/10.1007/978-3-030-01114-7_2

Classification, which is based on Japanese criteria [6]. Early cancers (Vienna categories 4 and 5) and precursor lesions in the gastrointestinal tract are best defined with these classifications.

2.2 Paris Classification and Malignant Potential of Neoplasms

2.2.1 Classification of Malignant Mucosal Neoplasms

The International Classification (macroscopic types; see Chap. 1, Fig. 1.2) is based on the histopathological definitions agreed upon in the Vienna classification (Table 2.1). Some disagreement remains between Japanese and Western pathologists as to the categorisation of lesions into high-grade intraepithelial neoplasias (HGIN) or definite cancer in situ (T0 m1), because diagnostic criteria of cancer in the West are based more on biopsy-proven tumor invasion into the lamina propria of the mucosa, whereas in Japan, criteria depend more on atypias (nuclear features and intraepithelial gland structure), similar to the intraepithelial spreading component of invasive carcinomas (Table 2.2). Therefore, up to 50% of carcinomas in situ diagnosed in Japan may be categorized as HGIN in the West [10, 11]. However, Japanese pathologists better predicted from single biopsies the correct categorization of the entire en-bloc resected neoplasias, because the majority of HGIN in the stomach were definite cancers in the resected specimens [11]. For the decision

Table 2.1 Vienna classification of gastrointestinal epithelial neoplasia [12]

Category	Description	Japanese viewpoint
Category 1	Negative for neoplasia/dysplasia	+[a]
Category 2	Indefinite for neoplasia/dysplasia	+[a]
Category 3	Non-invasive low-grade neoplasia (low-grade adenoma/dysplasia)	+[a]
Category 4	Non-invasive high-grade neoplasia	
	4.1 High-grade adenoma/dysplasia	Non-invasive carcinoma[c] (4.1 and 4.2)
	4.2 Non-invasive carcinoma (carcinoma in situ)[b]	
	4.3 Suspicion of invasive carcinoma	+[a]
Category 5	Invasive neoplasia	
	5.1 Intramucosal carcinoma[d]	+[a]
	5.2 Submucosal carcinoma or beyond	+[a]

[a]+ Identical terms in Japan

[b]Non-invasive indicates the absence of evident invasion

[c]High-grade adenoma/dysplasia could be regarded as non-invasive carcinoma according to Japanese criteria of atypia

[d]*Intramucosal* indicates invasion into the lamina propria or muscularis mucosae

Table 2.2 Japanese criteria for diagnosis of colorectal adenomas and differentiated cancers [13]

Criteria of atypia		Normal	Adenoma	Well-differentiated adenocarcinoma Low grade	Well-differentiated adenocarcinoma High grade
Cellular atypia	Nuclear size (μm)	4.5 × 1.5	⟶		≤20 × 10
	Chromatin (blue-violet)	Dotted	⟶		Coarse, bright
	Nuclear polarity	Basal	⟶		Nonpolarised
	Nucleus/gland ratio	Low	⟶		High
	Nucleus/cell height ratio	0.15–0.3	⟶		0.5–0.9
Structural atypia	Glandular structure	Tubular	Tubular/villous ± branching	Tubulovillous, ± snaking, branching	Tubulovillous and cribriform (por)
	Index of structural atypia	Normal	⟶	Increased	

whether an early malignant lesion should be resected en-bloc, this difference is irrelevant because both HGIN and carcinoma in situ should be removed en-bloc [1, 3, 6]. Minor differences may also exist in the categorization of low-grade versus high-grade intraepithelial neoplasias (LGIN vs. HGIN), but this decision is primarily a matter of individual expertise and should involve an expert reference pathologist [3, 6, 10].

2.2.2 *Malignant Potential*

The *likelihood of nodal metastasis* depends mainly on *histologic grading* and *depth of submucosal invasion* of any T1 carcinoma, as well as on *macroscopic type* and *anatomical localization* in the gastrointestinal tract. The macroscopic type of early cancer (Paris classification; *see* Fig. 1.2) relates to risk of lymphovascular spread [1–4, 16], probably reflecting morphogenic and molecular pathways of oncogenesis (Sect. 2.3).

Well-differentiated mucosal cancer shows a relatively structured and continuous infiltrative growth pattern of glandular crowding, branching, and budding, with clear histologic borders to normal tissue reflected by clear endoscopic margins of the neoplasia. Relative loss of polar structure of epithelial cell layers, enhanced nucleus/cytoplasm ratio, and bulky growth of the epithelial cell layer in the neoplasm alter the surface aspect of mucosal neoplasias, inducing a visible mucosal pattern on M-IEE. In massive submucosal invasion of coherently growing carci-

Table 2.3 Probability of lymph node metastasis of superficial cancers by extent of submucosal invasion (μm)

Carcinoma	Depth of invasion	Lymph node positive cases, %
Esophagus [3, 17, 19, 21, 22]		
SCC (type 0–II; grading G1, G2)	m1	0%
if *L0, V0, d < 5 cm, no ulcer, cN0*	m3 (muscularis mucosae)	8%
	sm1 (<200 μm and d < 5 cm)	4.2%
Overall	sm1 (<200 μm)	17%
AC (Barrett's CCLE)	pT1m	1.9% (CI 1.2–2.7%)
	pT1sm	21%
Stomach (if L0, V0) [2, 18]		
AC intestinal type G1–G2	pT1m (d < 30 mm)	0% (CI 0–0.3%)
	pT1sm1 (<500 μm)	0% (CI 0–2.5%)
AC undifferentiated G3–G4	pT1m (d < 20 mm, no ulcer)	<1% (CI 0–2.6%)
Colon (if *G1 or G2, L0, V0*) [1, 20]		
AC type 0–II	pT1 (sm <1000 μm)	1.4% (0–5%)
AC type Ip	pT1 (Ip-head, sm < 3000 μm)	0% (0–5%)

AC adenocarcinoma, *CCLE* columnar cell-lined esophagus, *CI* confidence intervall, *d* diameter, *SCC* squamous cell carcinoma, *sm* submucosal

noma, the surface gland structure (typical for differentiated mucosal cancer) becomes destroyed, yielding a highly irregular or even non-structured surface (amorphous pattern) on both stereomicroscopic observation and M-IEE. In addition, differentiated mucosal cancers require neoangiogenesis for deep submucosal invasion, so M-IEE shows irregular microvessels in the mucosal layer, as demonstrated by immunohistochemistry in resected early cancers and correlated with imaging features on M-IEE [1, 3, 5, 14, 15].

The likelihood of lymph node metastasis generally increases with *depth of invasion* of well-differentiated early cancer [2, 3, 16]. The best data on these correlations have been collected in large surgical series of resected early cancers with dissection of regional lymph nodes [2, 16–22], as summarized in Table 2.3. To predict risk of metastasis to locoregional lymph nodes for well-differentiated early cancers, T1 lesions of the colon are categorized into “low risk”, i.e. grading G1 or G2, no invasion of lymphatic vessels (L0) or submucosal veins (V0), and submucosal extension of less than 1000 μm, versus “high risk” in presence of any feature like tumor-cell budding (Bd > 1) at the invasive front (Fig. 2.1), submucosal invasion >1000 μm, lymphatic or venous vascular invasion, or grading G3 or G4 [20, 23, 24]. Tumor budding is defined as a single tumor cell or cluster up to 4 tumor cells – in contrast to poorly differentiated clusters (of ≥5 tumor cells) which could be related to enhanced epithelial-mesenchymal-transition properties and enhanced metastatic potency.

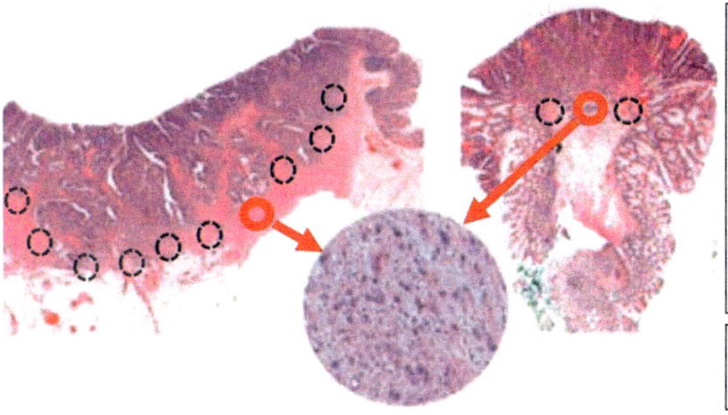

Object magnification: 20

Eyepiece FN diameter (mm)	Specimen area (mm^2)	Normalization factor
18	0.636	0.810
19	0.709	0.903
20	0.785	1.000
21	0.866	1.103
22	0.950	1.210
23	1.039	1.323
24	1.131	1.440
25	1.227	1.563
26	1.327	1.690

$$\text{Tumor bud count per } 0{,}785\ mm^2 = \frac{\text{Bud count (20 × objective)}}{\text{Normalization factor*}}$$

Bd1 (low)	0–4 buds	per 0.785 mm^2
Bd2 (intermediate)	5–9 buds	per 0.785 mm^2
Bd3 (high)	≥10 buds	per 0.785 mm^2

Reporting example:
Tumor budding:Bd3 (high), count 14 (per 0.785 mm^2)

Fig. 2.1 Procedure proposed by the International Tumor Budding Consensus Conference (ITBCC) [23] for reporting tumor budding in colorectal cancer. The area of 20-fold magnification of the microscope in use is normalized to 0.785 mm^2 (for 20 × objective lens 20 mm eyepiece field number [FN] diameter). Out of 10 separate fields (20 × objective), the "hotspot" with maximum budding at the invasive front is selected (indicated by *red circle*; H.E. stain, upper field) and all budding tumor cells are counted. The budding count normalized to the field area of 0.785 mm^2 is reported in *budding categories* Bd1–Bd3. (Modified from Lugli et al. [23] with permission of USCAP Inc)

Poorly differentiated or *undifferentiated* early cancers (G3/G4) show loss of cell-cell adhesion, discontinuous growth pattern, and high nucleus/cytoplasm ratio, paralleled by more rapid tumor cell replication/proliferation and higher metastatic potential (e.g. anoikis) on a cell biology level. Therefore, lymphatic vessel or blood vessel permeation is frequent even with small, poorly differentiated intramucosal early cancer, and rates of lymph node (or hematogenous) metastases are higher than with well-differentiated mucosal cancer [2, 16, 18]. The risk of metastatic spread to locoregional lymph nodes is increased for poorly differentiated early gastric cancer exceeding lateral extension of 20 mm [2, 18]. Also, margins of undifferentiated mucosal cancers tend to be less clear, the epithelial surface structure in the central part of the cancer may be destroyed by epithelial invasion with undifferentiated cancer cells, and the microcapillary pattern in the lamina propria mucosae tends to be very irregular on magnifying narrow band imaging (M-NBI) endoscopy.

Based on extensive quantitative histopathologic analysis of surgical resection specimens of early gastrointestinal cancers, the likelihood of cure from early cancer achievable by endoscopic en-bloc resection with free margins can now be predicted based on histologic characteristics, lateral size, depth of submucosal invasion, absence of lymphovascular invasion, and organ location in the GI tract (Table 2.4). Magnifying endoscopic analysis of early cancers attempts to predict whether the lesion allows endoscopic en-bloc resection for cure, based on characteristic alterations of the macroscopic type and the surface and microvascular structure.

Table 2.4 Criteria of curative endoscopic resection in esophagus, stomach, and colorectum

Organ	Criteria of curative en-bloc resection
Stomach	*Guideline criteria*
	m-ca, diff. type, ly (−), v (−), Ul (−), and ≤2 cm in size
	Expanded criteria
	m-ca, diff. type, ly (−), v (−), Ul (−), and any size >2 cm
	m-ca, diff. type, ly (−), v (−), Ul (+), and ≤3 cm in size
	sm 1-ca (invasion depth <500 μm), diff. type, ly (−), v (−)
	m-ca, undiff. type (G3), ly (−), v(−), Ul (−), and size <2 cm
Esophagus (squamous lesions only)	*Guideline criteria*
	pT1a-EP-ca, pT1a-LPM-ca
	Expanded criteria
	pT1a-MM-ca, diff. type, expansive growth, ly(−), v (−)
	cT1b/sm-ca (invasion depth <200 μm), infiltrative growth pattern, expansive, diff. type, ly (−), v (−)
Colorectum	*Guideline criteria*
	m-ca, diff. type, ly (−), v (−)
	sm-ca (<1000 μm), diff. type, ly (−), v (−)

Modified from Toyonaga et al. [25]
ca cancer, *diff* differentiated, *EP* epithelium, *LPM* lamina propria mucosae, *ly* lymphatic invasion, *m* mucosal, *MM* muscularis mucosae, *sm* submucosal, *Ul* ulceration, *v* vascular invasion

2.3 Characteristics of Colonic Neoplastic Lesions

On colonoscopy, most protruded or flat lesions classify as adenomatous or hyperplastic/serrated according to histomorphology (Fig. 2.2). Whereas strictly hyperplastic lesions are non-neoplastic, the similar-appearing serrated adenomas are (like classical polypoid adenomas) cancer precursor lesions.

The usual perception of morphological carcinogenesis still focuses on the classic "polyp–cancer sequence" [26], although at least four other precursor–cancer pathways exist in the colon: the depressed neoplasia pathway, the hereditary nonpolyposis colorectal cancer (HNPCC) pathway, the serrated adenoma pathway, and (in ulcerative colitis and in Crohn colitis) the "inflammation–dysplasia–carcinoma pathway" [1, 4, 26–28] (Table 2.5). Genetic analyses data of colorectal cancer (CRC) has now been grouped into four consensus molecular subtypes (CMS 1–4) plus a CMS "mixed features" group [28], and the immune cell, fibroblastic, and angiogenic microenvironment been described for the four subtypes [29]. The morphogenic types have not yet been systematically investigated for their relationship with the molecular CMS.

2.3.1 Classic Polypoid Adenoma-Carcinoma Pathway

Polyps have been snared in the colon since 1972, and histologic findings (Table 2.6) have led to the adenoma–dysplasia–cancer sequence [30], which was translated into molecular pathways of oncogenesis by Vogelstein et al. [26]. In addition, screening colonoscopy with clearing of all detectable adenomas by endoscopic polypectomy had reduced the incidence of CRC far below predicted rates [31]. This served as a rationale for approval of colonoscopy screening to prevent CRC in the United States and many other western countries. From an endoscopic vantage point, Kudo [4] and Uraoka [32] described a separate entity – superficially spreading adenomas of more than 10 mm diameter – as lateral spreading type (LST) neoplasia with its own ablative strategy.

2.3.2 Flat/Depressed Colonic Adenoma-Carcinoma Pathway

The majority of advanced CRC may develop from a non-polypoid precursor lesion [1, 4, 33, 34]. In the "depressed neoplasia–carcinoma sequence," Shimoda et al. described minute *de novo* cancers of 2- to 5-mm size, most with submucosal invasion [34]. In more than 1000 colonic neoplasms, they diagnosed 71 cancers, of which 78% originated from nonpolypoid precursor lesions and 22%, from polypoid adenomas. Ten (13%) of 75 cancers were minute (<5 mm), depressed-type cancers without adenomatous areas, all of which showed submucosal invasion [34]. Depressed-type (0-IIc) colorectal carcinomas are at a more advanced stage than non-depressed lesions (0-IIa or b) [4, 33]. Therefore, these depressed-type neoplasms have a high likelihood of malignant progression and show shorter evolution time to cancer.

2.3.3 Serrated Adenoma-Carcinoma Pathway

Sessile serrated adenomas show up like hyperplastic polyps with dilated pit pattern type II-O, whereas polypoid (i.e. "traditional") serrated adenomas exhibit an adenomatous pit pattern (pp IIIL or IV) mixed with type II-O (Table 2.6) However, these lesions are premalignant via the "serrated pathway" to adenocarcinoma [27, 36]. About 8% of all and 18% of proximal colorectal carcinomas originate from the "serrated pathway" involving the sequence hyperplastic aberrant crypt foci → sessile/polypoid serrated adenomas (SSA/P) → dysplastic serrated adenoma → serrated adenocarcinoma [27, 36]. Sessile serrated adenomas are located mainly in the proximal colon, whereas traditional polypoid serrated adenomas more often (>60%)

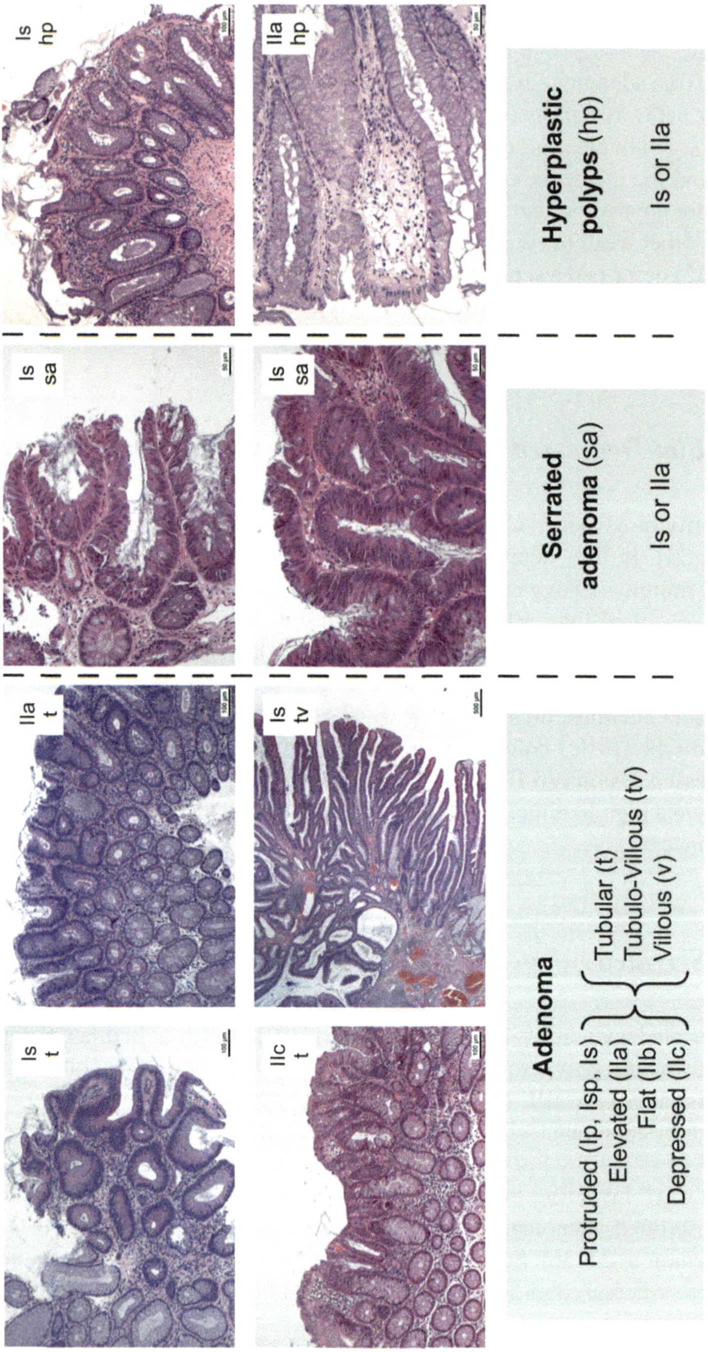

Fig. 2.2 Principles of histomorphology of adenomatous or hyperplastic mucosal lesions in the colon

Table 2.5 Morphogenic pathways of colorectal carcinogenesis [1, 4, 26–28, 34–36]

Superficial neoplasms	CRC risk estimates	Precursors of CRC estimated	Prevalence of CR neoplasia[a]
Classic adenoma	10 years 15–30%	50%	50%
Polypoid (type 0–Ip,s)			
Distal > proximal			
CIN (LoH, kRAS, APC)			
Serrated adenoma	5 years 60%	15–20%	30%
Serrated polyp (kRAS), distal			
Sessile SA (*BRAF*), proximal			5–8%
CIN (kRAS)			
MSI+++ (*BRAF*, CIMP)			
Serrated polyposis syndrome SPS	Lifetime 50%	< 1%	0.5%
Depressed NpI 0–IIc	1–5 years 75%	20–30%	< 3%
"De novo cancer"			
Proximal > distal			
MSI+++			
HNPCC adenoma	1–5 years 40–80%	~5%	< 5%
Flat adenoma 0–IIa/b/c			
Proximal (70%) > total colon			
MSI+++ (MLH mut, CIMP)			

[a]Estimates for CRC screening population. Abbreviations see text

Table 2.6 Histopathologic classification of adenomatous and serrated lesions

Histologic criteria of colorectal lesions 0-I & 0-II	Histologic criteria for SSA/P
Conventional adenomatous lesions	Criteria [diagnostic, when 2 of 4 (+) in ≥2 crypts[a]]
Tubular or villous growth pattern	1. Hyperserration of crypts, in lower third with/without branching
Grade of dysplasia (low vs. high)	2. T-shaped and L-shaped crypts above MM
Serrated lesions	3. Inverted crypts below MM (pseudoinversion)
Hyperplastic polyp	4. Columnar dilatation in the lower third
Sessile serrated adenoma/polyp	
SSA/P without dysplasia	
SSA/P with dysplasia (= MSA)	
Traditional serrated adenoma	

Modified from East et al. [27]

MM muscularis mucosae, *MSA* mixed serrated adenoma (previous nomenclature), *SSA/P* sessile serrated adenoma/polyp

[a]Two crypts need not be neighboring

occur in the left hemicolon [27, 37]. Serrated adenomas show malignant transition about twice as often as conventional adenomas. On a molecular basis, serrated adenomas are the precursors of type 1 CRC (CIMP-high/MSI-high/*BRAF* mutation) and type 2 CRC (CIMP-high/MSI-low or MSS/*BRAF* mutation) [8, 38]. Serrated precursor lesions were not described in the National Polyp Study and received attention in endoscopic studies after 2010 [27, 31].

2.3.4 Hereditary Non-polyposis Colon Cancer Pathway

HNPCC shows a right-sided (~70% of cases) or even (30%) colonic distribution of cancer and mainly non-polypous precursor lesions (0-IIa and 0-IIb) with predominant villous architecture, containing high-grade dysplasia as well as mucinous differentiation [39–45]. On initial and follow-up surveillance colonoscopy, the detection rate for non-polypoid adenomas is about 1.1 per HNPCC patient [40, 42]. The progression to high-grade dysplasia is more common in proximal than in distal HNPCC adenomas [45]. A high proportion of these non-polypoid adenomas will rapidly progress to cancer that is CpG island methylator phenotype (CIMP)–negative with microsatellite instability (MSI-high) or chromosomal instability (and MS-stable) [39].

2.3.5 Inflammation–Dysplasia–Cancer Pathway in Inflammatory Bowel Disease

Patients with ulcerative colitis or colitis Crohn may exhibit three different types of neoplastic lesions: *sporadic adenoma, visible dysplasia*, and *invisible dysplasia.* Sporadic adenoma occurs only in mucosa uninvolved with inflammatory bowel disease (IBD). The term *DALM* (dysplasia-associated lesion or mass) was created in 1981, but was imprecise and often interpreted as needing colectomy. It has been abandoned in the new SCENIC guidelines [46, 47]. This new classification fits the Paris classification and uniform histologic criteria [48]. Systematic random biopsy protocols, such as the Seattle protocol, no longer are recommended. Instead, the mucosa is examined with high-definition colonoscopy and chromoendoscopy for visible dysplastic lesions, which are reported according to the Paris classification. Targeted biopsies are taken from areas suspicious for dysplasia.

Dysplasia shows in colonic epithelium nuclear enlargement crowding, and stratification, hyperchromasia, and prominent nucleoli in both crypts and surface epithelium (i.e., loss of surface epithelial maturation). IBD-associated HGIEN and CRC stain pos. for p53 on IHC (but sporadic HGIEN/CRC in IBD is p53 negative). Dysplasia is systematically reported as high-grade intraepithelial neoplasia (HGIEN), low-grade intraepithelial neoplasia (LGIEN), or "indefinite" or "negative" [12, 48]. *Visible dysplasia* (HGIEN and LGIEN) is an indication for endoscopic resection (preferably en-bloc) if the lesion is delineated and resectable; otherwise, it is an indication for colectomy. The risk of associated cancer is very high (42–67%) for HGIEN, and also high (22%) for multifocal LGIEN [49–51]; colectomy is recommended for either one [46, 47]. Solitary LGIEN should be examined with repeat endoscopy and resection when well feasible; management is individualized. A prospective study on flat low-grade dysplasia (LGD) found only a 3% initial rate of progression to CRC, and a 10% rate of subsequent progression within 10 years [49]. However, a later meta-analysis (477 patients) indicated that flat LGD had a risk of 22% for synchronous cancer and a 5-year progression rate of 33–53% to advanced neoplasia (CRC or HGD) [51].

Invisible dysplasia results from untargeted random biopsy in IBD-involved mucosa. Random biopsies are justified in the presence of multiple pseudopolyps, postinflammatory narrowing or near visible lesions, but otherwise are no longer recommended [46, 47]. A finding of *indefinite for dysplasia* can be the result of active regenerative signs. Regenerative mucosal alterations can be difficult to differentiate endoscopically and histologically from dysplasia in ulcerative colitis. Hence, therapy for IBD should be intensified to eliminate inflammation before repeat endoscopy to exclude or confirm dysplasia. In general, surveillance colonoscopy should be planned when the IBD is in clinical remission [46, 47].

2.4 Characteristics of Gastric Carcinomas

Gastric adenocarcinomas (GC) occur sporadically in approximately 90% of cases; 10% are inherited. The latter comprise at least three forms: familial diffuse gastric cancer (FDGC), familial intestinal gastric cancer (FIGC), and hereditary diffuse gastric cancer (HDGC), which is caused by *CDH1* germline mutations encoding the cell-adhesion protein e-cadherin [52]. Four molecular subgroups of GC have been defined: *EBV induced GC* (9%, with a high frequency of *PIK3CA* mutations, hypermethylation and amplification of *JAK2*, PD-L1, and PD-L2), often analogous in HP induced GC; *MSI pos.* (22%, with a high rate of mutation, also often in HP induced GC); *genomically stable GC* with diffuse histology (20%, mutations of *RAS* and genes encoding integrins and adhesion proteins, including *CDH1*); and *chromosomal instabile GC (CIN & aneuploidy)* [53]. However, therapeutic considerations are still based on histomorphological classification. The two main *histogenetic types* of gastric cancer are the intestinal type, forming gland-like tubular structures (most with grading G1 or G2), and the *diffuse type*, lacking cell cohesion and infiltrating the gastric wall by spreading of single cancer cells (grading G3) (Fig. 2.3) [9, 54, 55].

2.4.1 Intestinal-Type Gastric Adenocarcinoma

Intestinal-type cancer comprises two major histogenetic phenotypes: the *intestinal* phenotype and the *gastric* phenotype [56, 57]. The classic intestinal phenotype arises in chronic atrophic gastritis (either autoimmune type A or *Helicobacter pylori*–induced type B gastritis) via the "immature" intestinal metaplasia to flat or adenomatous intraepithelial neoplasia, and finally to the gland-forming intestinal-type carcinoma, which frequently shows solid tumor growth and less invasion [56–58]. Intestinal metaplasia with HGIN has a 33–85% chance to progress to gastric cancer [59]. Sporadic gastric adenomas occur infrequently; they carry a 35% chance of carcinomatous foci [59].

Early gastric cancers of the intestinal type may exhibit any of the macroscopic lesions (0-Ip/s, 0-IIa/b/c, 0-III). Polypoid adenomas play a minor role as precursor lesions for gastric cancer, as less than 5% of gastric cancers originate from 0-Is adenomas. The risk of submucosal invasion is high in type 0-Is and even higher in type 0-IIc [6]. The risk of lymph node metastasis is low (<5%) when submucosal invasion is <500 μm (Ly 0, V 0), but is 21% for invasion of sm2 >500 μm [2, 18].

2.4.2 Gastric Phenotype Adenocarcinoma

Gastric phenotype carcinoma, frequently with microsatellite instability, develops from non-metaplastic gastric epithelium, either *de novo* or from small adenomas of pyloric mucoid glands [58, 60]. Gastric-type differentiated carcinoma represents 8–24% of early gastric cancers, often type II-b or II-c lesions with less discoloured surface [56]. This type of cancer tends to be larger and exhibits submucosal invasion more often than the intestinal type [56–58]. Advanced gastric-type and intestinal-type cancers often express a mixed phenotype, including a diffuse growth component caused by inactivation of the e-cadherin gene *CDH1*, perhaps by biallelic hypermethylation [58]. Individualized therapeutic decisions rest mainly on grading G3.

2.4.3 Diffuse/Signet-Ring Type (De Novo) Gastric Cancer

Early diffuse-type cancer shows either flat lesions (type 0-IIb) or depressed lesions (0-IIc), with diffusely infiltrating single cancer cells in the mucosa and submucosa, which exhibit massive cellular atypia (most with grading G3) [6, 14, 61]. Minute diffuse-type cancers (diameter <5 mm) are difficult to detect; they most often appear as a small, pale spot in the gastric mucosa [62].

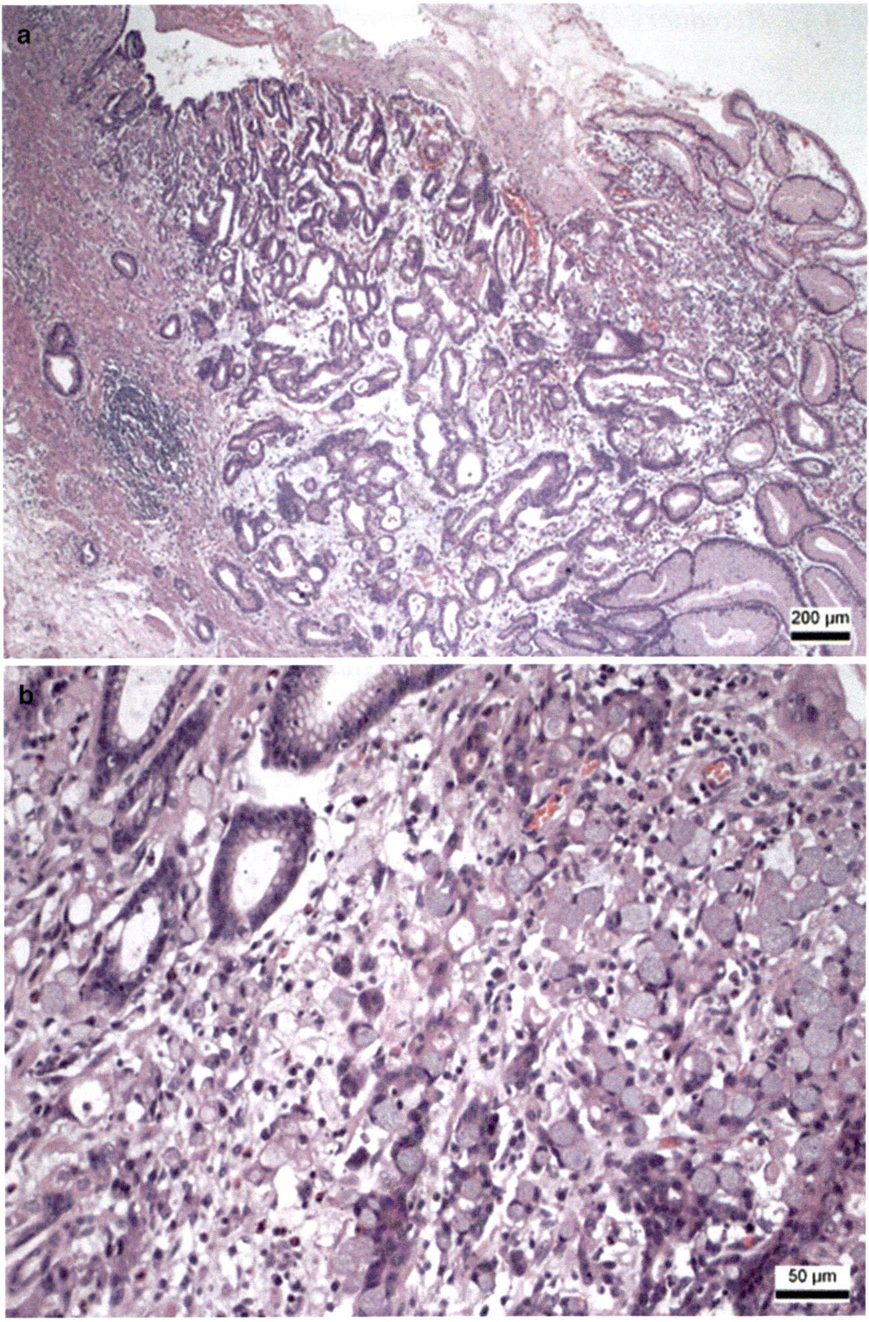

Fig. 2.3 Typical histomorphology of (**a**) intestinal-type gastric cancer and (**b**) diffuse/signet-ring gastric adenocarcinoma. The growth pattern in the intestinal type shows well-defined glands, in contrast to the discohesive tumor sheet in the diffuse type

2.4.4 *Hereditary Diffuse-Type Gastric Cancer (HDGC)*

In patients less than 60 years old, this cancer (caused by *CDH1* germline mutations) usually is multifocal and synchronous; the neoplastic foci are very difficult to detect. Therefore, the diagnosis in suspected cases must be established by molecular genetic analysis, starting with the index case in the kindred. Individuals with a proven inherited genetic defect must undergo prophylactic gastrectomy [52].

2.5 Characteristics of Esophageal Neoplastic Lesions

For both types of esophageal cancer—squamous cell carcinoma (SCC) and adenocarcinoma (AC) in the columnar cell–lined esophagus (Fig. 2.4)—chronic inflammation of the esophageal epithelium is the trigger of carcinogenesis. The chronic esophagitis–dysplasia–cancer sequence is maintained by a host of noxious agents in SCC and mainly by gastroesophageal reflux of acid and pepsin or bile in AC [63].

2.5.1 *Cylinder Epithelial Dysplasia: Cancer Pathway (Barrett's Cancer)*

Barrett's adenocarcinoma arises in columnar epithelial metaplasia of previously SC-lined esophagus. Because of chronic inflammation with reflux disease and regeneration, dysplasia evolves from columnar metaplasia, which by itself is considered a precursor for neoplasia. Therefore, the terms *columnar intraepithelial neoplasia* (CIN) in the Vienna classification, or *intraepithelial neoplasia* (IEN) in the WHO classification, are preferred to the term *adenoma* as the precursor lesion for cancer [7, 12]. In a high proportion of HGIEN, the Wnt-β-catenin pathway is activated and *p53* is mutated [64]. Low-grade dysplasia may either regress again or progress to HGIN, which carries on the average a 30% chance of concurrent carcinomatous foci [65]. The flat lesions (0-IIa-c) are harder to detect and by far the most frequent macroscopic types of neoplastic lesion [7].

The mucosal smooth muscle (MM) layer becomes duplicated in Barrett's mucosa, because chronic inflammation stimulates myofibroblasts to form a superficial muscle layer (SMM) in the lamina propria mucosae (LPM). The original deep MM layer (DMM) serves as the reference for depth of submucosal invasion (Fig. 2.5). The risk for lymph node metastasis (LN 1) is about 1% for intramucosal AC pT1a-LPM (the classic limit for curative resection), and starts to rise with invasion of MM (<4%) and even more with pT1b-SM1 (9%, but for low-risk criteria <4%) [17, 66]. Mucosal Barrett's cancers pT1a show mainly low-risk criteria (95%). With deeper infiltration of the submucosal layer T1b-SM2-3, high budding grade

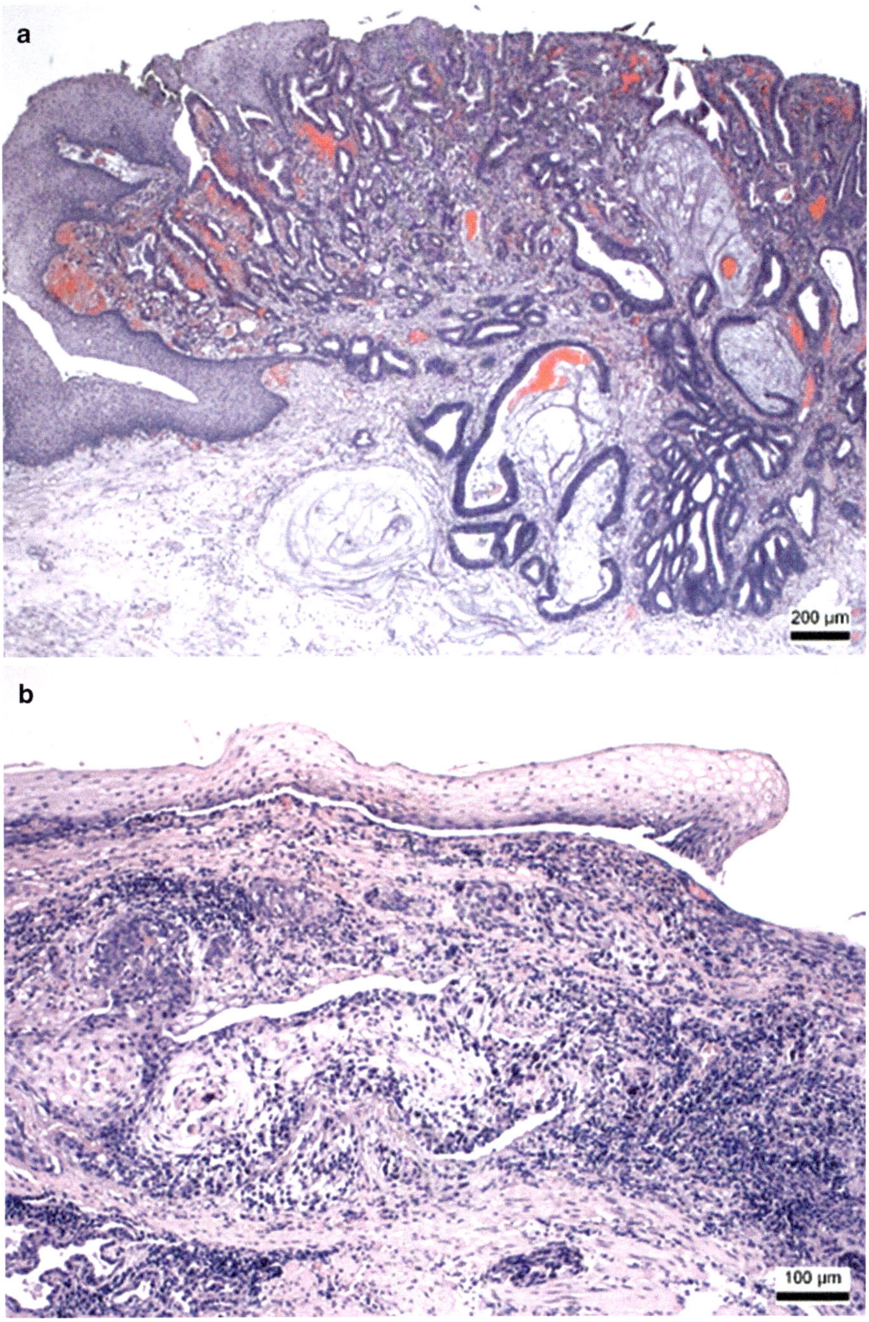

Fig. 2.4 Histomorphology of (**a**) Barrett's cancer and (**b**) squamous epithelial cancer of the esophagus, revealing atypical tubular glands of the Barrett esophagus, as well as irregular, formed squamous cell nests with keratin pearls with extension of the squamous epithelium above it in both cases

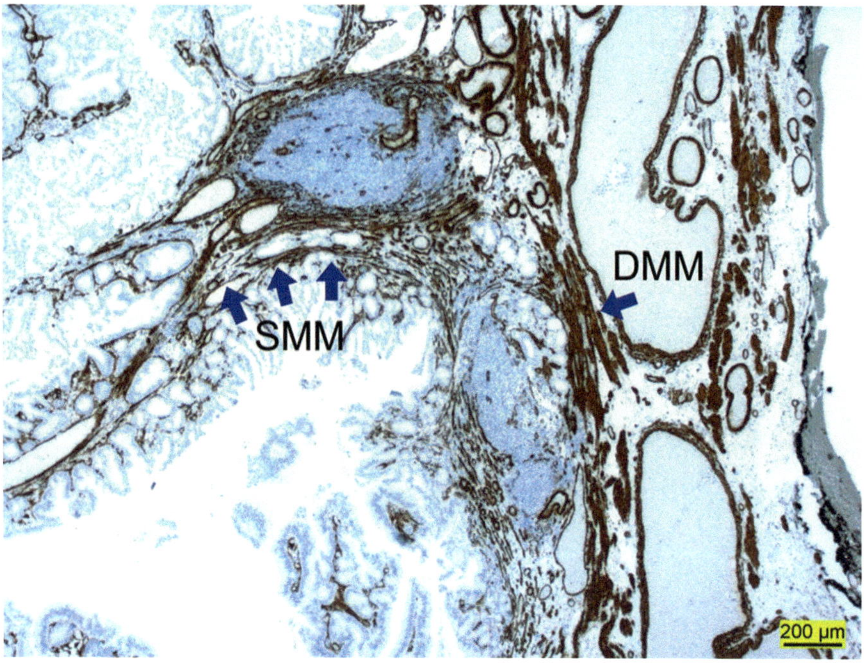

Fig. 2.5 Margin of Barrett well-differentiated adenocarcinoma (WDAC) pT1a-MM G1 L0 V0 with adjacent Barrett mucosa that shows characteristic doubling of the MM layer into a superficial newly formed layer (SMM), and original deep MM layer (DMM). (Desmin IHC stain, smooth muscle). AC infiltrates into MM. Endoscopic submucosal dissection (ESD) was curative

Bd $\geq$ 2 and grading G3 become more prevalent (up to ~30%), and risk of lymph node metastasis rises up to 10% in sm1, and 30–50% with T1b-SM2-3 [66–68].

2.5.2 *Squamous Epithelial Cell Dysplasia: Cancer Pathway*

Chronic esophagitis may be caused by a variety of irritants of the squamous cell epithelium such as caustic damage by hot drinks or food or chronic alcohol use, often combined with carcinogens from tobacco use; nutritional deficiencies (vitamins A, B1–B6, or C; zinc); and chronic viral infection (e.g. human papillomavirus) [59, 63]. Chronic inflammation combined with carcinogen exposure leads to squamous epithelial dysplasia that is graded in a two-tier system of low-grade and high-grade [6, 12].

Early lesions appear as reddish spots or small grey-white or plaque-like elevations of the mucosa, apparent intraepithelial neoplasms (HGIN), or carcinoma in situ [3, 15, 69]. About half of these lesions are located in the middle third of the esophagus, with the remainder equally in the upper and lower thirds; about 10% are synchronous multifocal [3, 69]. Most of the lesions are well-differentiated or moderately differentiated squamous cell carcinomas (grading G1 or G2), but owing to the thin submucosal layer rich in lymphatic vessels, the risk of early local spread is high [3].

2.6 Processing of En Bloc Specimens from Endoscopic Mucosal Resection (EMR) or Endoscopic Submucosal Dissection (ESD)

The resected specimen soaked with 0.9% saline must be pinned (every 1.5 mm, 0.5 mm from the margin) onto cork or rubber board in distended [→ to original size] and orientated fashion, so that the surrounding mucosa is evident. Then the specimen is image documented and rapidly immersed, fixed for 24 h in 4% buffered formaldehyde solution. Then specimens are cut into slices 2–3 mm thick and image-documented for subserial microscopic examination [3, 70] (Fig. 2.6).

Note The histology of the mucosectomy specimen (EMR en bloc or ESD) must evaluate

- Macroscopic type 0 and subtypes
- Low-grade or high-grade intraepithelial neoplasia or grading of carcinoma
- Budding of tumor at the invasion front
- Lymphovascular or perineural invasion of cancer
- Invasion of the submucosa as depth beyond the muscularis mucosae
- Completeness of resection at the margins of the specimen

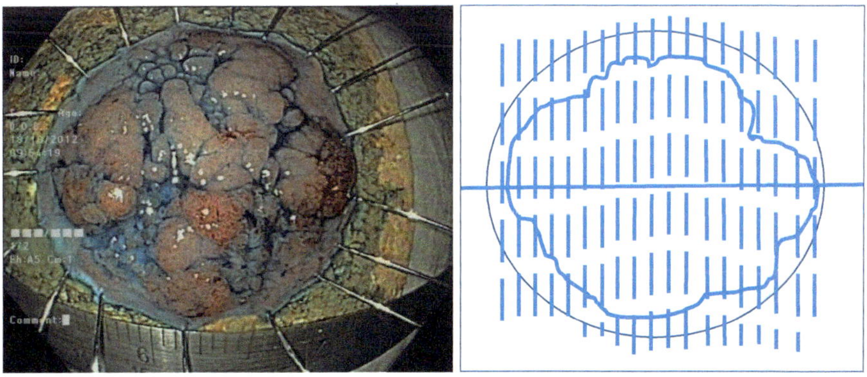

Fig. 2.6 *Left panel*: Endoscopic submucosal dissection (ESD) specimen (4.5 × 5 cm; WLI, indigo carmine chromoendoscopy [CE]) fixed on cork. (Indicate malignant/invasive looking spots in report.) *Right panel*: Scheme of actual cutting procedure: Serial cuts perpendicular to long tumor axis, starting at the closest tumor edge (right side), after 24 h fixation in formalin. Rectosigmoid LST-mixed, tubulovillous adenoma, focal pTis, resection R0

The diagnosis of invasiveness (including lymphovascular infiltration and infiltrative depth of the malignant gastrointestinal tumor) inside the ESD specimen should be supported by auxiliary immunohistochemical analysis. Therefore, immunohistochemical markers such as smooth muscle actin, CD34, and podoplanin could be helpful to highlight the muscularis mucosae and vascular and lymphatic structures in the tumor specimen. Additionally, an image analysis system quantifies the infiltrative depth (in micrometers) for further therapeutic stratifications. Finally, the application of immunohistochemistry could clarify the tumor differentiation (intestinal, squamous, mucinous, neuroendocrine) as well as the oncogenic potency (e.g. proliferation and tumor budding) in the ESD specimen for considerations of hematogenic and lymphatic metastatic potency. All this information should be integrated in the final pathological examination/assessment of the ESD specimen.

Note The *pathology report* confirms the curative safety of a local excision or recommends the need for additional surgical resection or adjuvant treatment, based on

- qualitative criteria (grading, L or V invasion, budding, cribriform pattern) and
- quantitative criteria (width and depth of invasion into the submucosa).

As mentioned, the depth of invasion correlates with the risk of lymph node metastasis (*see* Table 2.1). Quantitative micrometer (μm) measurements are reported from the lower limit of the muscularis mucosae, when the position of the muscularis mucosae can be determined precisely in the area of the tumor invasion. Rigorous analysis of the excised lesion provides a quality standard for therapeutic endoscopy and serves as a safeguard against erroneous decisions, such as unnecessary surgical resection of a non-neoplastic lesion or the inappropriate endoscopic resection (R1 or R2) of a carcinoma with submucosal invasion.

Acknowledgments The authors gratefully acknowledge Susanna Mueller, M.D., Department of Pathology, Ludwig-Maximilians-University Munich, Munich, Germany; and Manfred Stolte, M.D., Institut für Pathologie, Kulmbach, for proofreading of the chapter and focusing on the formal differences in histopathologic criteria of cancer diagnosis used by Japanese and Western pathologists.

References

1. Fujimori T, et al. Pathological diagnosis of early colorectal carcinoma and its clinical implications. Digestion. 2009;79(Suppl 1):40–51.
2. Gotoda T, et al. Incidence of lymph node metastasis from early gastric cancer: estimation with a large number of cases at two large centers. Gastric Cancer. 2000;3:219–25.
3. Takubo K, et al. Early squamous cell carcinoma of the oesophagus: the Japanese viewpoint. Histopathology. 2007;51:733–42.
4. Kudo S, et al. Nonpolypoid neoplastic lesions of the colorectal mucosa. Gastrointest Endosc. 2008;68:S3–47.
5. Sano Y, et al. Narrow-band imaging (NBI) magnifying endoscopic classification of colorectal tumors proposed by the Japan NBI Expert Team. Dig Endosc. 2016;28:526–33.
6. The Paris endoscopic classification of superficial neoplastic lesions: esophagus, stomach, and colon: November 30 to December 1, 2002. Gastrointest Endosc. 2003;58:S3–43.

7. Paris workshop on columnar metaplasia in the esophagus and the esophagogastric junction, Paris, France, December 11–12, 2004. Endoscopy. 2005;37:879–920.
8. Jass JR. Classification of colorectal cancer based on correlation of clinical, morphological and molecular features. Histopathology. 2007;50:113–30.
9. Lauren P. The Two histological main types of gastric carcinoma: diffuse and so-called intestinal-type carcinoma. An attempt at a histo-clinical classification. Acta Pathol Microbiol Scand. 1965;64:31–49.
10. Schlemper RJ, et al. Differences in the diagnostic criteria used by Japanese and Western pathologists to diagnose colorectal carcinoma. Cancer. 1998;82:60–9.
11. Schlemper RJ, et al. Differences in diagnostic criteria for gastric carcinoma between Japanese and western pathologists. Lancet. 1997;349:1725–9.
12. Schlemper RJ, et al. The Vienna classification of gastrointestinal epithelial neoplasia. Gut. 2000;47:251–5.
13. Kudo SE. Early colorectal cancer. In: Detection of depressed types of colorectal carcinoma. Tokyo: IGAKU-SHOIN Ltd; 1996.
14. Muto M, et al. Magnifying endoscopy simple diagnostic algorithm for early gastric cancer (MESDA-G). Dig Endosc. 2016;28:379–93.
15. Oyama T, et al. Prediction of the invasion depth of superficial squamous cell carcinoma based on microvessel morphology: magnifying endoscopic classification of the Japan Esophageal Society. Esophagus. 2017;14:105–12.
16. Ueno H, et al. Risk factors for an adverse outcome in early invasive colorectal carcinoma. Gastroenterology. 2004;127:385–94.
17. Dunbar KB, et al. The risk of lymph-node metastases in patients with high-grade dysplasia or intramucosal carcinoma in Barrett's esophagus: a systematic review. Am J Gastroenterol. 2012;107:850–62. quiz 863
18. Hirasawa T, et al. Incidence of lymph node metastasis and the feasibility of endoscopic resection for undifferentiated-type early gastric cancer. Gastric Cancer. 2009;12:148–52.
19. Holscher AH, et al. Prognostic impact of upper, middle, and lower third mucosal or submucosal infiltration in early esophageal cancer. Ann Surg. 2011;254:802–7; discussion 807–808.
20. Kitajima K, et al. Correlations between lymph node metastasis and depth of submucosal invasion in submucosal invasive colorectal carcinoma: a Japanese collaborative study. J Gastroenterol. 2004;39:534–43.
21. Stein HJ, et al. Early esophageal cancer: pattern of lymphatic spread and prognostic factors for long-term survival after surgical resection. Ann Surg. 2005;242:566–73; discussion 573–565.
22. Tajima Y, et al. Histopathologic findings predicting lymph node metastasis and prognosis of patients with superficial esophageal carcinoma: analysis of 240 surgically resected tumors. Cancer. 2000;88:1285–93.
23. Lugli A, et al. Recommendations for reporting tumor budding in colorectal cancer based on the International Tumor Budding Consensus Conference (ITBCC) 2016. Mod Pathol. 2017;30:1299–311.
24. Watanabe T, et al. Japanese Society for Cancer of the Colon and Rectum (JSCCR) guidelines 2016 for the treatment of colorectal cancer. Int J Clin Oncol. 2018;23:1–34.
25. Toyonaga T, et al. Principles of quality controlled endoscopic submucosal dissection with appropriate dissection level and high quality resected specimen. Clin Endosc. 2012;45:362–74.
26. Vogelstein B, et al. Genetic alterations during colorectal-tumor development. N Engl J Med. 1988;319:525–32.
27. East JE, et al. Serrated lesions in colorectal cancer screening: detection, resection, pathology and surveillance. Gut. 2015;64:991–1000.
28. Guinney J, et al. The consensus molecular subtypes of colorectal cancer. Nat Med. 2015;21:1350–6.
29. Becht E, et al. Immune and stromal classification of colorectal cancer is associated with molecular subtypes and relevant for precision immunotherapy. Clin Cancer Res. 2016;22:4057–66.
30. Hermanek P. Polypectomy in the colorectum histological and oncological aspects. Endoscopy. 1983;15(Suppl 1):158–61.

31. Lieberman DA. Clinical practice. Screening for colorectal cancer. N Engl J Med. 2009;361:1179–87.
32. Uraoka T, et al. Endoscopic indications for endoscopic mucosal resection of laterally spreading tumours in the colorectum. Gut. 2006;55:1592–7.
33. Goto H. Proportion of de novo cancers among colorectal cancers in Japan. Gastroenterology. 2006;131:40–6.
34. Shimoda T, et al. Early colorectal carcinoma with special reference to its development de novo. Cancer. 1989;64:1138–46.
35. Ijspeert JEG, et al. Detection rate of serrated polyps and serrated polyposis syndrome in colorectal cancer screening cohorts: a European overview. Gut. 2017;66:1225–32.
36. Makinen MJ. Colorectal serrated adenocarcinoma. Histopathology. 2007;50:131–50.
37. Oka S, et al. Clinicopathologic and endoscopic features of colorectal serrated adenoma: differences between polypoid and superficial types. Gastrointest Endosc. 2004;59:213–9.
38. Leggett B, et al. Role of the serrated pathway in colorectal cancer pathogenesis. Gastroenterology. 2010;138:2088–100.
39. De Jong AE, et al. The role of mismatch repair gene defects in the development of adenomas in patients with HNPCC. Gastroenterology. 2004;126:42–8.
40. East JE, et al. Narrow band imaging for colonoscopic surveillance in hereditary non-polyposis colorectal cancer. Gut. 2008;57:65–70.
41. Huneburg R, et al. Chromocolonoscopy detects more adenomas than white light colonoscopy or narrow band imaging colonoscopy in hereditary nonpolyposis colorectal cancer screening. Endoscopy. 2009;41:316–22.
42. Lecomte T, et al. Chromoendoscopic colonoscopy for detecting preneoplastic lesions in hereditary nonpolyposis colorectal cancer syndrome. Clin Gastroenterol Hepatol. 2005;3:897–902.
43. Lynch HT, et al. Hereditary colorectal cancer. N Engl J Med. 2003;348:919–32.
44. Rijcken FE, et al. Proximal adenomas in hereditary non-polyposis colorectal cancer are prone to rapid malignant transformation. Gut. 2002;50:382–6.
45. Watanabe T, et al. Flat adenoma as a precursor of colorectal carcinoma in hereditary nonpolyposis colorectal carcinoma. Cancer. 1996;77:627–34.
46. Laine L, et al. SCENIC international consensus statement on surveillance and management of dysplasia in inflammatory bowel disease. Gastrointest Endosc. 2015;81:489–501. e426.
47. Magro F, et al. Third European evidence-based consensus on diagnosis and management of ulcerative colitis. Part 1: definitions, diagnosis, extra-intestinal manifestations, pregnancy, cancer surveillance, surgery, and Ileo-anal pouch disorders. J Crohns Colitis. 2017;11:649–70.
48. Chiu K, et al. DALM, rest in peace: a pathologist's perspective on dysplasia in inflammatory bowel disease in the post-DALM era. Mod Pathol. 2018;31:1080–90.
49. Lim CH, et al. Ten year follow up of ulcerative colitis patients with and without low grade dysplasia. Gut. 2003;52:1127–32.
50. Soetikno R, et al. Paradigm shift in the surveillance and management of dysplasia in inflammatory bowel disease (West). Dig Endosc. 2016;28:266–73.
51. Thomas T, et al. Meta-analysis: cancer risk of low-grade dysplasia in chronic ulcerative colitis. Aliment Pharmacol Ther. 2007;25:657–68.
52. Blair V, et al. Hereditary diffuse gastric cancer: diagnosis and management. Clin Gastroenterol Hepatol. 2006;4:262–75.
53. Cislo M, et al. Distinct molecular subtypes of gastric cancer: from Lauren to molecular pathology. Oncotarget. 2018;9:19427–42.
54. Japanese Gastric Cancer Association. Japanese gastric cancer treatment guidelines 2014 (ver. 4). Gastric Cancer. 2017;20:1–19.
55. Sobin LH, et al. TNM classification of malignant tumours. Oxford: Wiley-Blackwell; 2009.
56. Namikawa T, et al. Mucin phenotype of gastric cancer and clinicopathology of gastric-type differentiated adenocarcinoma. World J Gastroenterol. 2010;16:4634–9.
57. Yamazaki K, et al. Tumor differentiation phenotype in gastric differentiated-type tumors and its relation to tumor invasion and genetic alterations. World J Gastroenterol. 2006;12:3803–9.

58. Tajima Y, et al. Gastric and intestinal phenotypic marker expression in early differentiated-type tumors of the stomach: clinicopathologic significance and genetic background. Clin Cancer Res. 2006;12:6469–79.
59. Hirota WK, et al. ASGE guideline: the role of endoscopy in the surveillance of premalignant conditions of the upper GI tract. Gastrointest Endosc. 2006;63:570–80.
60. Vieth M, et al. Pyloric gland adenoma: a clinico-pathological analysis of 90 cases. Virchows Arch. 2003;442:317–21.
61. Endoscopic Classification Review Group. Update on the Paris classification of superficial neoplastic lesions in the digestive tract. Endoscopy. 2005;37:570–8.
62. Yao K, et al. Magnifying endoscopy for diagnosing and delineating early gastric cancer. Endoscopy. 2009;41:462–7.
63. Engel LS, et al. Population attributable risks of esophageal and gastric cancers. J Natl Cancer Inst. 2003;95:1404–13.
64. Quante M, et al. Insights into the pathophysiology of esophageal adenocarcinoma. Gastroenterology. 2018;154:406–20.
65. Buttar NS, et al. Extent of high-grade dysplasia in Barrett's esophagus correlates with risk of adenocarcinoma. Gastroenterology. 2001;120:1630–9.
66. Leers JM, et al. The prevalence of lymph node metastases in patients with T1 esophageal adenocarcinoma a retrospective review of esophagectomy specimens. Ann Surg. 2011;253:271–8.
67. Landau MS, et al. Tumor budding is associated with an increased risk of lymph node metastasis and poor prognosis in superficial esophageal adenocarcinoma. Mod Pathol. 2014;27:1578–89.
68. Zemler B, et al. Early Barrett's carcinoma: the depth of infiltration of the tumour correlates with the degree of differentiation, the incidence of lymphatic vessel and venous invasion. Virchows Arch. 2010;456:609–14.
69. Yokoyama A, et al. Risk appraisal and endoscopic screening for esophageal squamous cell carcinoma in Japanese populations. Esophagus. 2007;4:135–43.
70. Nagata K, Shimizu M. Pathological evaluation of gastrointestinal endoscopic submucosal dissection materials based on Japanese guidelines. World J Gastrointest Endosc. 2012;4:489–99.

Chapter 3
Principles of Endoscopic Resection: Diagnostic and Curative Resection of Mucosal Neoplasias

Tsuneo Oyama and Naohisa Yahagi

3.1 Introduction

Endoscopic analysis now can quite accurately predict precursor lesions and the likely grading and pT category of superficial cancer of the gastrointestinal (GI) tract. These lesions are removed by endoscopic mucosa resection (EMR), endoscopic submucosal dissection (ESD), or minimally invasive laparoscopic resection (LR). ESD has been developed to comply with the principle of en-bloc resection for lesions endoscopically suspect for early cancer. Indication criteria for ESD, as well as benchmark criteria for ESD performance as established in Japan, are widely accepted as state-of-the-art [1–4]. In the West, ESD has achieved similar rates of en-bloc resection but fewer curative resections, mainly owing to poorer differential indication for resection techniques [5, 6]. This chapter aims to provide basic understanding of these techniques necessary to make correct indications for the appropriate resection technique. It does not give instructions on how to perform EMR or ESD, as these techniques have been published elsewhere [3, 4, 7–10].

T. Oyama
Department of Endoscopy, Saku Central Hospital Advanced Care Center, Saku, Nagano, Japan

N. Yahagi (✉)
Division of Research and Development for Minimally Invasive Treatment, Cancer Center, Keio University School of Medicine, Shinjuku-ku, Tokyo, Japan
e-mail: yahagi-tky@umin.ac.jp

F. Berr et al. (eds.), *Atlas of Early Neoplasias of the Gastrointestinal Tract*,
https://doi.org/10.1007/978-3-030-01114-7_3

3.2 Basic Resection Techniques for Superficial Epithelial Neoplasias

3.2.1 Snaring Techniques: Polypectomy, EMR, and EFTRD

Cancer precursor neoplasias should be completely resected, usually with snaring techniques, which achieve en-bloc resection of sub-/pedunculated neoplasms (0-Ip/Isp) and small flat neoplastic lesions (0-IIa-b). In the West, for two decades, even malignant intraepithelial flat lesions (0-II, HGIEN or T0 cancer) with 5–10% risk of submucosal (sm) invasive cancer have been resected with hot-snare EMR in columnar epithelial esophagus and colorectum [7, 11] (Fig. 3.1). Preconditions for EMR techniques were low histological grading of differentiated mucosal cancer (G1 or G2) and suspected absence of submucosal invasion. However, flat lesions 0-IIa/b beyond the size of 20 mm and depressed lesions 0-IIc beyond 10 mm are resectable

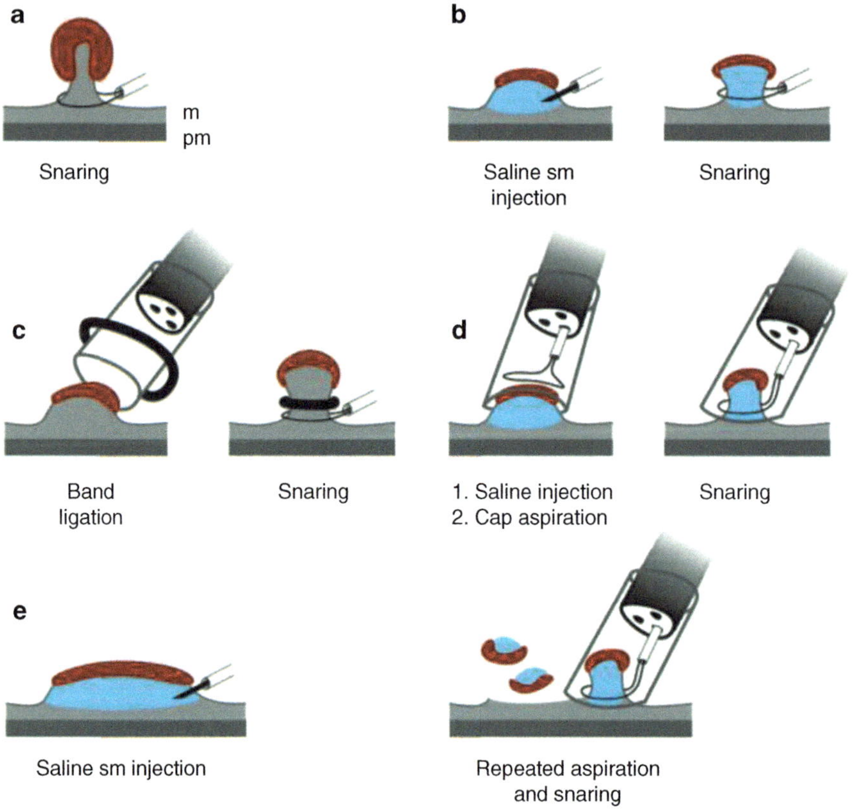

Fig. 3.1 Basic resection techniques of mucosal neoplasias by electrosnaring (**a**) or expanded snaring techniques (**b–d**, endoscopic mucosal resection, EMR). Larger lesions (>20 mm) are only resectable in piecemeal fashion (**e**)

only by snaring techniques using endoscopic piecemeal mucosal resection (EPMR), and EPMR cannot prove whether horizontal resection margins are free of tumor cells [12]. We use en-bloc resection for lesions suspect for intraepithelial (HGIN) or mucosal cancer [1, 13, 14]. Recent studies have shown cold-snare polypectomy (CSP) to be superior to hot-snare polypectomy (HSP) on small polyps and probably even for EPMR on larger flat lesions for histologic assessment and lower risk of thermal organ injury; European guidelines now recommend CSP or CS-EMR as the preferred technique over HSP for smaller or flat lesions [15].

The endoscopic *full-thickness resection device* (FTRD) uses an over-the-scope clip device for an en-bloc snaring technique useful for full-wall resection of relatively small lesions (diameter less than about 2.5 cm). The device, a long-size cap with inserted hot snare and an over-the-scope clip on the outside, is mounted onto the tip of the scope. The entire wall of the colon with the lesion on top is retracted into the cap with a grasper, before deploying the clip and snaring the clipped wall in full thickness. The result is optimum control of vertical invasion, but no visual control of lateral margins during the resection. Endoscopic full-thickness resection (EFTR) was accomplished in 89.5% of 181 colonic lesions (size 2.4 [1.2–4.0] cm) with 76% R0 resection, but the curative resection rate of early cancer (n = 15) was too low to recommend its first-line use [16]. As approved for the colorectum in Europe, indications are moderate-size (<2 cm), sm-fibrotic colorectal superficial early cancer.

3.2.2 Endoscopic En-bloc Resection Techniques

ESD enables margin-free en-bloc resection of large, flat mucosal lesions (diameter >20 mm) or depressed lesions 0-IIc (diameter >10 mm) [3, 17–19] (Fig. 3.2). Endoscopic en-bloc resection is indicated for suspected malignant intraepithelial

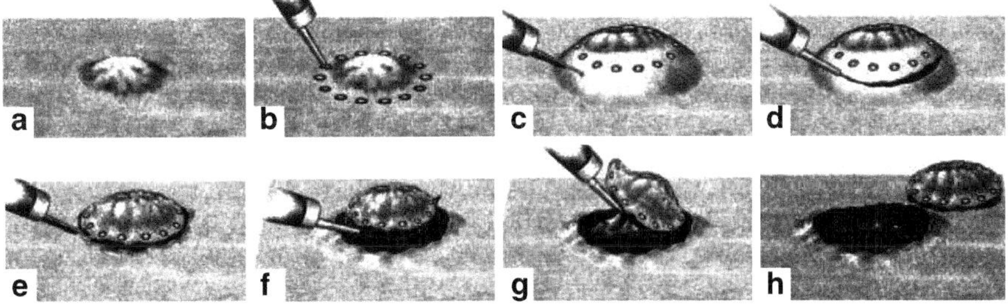

Fig. 3.2 Basic technique of endoscopic submucosal dissection (ESD) – initial complete circumferential incision method. (**a**) Small flat neoplasm without ulceration. (**b**) Circumferential marking dots using coagulation current. (**c**) Lifting of the lesion by submucosal injection. (**d**) Circumferential mucosal incision around the marking dots. (**e**) Re-inject and (**f**) visualize the submucosal space under the lesion using a transparent cap. (**g**) Dissect submucosal tissue until the lesion is removed. (**h**) The resection bed is examined for perforating vessels or injury to the proper muscle layer. (From Yahagi N, et al. [20], permission granted by John Wiley & Sons Inc)

lesion (HGIN / carcinoma T0) to confirm the optical diagnosis by histopathology of the intact specimen, because such malignant lesions may include invasive cancer. This point is controversial for the colorectum and columnar-lined esophagus, where some Western countries still use EPMR [7, 11]. However, superficial mucosal or incipient submucosa (sm) invasive cancer (T1a, T1b-sm1) must be resected en-bloc with EMR or ESD to enable precise staging and assessment of oncological cure. By contrast, deep sm invasive early cancer (T1b-sm2–3) needs first-line LR, except ESD for *diagnostic* purpose at gastric cardia or anorectum, or in patients who are a poor surgical risk.

Note Development of ESD has led to major clinical benefits:

- Enhanced endoscopic detection / analysis of early-stage neoplasias
- Organ-sparing curative tumor resection, especially in the elderly
- Precise histopathological staging of pT category and resection status
- En-bloc resection (curative) with very low risk of recurrence.

Methods of ESD, outcome, and complication management are discussed further in Sect. 3.4.

3.2.3 Laparoscopic Resection Techniques for Early Cancer

Thoracoscopic esophagectomy and laparoscopic hemicolectomy with lymph node dissection are the preferred least-invasive procedures for deep sm-invasive cancer [1, 14]. Advanced or sentinel node–positive gastric cancer (T1b) must undergo at least partial gastrectomy with extended LN dissection [13].

In the stomach, the risk of lymph node metastasis is less than 20–25% for deep sm-invasive differentiated gastric cancer with otherwise low-risk criteria [21]. Conversely, with subtotal gastrectomy, about 75–80% of patients who do not have LN metastasis would be over-treated with radical surgery, risking higher mortality, morbidity, and reduced quality of life. For patients with sm-invasive gastric differentiated adenocarcinoma of size <4 cm, the Japan Society of Sentinel Node Navigation Surgery showed in a prospective trial that sentinel node mapping is feasible to confirm or exclude LN metastasis [22], so that treatment can proceed with either gastrectomy or wedge resection only.

In classic *laparoscopic-endoscopic cooperative surgery (LECS)*, endoscopic full-thickness resection of the gastric wall is performed around the cancer under laparoscopic observation, and the wall defect is closed by laparoscopic linear stapling or sewing. The open gastric wall defect allowed leakage of fluid contaminated with bacteria or even tumor cells into the peritoneum, with risk of peritonitis and peritoneal dissemination. *Non-exposed endoscopic wall inversion surgery (NEWS)* avoids opening of the gastric wall [23] (Fig. 3.3). After sentinel node navigation surgery (SNNS) has proved sentinel node–negative status, clinical sm-invasive differentiated cancer cT1N0 of moderate size (diameter <4 cm) can undergo

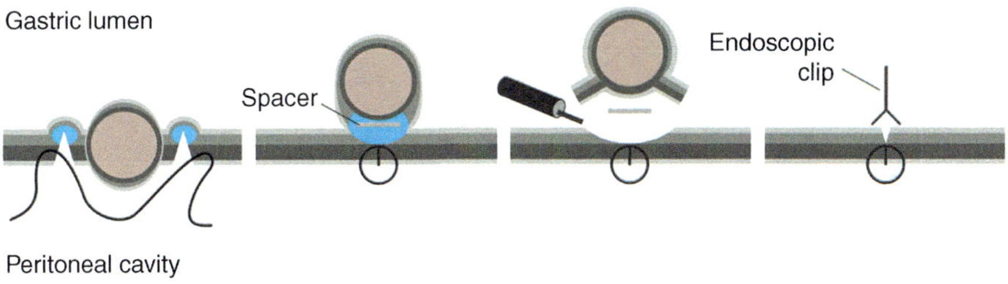

Fig. 3.3 Non-exposed endoscopic wall inversion surgery (NEWS) technique. After endoscopic sm-injection, circumferential laparoscopic seromuscular incision (panel left side) is performed. Seromuscular layers are linearly sutured, with the lesion inverted into the stomach lumen. A surgical sponge (*grey*) is inserted as a spacer between the serosal layer and suture layer (2nd panel). Circumferential mucosal incision and remnant submucosal incisions are made in ESD technique (3rd panel). Peroral retrieval of the specimen is limited by specimen size. The defect is closed with endoscopic clips (right panel). (Based on Maehata T, et al. [24])

limited resection with NEWS, with the advantage of full-thickness resection in a non-exposure technique under precise endoscopic localization of resection lines (the least invasive technique). The concept is feasible and attractive [23]; prospective series on SNNS and NEWS for curative outcome of such early gastric T1b adenocarcinomas are still pending [24].

3.3 Indications for Endoscopic En-bloc Resection in the GI Tract

The indications for ESD are based on pathohistological staging of large series of resected tumors, and define lesions with minimal risk of metastatic spread to regional lymph nodes [25–28]. Indications established in Japan for en-bloc ESD are listed in Table 3.1.

Note *General indication* for ESD is any *mucosal* neoplasia (pre-/malignant)

- suitable by electro-snaring only for piecemeal EMR, but
- demanding *en-bloc resection* (for pT-staging and cure),

in absence of the contraindication:

- evidence of deep invasion of submucosa layer (sm2–3).

Guideline (classic) indications aim for *curative* endoscopic resection.

En-bloc EMR or ESD of differentiated early cancer (G1 or G2) is *curative* (*see* Table 2.4) when cancer does not show scatter infiltration (budding Bd $\leq$ 1) nor invasion of lymph or blood vessels (L0, V0), and when vertical invasion beyond the muscularis mucosae does not exceed 200 μm in squamous epithelial esophagus, 500 μm in the stomach (and probably Barrett's esophagus [29]), and 1000 μm in the

Table 3.1 Indications for endoscopic en-bloc resection of GI neoplasias

Organ	Indications for …	References
Stomach	ESD – Classic indications Mucosal adenocarcinoma; intestinal type G1 or G2, size d ≤ 2 cm, no ulcer ESD – Expanded indications Adenocarcinoma, intestinal type, G1 or G2, any size without ulcer, Adenocarcinoma, intestinal type, G1 or G2, sm-invasive <500 μm, Adenocarcinoma, intestinal type, G1 or G2, d ≤ 3 cm, with ulcer, Adenocarcinoma, diffuse type, G3 or G4, d ≤ 2 cm, no ulcer.	[2, 17]
Esophagus	ESD – Classic indications SCC type 0-IIb (HGIN or G1, G2), intramucosal (m1, m2), any size Barrett adenocarcinoma. type 0-II (G1, G2), intramucosal (m1, LPM), no ulcer. ESD – Expanded indications SCC type 0-II (G1, G2) slightly invasive (m3, sm <200 μm), any size[a], clinical N0 Barrett adenocarcinoma type 0-II (HGIN or G1,G2), mucosal (≤ MM),clinical N0	[1, 28, 29]
Colorectum	ESD – Indications according to Japan Gastroenterological Endoscopy Society (JGES)[b] Lesions for which endoscopic en-bloc resection is required: 1. Lesions for which en-bloc resection with snare-EMR is difficult to apply LST-NG, particularly LST-NG(PD) Lesions showing V_I (irregular)–type pit pattern Mucosal carcinoma with shallow T1 (SM) invasion Large depressed-type tumors (0-IIc) Large protruded-type lesions suspected to be carcinoma[c] 2. Mucosal tumors with submucosal fibrosis [d] 3. Sporadic localized tumors in conditions of chronic inflammation such as ulcerative colitis 4. Local residual or recurrent early carcinomas after endoscopic resection	[4, 27, 30]

HGIN high-grade intraepithelial neoplasia, *LST* laterally spreading type, *MM* muscularis mucosae, *NG(PD)* non-granular (pseudo-depressed), *SCC* squamous cell carcinoma

[a]Increased risk for stricture formation, when ESD extends for ≥70% of circumference

[b]Partially modified from the draft of the Colorectal ESD Standardization implementation Working Group

[c]Including LST-G, nodular mixed type. LST-granular type may also be resected in piecemeal fashion, the larger nodule resected first [30]

[d]As a result of previous biopsy or prolapse caused by peristalsis of the intestine

colorectum [18]. After *curative* ESD of mucosal neoplasm fulfilling guideline ESD criteria, the probability of lymph node metastasis is zero (range 0–3%) and of local recurrence is close to zero.

Note *Surgery* is indicated *after* ESD of early cancer for any of the following:

- Vertical (deep) margin is tumor-positive (R1).
- Deep submucosal invasion (sm2-sm3, exceeding organ-specific depth)

- Lympho/vascular tumor infiltration is positive (Ly 1 or V 1).
- Tumor budding (Bd 2 or 3) is seen at the deepest front of invasion.
- Cancer is poorly differentiated or undifferentiated (G3, G4), except in stomach for cancer G3, G4 of size <2 cm without ulceration.

3.4 Endoscopic Submucosal Dissection: Basic Techniques

Diagnostic assessment for lateral extension and absence of signs of deep submucosal invasion – *proving the indication criteria* – and decision on *strategy of dissection* come first. Strategy of ESDdepends on the location of the lesion in relation to gravity (water level = bottom) and decubitus position of the patient, and special risk factors of the lesion, such as straddling of haustral folds or inaccessibility of margins. The diagnostic assessment and decision on strategy are best done during prior diagnostic endoscopy.

ESD starts with faint electrocoagulation markings around the lesion in safety distance (3–5 mm; at Barrett's lesion, 10 mm), except for colonic lesions with distinct margins, and submucosal injection. Dissection strategy follows the best plan for sequential mucosal cutting and submucosal dissection, so that the gravity of the specimen will help to open with the cap the dissected submucosal space and expose the site targeted for further dissection. Stepwise rotation of the patient's position around the longitudinal axis is an option to facilitate access to submucosa (sm). Another option is placing a clip with a traction line to the edge of the lesion for counter-traction [31].

Several considerations are basic for the dissection strategy [3, 9, 10, 31]:

- The *tangential approach* of the knife towards the proper muscle layer (and mucosal surface) is preferable to the *perpendicular approach*, as the former allows better access to the submucosal layer beneath the lesion, carries less risk of perforation, and is quicker.
- *Partial circumferential incision* (PCI method) usually facilitates subsequent submucosal dissection better than *initial complete circumferential incision* of mucosa (ICCI method, Fig. 3.2), because the PCI method better maintains the fluid cushion injected into the submucosa beneath the lesion (Fig. 3.4a).
- *Tunnelling technique* starts with mucosal incision at both ends of the planned tunnel, followed by prograde sm tunnelling dissection under the entire length of the lesion, and finally dissects the lateral margins and lateral sm-bridges.
- *Pocket creating method (PCM)* ESD means a small mucosal incision and tunnelling under the entire lesion, before stepwise the circumferential cut is extended and the lateral sm-bridge is dissected starting at the inlet of the pocket (Fig. 3.4b). PCM-ESD has facilitated resection of challenging and risky lesions [32].
- *Hybrid ESD* with snaring of the final central sm tissue bridge after circumferential incision and widespread sm dissection was originally designed to speed up

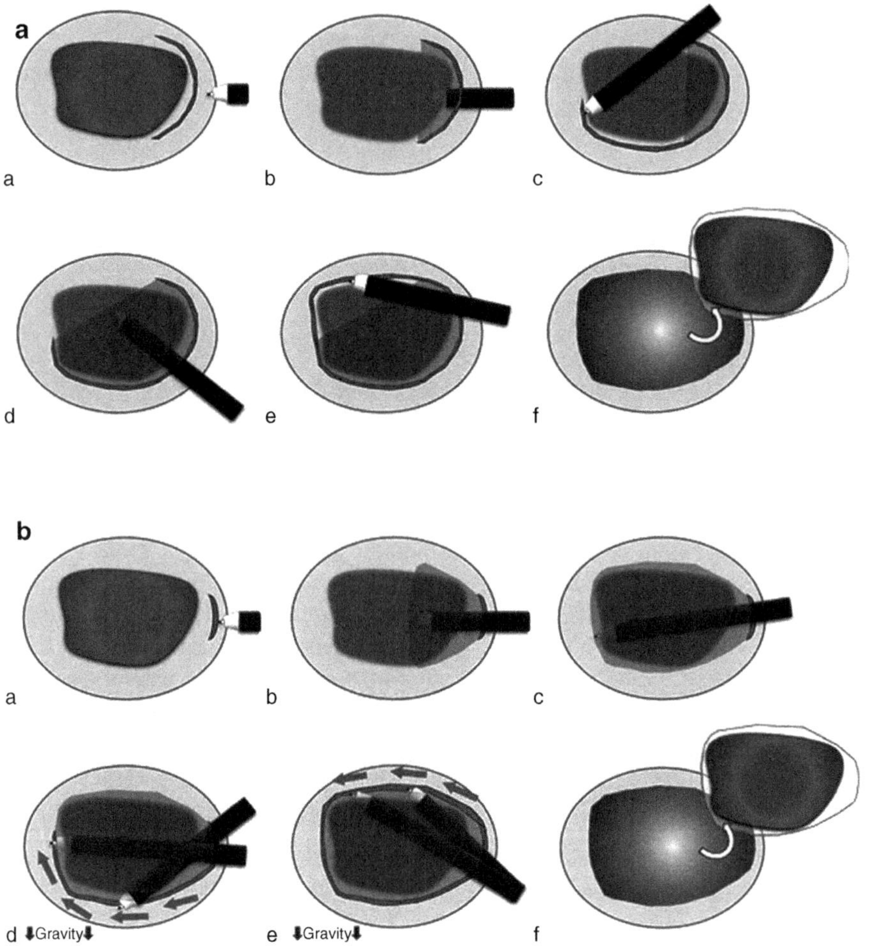

Fig. 3.4 Endoscopic submucosal dissection strategies for submucosa (sm) lifting. (**a**) *Partial circumferential incision (PCI)* method: *(a)* Sm-injection and minor circumferential m-incision. *(b)* Deeper cut (→mucosa-flap). *(c)* Extend m-cut (on "lower" gravity side). *(d)* Further smd. *(e)* Complete m-cut. *(f)* Complete smd (en-bloc ESD). (**b**) *Pocket creating (PCM)* method: *(a)* Sm-injection and small m-incision. *(b)* Access to deep sm-layer. *(c)* Create smd-pocket under entire lesion (by repeated injection & dissection). *(d)* Step-by-step m-cut along lower gravity side and *(e)* along "upper side." (Modified from Sakamoto H et al. [32], reprint according to Open Access Regulations under the Creative Commons Public Domain Mark 1.0)

ESD (*see* Fig. 11.27). When the lesion was snared en bloc or in two or three pieces, the outcome was "clinically curative" (<3% recurrence rate) [33, 34]. During un-supervised implementation of ESD technique, hybrid ESD served for self-completion after prolonged procedure time or rescue after a complication (perforation, acute bleeding), yielding poorer outcomes than en-bloc ESD [5].

ESD technique of submucosal injection, mucosal incision, and submucosal dissection is beyond the scope of this chapter. For details, we refer to literature [4, 8–10, 35] and e-learning sources on ESD (www.early-cancer.eu; www.olympusprofed.com).

3.5 Outcome of ESD and Management of Complications

3.5.1 Outcome of ESD

ESD for cure yields en-bloc resection in 84–98% of cases and is complicated by perforation in up to 10% (up to 20% during untutored learning). Gastric, esophageal, and colorectal ESD procedures have been standardized in Japan [1–4]. Current outcomes of ESD in the GI tract are listed in Table 3.2.

Note Benchmark criteria (rate in %) for ESD with curative intention [3, 5, 46, 51, 54]:

- En-bloc resection rate >90%
- Oncological curative resection ≥80% (R0 resection ≥85%)
- Complications <5%, surgical repair <2%, mortality <0.1%
- Local recurrence <3% after R0 resection

Table 3.2 Organ-specific outcome of curative ESD for classic indications

	Esophagus (% of ESDs)[a]		Stomach[a] (% of ESDs)	Colorectum (% of ESDs)[b]	
	SCL-E	CCL-E		Asian	Non-Asian[c]
En-bloc resection	100 [95–100]	91 [90–100]	92 [83–98]	93 (91–94)	81 (77–85)
Curative resection	90 [79–97]	66 [39–84]	83 [74–93]	84 (79–88)	67 (58–76)
Local recurrence[d]	0 [0–4][e]	0 [0–2.4][f]	1.5 [0–3.2]	1.1 (0.7–1.8)	5.2 (3.3–8.1)
Recurrence-free OS	100 [96–100][e]	99 [97–100][f]	98[f][94[e]–100[g]]	99.6 [98–100][b, h]	n.g.
Perforation	0 [0–5]	2 [0–7]	4 [3–11]	4.5 (3.9–5.3)	8.6 (6–12)
Delayed bleeding	0 [0–2]	4 [0–9]	1.6 [0–23]	2.4 (1.9–3.0)	4.2 (1.9–5.9)
Surgical repair	0	0	0 [0–3.5]	0.3 [0–4.3][h]	n.g.
ESD mortality	0	0 [0–3.8]	0	0[h]	0

CCL-E columnar cell–lined esophagus, *n.g* not reported, *OS* overall survival, *SCL* squamous cell–lined
[a]Compiled rates (median [range]) for SCL-E [3, 36–39], CCL-E [40–45], Stomach [12, 46–50]
[b]Meta-analysis of studies from Asian and non-Asian countries (median, 95% CI) according to [5]
[c]Including studies on ESD learning curve
[d]All after curative ESD resection
[e]Per 1.7 yrs
[f]Per 3 yrs
[g]Per 5 yrs
[h]Compiled rates (median, 95% CI) for colorectum [49, 51–53]

In Western countries, outcome of ESD is similar for en-bloc resection but inferior for curative resection and local recurrence, at least in SC-lined esophagus and colorectum [5, 6]. So far, endoscopic analysis for ESD indications is less accurate, and deep sm invasive cancer is often underdiagnosed. Most Western series present less than 10–20% of the case volume of Asian studies [5, 6].

ESD for the purpose of diagnosis of sm invasive early cancer does not impair oncological outcome of subsequent curative surgery for esophageal SCC, nor for gastric or colorectal adenocarcinoma [55, 56]. Approximately 20% of patients with esophageal SCC clinically staged cT1-m3-sm2 N0 M0 can avoid esophagectomy using diagnostic ESD with curative outcome [56]. Even non-curative ESD (which has low morbidity and mortality) may better combine with adjuvant chemoradiotherapy in candidates with poor surgical risk, and has in combination shown better survival and quality of life than definitive chemoradiotherapy alone [57, 58]. This may open a new field of adjuvant and first-line palliative treatment concepts for local control of GI tract cancers, in order to prevent advanced local tumor stages during progression to stage IV cancer [58].

3.5.2 Complications of ESD and Management of Complications

The *risk of perforation* increases with low experience and poor skill of the operator, and with larger size, submucosal fibrosis, and challenging location of the lesion. The risk is lowest in the gastric corpus and oral antrum; in other sites and organs, it increases in the following order: prepyloric antrum; fundic and subcardiac stomach; and thin-walled organs such as the rectum, esophagus, descending and transverse colon, ascending colon, cecum, sigmoid colon, splenic and hepatic flexure, and especially the duodenum [59, 60]. In the colon and duodenum, even cautious contact coagulation of small vessels overlying the thin (~1 mm) proper muscle layer may cause free mini-perforation. In the duodenum, mucosal ulcer after ESD carries a high risk of delayed bleeding or perforation owing to aggressive pancreatobiliary secretions; it should be closed by adaption and clipping of mucosal margins [60].

Acute perforations usually are small. In experienced hands, they are closed by clipping and are treated with intravenous antibiotics, parenteral nutrition, and clinical follow-up for few days, without surgery [61]. There are some tricks and devices to close even larger perforations [61–63]. Frank pneumoperitoneum or thoracic compartment syndrome (pneumomediastinum or pneumothorax) due to delayed clipping of perforation can be a life-threatening cardiorespiratory emergency and must be relieved by peritoneal puncture with a 20-gauge Teflon cannula, or even emergency repair surgery [61, 63]. Organ perforation during ESD of differentiated early gastric cancer did not increase the risk of peritoneal dissemination [64].

Delayed perforation (after 2–10 days) is rare, occurring after 0.3–0.7% of colonic ESDs, but it carries a high risk of peritonitis because abdominal pain is *slowly* increasing. *Electrocoagulation syndrome* (rebound tenderness and fever or marked leukocytosis) may occur, and even larger-size delayed perforation, when too much coagulation current has been applied to proper muscle. Repair is by open surgery [61, 65, 66].

Risk of bleeding is increased at major curvature, antrum, and cardia in the stomach, in the duodenum, and in the distal rectum. Late re-bleeding is best prevented by prophylactic electrocoagulation or clipping of any coagulated perforating vessels after ESD.

Severe stenosis ensues after ESD involving more than 70% of the circumference of the esophagus, prepyloric antrum, or anorectal channel [67, 68]. Repeated topical application of corticosteroid and balloon dilation after circumferential ESD can prevent stricturing of the esophagus or anorectal channel. Circumferential ESD is contraindicated in the prepyloric antrum and pylorus, because severe gastric outlet stenosis is unavoidable and balloon dilation carries a high risk of perforation [69]. Gastric mucosa must remain intact on at least 40% of the circumference in the prepyloric antrum.

Mucosal closure of the ESD resection bed with continuous endoscopic suture is feasible, can shorten the hospital stay to a single-day procedure, and may enhance complication-free recovery, but prospective data for lack of covert recurrence are pending [62].

Note ESD in high-risk locations requires high skill and competence in performing ESD (see below). Operators must be cautious and slowly raise their level of challenge, continuing to update their knowledge and skills with ESD experts.

3.6 Learning ESD: Minor Invasive Endoscopic Surgery

ESD is a low-tech but highly skilled procedure demanding *two learning curves* for the principal skills that need to be acquired:

- *Endoscopic diagnosis* by accurate assessment of early neoplasias
- *Endoscopic electrosurgical skills*
  - Superior maneuvering of the endoscope for "single-handed" surgery
  - Planning of the best gravity-dependent resection strategy
  - Distinction of submucosal tissues (fibers/proper muscle/MM/neoplasia)
  - Upgrades in electro-knife handling and endoscopic surgical assistance
  - Upgrades in how to manage complications (e.g., bleeding, perforation).

The ESD procedure requires a team approach. A skilled person needs 30–50 ESDs to achieve and prove the *Level of Competence* for safe ESD (i.e., combined rate of mini-perforations and frank bleeding <10%). The aim (after another 50–100 ESDs) is to progress to *Professional Level* [6, 70–72]:

- Safety (<5% rate of perforations)
- High rate of en-bloc resection (95%) and R0 resection (85%)
- Short ESD procedure time (<60 min for 3 × 3-cm gastric lesion).

Basic equipment for ESD:

- Endoscopes – full-angles maneuverable and with short-pulsed water-jet
- CO_2 insufflation, electrosurgical generator for an array of current modes
- Electric knives, coagraspers, injection sets, snares, injection solution, etc.
- Transparent distal attachments for scopes

Altogether this procedure requires expertise of operator and assistant team, a referral hospital (for case volume), and commitment of medical disciplines and administration.

For implementing ESD technique, Japanese experts recommended several steps to Western endoscopists:

- To gather theoretical experience and follow at least 15 entire ESD procedures done by experts in different locations of the GI tract
- To acquire basic skills for electric knife techniques in isolated porcine stomach or bovine colon (courses and ~30 independent procedures)
- To complete at least five experimental ESD procedures in living piglets, with tutoring by experts
- To follow a step-up of technical challenge (stomach → rectum → esophagus → colon) for clinical ESD [73, 74].

Most participants in such an experimental ESD training successfully performed untutored clinical ESD in different organs with an acceptable rate of complications (perforation, 9.7%; surgical repair, 3.5%) without long-term morbidity [75]. After a decade of such annual courses, feedback by previous participants now indicates that more than 45 centers with substantial case volume (>50 ESD per center, 60% colorectal) implemented the procedure with few serious complications (surgical repair rate, <2%; 30-day mortality, 0.04%) [76]. Apart from the step-up approach, ESD has also been implemented mainly in the entire colorectum, reaching competence after 30 ESD procedures and professional level after 80 procedures [77–79].

At least 20 centers in Europe exceed a case volume of 150 ESD procedures and probably are on the professional level [38, 45, 76–80]. An effort is now needed to offer quality of endoscopic diagnosis everywhere and ESD on benchmark levels in the centers.

Key points for *curative endoscopic resection* of early neoplasias:

- Early endoscopic detection
- Accurate endoscopic evaluation for correct indication of resection technique
- Ruling out of deeply submucosa-invasive cancer
- En-bloc resection as the goal for histopathological evaluation
- ESD is promising even for large and difficult lesions.

References

1. Kuwano H, et al. Guidelines for diagnosis and treatment of carcinoma of the esophagus April 2012 edited by the Japan Esophageal Society. Esophagus. 2015;12:1–30.
2. Ono H, et al. Guidelines for endoscopic submucosal dissection and endoscopic mucosal resection for early gastric cancer. Dig Endosc. 2016;28:3–15.
3. Oyama T, et al. Endoscopic submucosal dissection of early esophageal cancer. Clin Gastroenterol Hepatol. 2005;3:S67–70.
4. Tanaka S, et al. JGES guidelines for colorectal endoscopic submucosal dissection/endoscopic mucosal resection. Dig Endosc. 2015;27:417–34.
5. Fuccio L, et al. Clinical outcomes after endoscopic submucosal dissection for colorectal neoplasia: a systematic review and meta-analysis. Gastrointest Endosc. 2017;86:74–86. e17.
6. Oyama T, et al. How to establish endoscopic submucosal dissection in Western countries. World J Gastroenterol. 2015;21:11209–20.
7. Pech O, et al. Long-term efficacy and safety of endoscopic resection for patients with mucosal adenocarcinoma of the esophagus. Gastroenterology. 2014;146:652–60.
8. Tanaka S, et al. Endoscopic submucosal dissection for colorectal neoplasia: possibility of standardization. Gastrointest Endosc. 2007;66:100–7.
9. Toyonaga T. Endoscopic submucosal dissection using the Flush knife and Flush knife BT. Tech Gastrointest Endosc. 2011;13:84–90.
10. Yahagi N, et al. Endoscopic submucosal dissection using the flex and the dual knives. Tech Gastrointest Endosc. 2011;13:74–8.
11. Lee EY, et al. EMR should be the first-line treatment for large laterally spreading colorectal lesions. Gastrointest Endosc. 2016;84:326–8.
12. Watanabe K, et al. Clinical outcomes of EMR for gastric tumors: historical pilot evaluation between endoscopic submucosal dissection and conventional mucosal resection. Gastrointest Endosc. 2006;63:776–82.
13. Japanese Gastric Cancer Association. Japanese gastric cancer treatment guidelines 2014 (ver. 4). Gastric Cancer. 2017;20:1–19.
14. Watanabe T, et al. Japanese Society for Cancer of the Colon and Rectum (JSCCR) guidelines 2016 for the treatment of colorectal cancer. Int J Clin Oncol. 2018;23:1–34.
15. Ferlitsch M, et al. Colorectal polypectomy and endoscopic mucosal resection (EMR): European Society of Gastrointestinal Endoscopy (ESGE) Clinical Guideline. Endoscopy. 2017;49:270–97.
16. Schmidt A, et al. Colonoscopic full-thickness resection using an over-the-scope device: a prospective multicentre study in various indications. Gut. 2018;67:1280–9.
17. Gotoda T, et al. Extending and limitation of the indication for endoscopic mucosal resection of gastric mucosal cancer. The importance of histological evaluation and the necessity of one-piece resection for endoscopic gastric mucosal resection. Stomach Intestine. 2002;37:1145–54.
18. Toyonaga T, et al. Principles of quality controlled endoscopic submucosal dissection with appropriate dissection level and high quality resected specimen. Clin Endosc. 2012;45:362–74.
19. Yahagi N, et al. Endoscopic submucosal dissection for the reliable en bloc resection of colorectal mucosal tumors. Dig Endosc. 2004;16:s89–92.
20. Yahagi N, et al. Endoscopic submucosal dissection for early gastric cancer using the tip of an electrosurgical snare (thin type). Dig Endosc. 2004;16:34–8.
21. Matsuda T, et al. Laparoscopic endoscopic cooperative surgery (LECS) for the upper gastrointestinal tract. Transl Gastroenterol Hepatol. 2017;2:40.
22. Kitagawa Y, et al. Sentinel node mapping for gastric cancer: a prospective multicenter trial in Japan. J Clin Oncol. 2013;31:3704–10.

23. Goto O, et al. First case of non-exposed endoscopic wall-inversion surgery with sentinel node basin dissection for early gastric cancer. Gastric Cancer. 2015;18:434–9.
24. Maehata T, et al. Cutting edge of endoscopic full-thickness resection for gastric tumor. World J Gastrointest Endosc. 2015;7:1208–15.
25. Gotoda T, et al. Incidence of lymph node metastasis from early gastric cancer: estimation with a large number of cases at two large centers. Gastric Cancer. 2000;3:219–25.
26. Hirasawa T, et al. Incidence of lymph node metastasis and the feasibility of endoscopic resection for undifferentiated-type early gastric cancer. Gastric Cancer. 2009;12:148–52.
27. Kitajima K, et al. Correlations between lymph node metastasis and depth of submucosal invasion in submucosal invasive colorectal carcinoma: a Japanese collaborative study. J Gastroenterol. 2004;39:534–43.
28. Oyama T, et al. Diagnosis and long-term results and prognosis of m3 and sm1 esophageal cancer. Lymph nodal metastasis of m3, sm1 esophageal cancer. Stomach Intestine. 2002;37:71–4.
29. Paris workshop on columnar metaplasia in the esophagus and the esophagogastric junction, Paris, France, December 11–12 2004. Endoscopy. 2005;37:879–920.
30. Uraoka T, et al. Endoscopic indications for endoscopic mucosal resection of laterally spreading tumours in the colorectum. Gut. 2006;55:1592–7.
31. Oyama T. Counter traction makes endoscopic submucosal dissection easier. Clin Endosc. 2012;45:375–8.
32. Sakamoto H, et al. Pocket-creation method facilitates endoscopic submucosal dissection of colorectal laterally spreading tumors, non-granular type. Endosc Int Open. 2017;5:E123–9.
33. Sakamoto T, et al. Learning curve associated with colorectal endoscopic submucosal dissection for endoscopists experienced in gastric endoscopic submucosal dissection. Dis Colon Rectum. 2011;54:1307–12.
34. Toyonaga T, et al. The new resources of treatment for early stage colorectal tumors: EMR with small incision and simplified endoscopic submucosal dissection. Dig Endosc. 2009;21(Suppl 1):S31–7.
35. Pioche M, et al. Randomized comparative evaluation of endoscopic submucosal dissection self-learning software in France and Japan. Endoscopy. 2016;48:1076–83.
36. Esaki M, et al. Risk factors for local recurrence of superficial esophageal cancer after treatment by endoscopic mucosal resection. Endoscopy. 2007;39:41–5.
37. Ishihara R, et al. Comparison of EMR and endoscopic submucosal dissection for en bloc resection of early esophageal cancers in Japan. Gastrointest Endosc. 2008;68:1066–72.
38. Repici A, et al. Endoscopic submucosal dissection in patients with early esophageal squamous cell carcinoma: results from a prospective Western series. Gastrointest Endosc. 2010;71:715–21.
39. Teoh AY, et al. Outcomes of endoscopic submucosal dissection versus endoscopic mucosal resection in management of superficial squamous esophageal neoplasms outside Japan. J Clin Gastroenterol. 2010;44:e190–4.
40. Chevaux JB, et al. Clinical outcome in patients treated with endoscopic submucosal dissection for superficial Barrett's neoplasia. Endoscopy. 2015;47:103–12.
41. Coman RM, et al. Prospective evaluation of the clinical utility of endoscopic submucosal dissection (ESD) in patients with Barrett's esophagus: a Western center experience. Endosc Int Open 2016;4:E715–21.
42. Hirasawa K, et al. Superficial adenocarcinoma of the esophagogastric junction: long-term results of endoscopic submucosal dissection. Gastrointest Endosc. 2010;72:960–6.
43. Hobel S, et al. Single center experience of endoscopic submucosal dissection (ESD) in early Barrett's adenocarcinoma. Surg Endosc. 2015;29:1591–7.
44. Kagemoto K, et al. Clinical outcomes of endoscopic submucosal dissection for superficial Barrett's adenocarcinoma. Gastrointest Endosc. 2014;80:239–45.
45. Probst A, et al. Early esophageal cancer in Europe: endoscopic treatment by endoscopic submucosal dissection. Endoscopy. 2015;47:113–21.

46. Gotoda T, et al. Endoscopic resection of early gastric cancer treated by guideline and expanded National Cancer Centre criteria. Br J Surg. 2010;97:868–71.
47. Nakamoto S, et al. Indications for the use of endoscopic mucosal resection for early gastric cancer in Japan: a comparative study with endoscopic submucosal dissection. Endoscopy. 2009;41:746–50.
48. Probst A, et al. Endoscopic submucosal dissection in gastric neoplasia – experience from a European center. Endoscopy. 2010;42:1037–44.
49. Toyonaga T, et al. 1,635 endoscopic submucosal dissection cases in the esophagus, stomach, and colorectum: complication rates and long-term outcomes. Surg Endosc. 2013;27:1000–8.
50. Yamamoto Y, et al. Therapeutic outcomes of endoscopic submucosal dissection of undifferentiated-type intramucosal gastric cancer without ulceration and preoperatively diagnosed as 20 millimetres or less in diameter. Dig Endosc. 2010;22:112–8.
51. Saito Y, et al. A prospective, multicenter study of 1111 colorectal endoscopic submucosal dissections (with video). Gastrointest Endosc. 2010;72:1217–25.
52. Niimi K, et al. Long-term outcomes of endoscopic submucosal dissection for colorectal epithelial neoplasms. Endoscopy. 2010;42:723–9.
53. Nishiyama H, et al. Endoscopic submucosal dissection for laterally spreading tumours of the colorectum in 200 consecutive cases. Surg Endosc. 2010;24:2881–7.
54. Bang CS, et al. Endoscopic submucosal dissection for early gastric cancer with undifferentiated-type histology: a meta-analysis. World J Gastroenterol. 2015;21:6032–43.
55. Goto O, et al. Endoscopic submucosal dissection as a staging measure may not lead to worse prognosis in early gastric cancer patients with additional gastrectomy. Dig Liver Dis. 2008;40:293–7.
56. Takeuchi M, et al. Technical feasibility and oncological safety of diagnostic endoscopic resection for superficial esophageal cancer. Gastrointest Endosc. 2018;88:456–65.
57. Ikeda A, et al. Endoscopic submucosal dissection (ESD) with additional therapy for superficial esophageal cancer with submucosal invasion. Intern Med. 2015;54:2803–13.
58. Kawaguchi G, et al. The effectiveness of endoscopic submucosal dissection followed by chemoradiotherapy for superficial esophageal cancer. Radiat Oncol. 2015;10:31.
59. Uraoka T, et al. Colorectal endoscopic submucosal dissection: is it suitable in western countries? J Gastroenterol Hepatol. 2013;28:406–14.
60. Yahagi N, et al. Outcomes of endoscopic resection for superficial duodenal epithelial neoplasia. Gastrointest Endosc. 2018;88:676–82.
61. Hotta K, et al. Criteria for non-surgical treatment of perforation during colorectal endoscopic submucosal dissection. Digestion. 2012;85:116–20.
62. Kantsevoy SV, et al. Endoscopic suturing closure of large mucosal defects after endoscopic submucosal dissection is technically feasible, fast, and eliminates the need for hospitalization (with videos). Gastrointest Endosc. 2014;79:503–7.
63. Minami S, et al. Complete endoscopic closure of gastric perforation induced by endoscopic resection of early gastric cancer using endoclips can prevent surgery (with video). Gastrointest Endosc. 2006;63:596–601.
64. Ikehara H, et al. Gastric perforation during endoscopic resection for gastric carcinoma and the risk of peritoneal dissemination. Br J Surg. 2007;94:992–5.
65. Jung D, et al. Risk of electrocoagulation syndrome after endoscopic submucosal dissection in the colon and rectum. Endoscopy. 2013;45:714–7.
66. Toyonaga T, et al. Retrospective study of technical aspects and complications of endoscopic submucosal dissection for laterally spreading tumors of the colorectum. Endoscopy. 2010;42:714–22.
67. Coda S, et al. Risk factors for cardiac and pyloric stenosis after endoscopic submucosal dissection, and efficacy of endoscopic balloon dilation treatment. Endoscopy. 2009;41:421–6.
68. Ono S, et al. Predictors of postoperative stricture after esophageal endoscopic submucosal dissection for superficial squamous cell neoplasms. Endoscopy. 2009;41:661–5.

69. Tsunada S, et al. Case series of endoscopic balloon dilation to treat a stricture caused by circumferential resection of the gastric antrum by endoscopic submucosal dissection. Gastrointest Endosc. 2008;67:979–83.
70. Hotta K, et al. Learning curve for endoscopic submucosal dissection of large colorectal tumors. Dig Endosc. 2010;22:302–6.
71. Oda I, et al. Learning curve for endoscopic submucosal dissection of early gastric cancer based on trainee experience. Dig Endosc. 2012;24(Suppl 1):129–32.
72. Yoshida M, et al. Learning curve and clinical outcome of gastric endoscopic submucosal dissection performed by trainee operators. Surg Endosc. 2017;31:3614–22.
73. Deprez PH, et al. Current practice with endoscopic submucosal dissection in Europe: position statement from a panel of experts. Endoscopy. 2010;42:853–8.
74. Gotoda T, et al. A learning curve for advanced endoscopic resection. Gastrointest Endosc. 2005;62:866–7.
75. Berr F, et al. Experimental endoscopic submucosal dissection training in a porcine model: learning experience of skilled Western endoscopists. Dig Endosc. 2011;23:281–9.
76. Oyama T, et al. Implementation of endoscopic submucosal dissection (ESD) in Europe: survey after ESD Expert Training Workshops 2009–2018. (ESGE abstr OP300) Endosc. 2019;51(4), in press.
77. Sauer M, et al. Endoscopic submucosal dissection for flat or sessile colorectal neoplasia >20 mm: a European single-center series of 182 cases. Endosc Int Open. 2016;4:E895–900.
78. Spychalski M, et al. Colorectal endoscopic submucosal dissection (ESD) in the west – when can satisfactory results be obtained? A single-operator learning curve analysis. Scand J Gastroenterol. 2017;52:1442–52.
79. Wagner A, et al. Single-center implementation of endoscopic submucosal dissection (ESD) in the colorectum: low recurrence rate after intention-to-treat ESD. Dig Endosc. 2018;30:354–63.
80. Pimentel-Nunes P, et al. Long-term follow-up after endoscopic resection of gastric superficial neoplastic lesions in Portugal. Endoscopy. 2014;46:933–40.

Chapter 4
Subepithelial Gastrointestinal Tumors: Diagnosis and Indications for Resection

Frieder Berr, Jürgen Hochberger, and Tsuneo Oyama

4.1 Introduction

Subepithelial lesions (SEL) are incidentally observed in the stomach of about 0.3% of middle-aged men and women; half of these are neoplastic [1, 2]. In the esophagus, small intestine, and colorectum, their incidence seems to be less but is not precisely known. The incidence of subepithelial tumors (SET) of gastrointestinal (GI) origin has risen twofold to fivefold within the past 30 years [3, 4]. About a third of solid SET are malignant (mainly lymphomas, malignant gastrointestinal stromal tumor [GIST], or neuroendocrine carcinoma) or have malignant potential, like GIST and neuroendocrine tumors (NET). After exclusion of insignificant SEL by endoscopic gross aspect and endosonographic ultrasound (EUS), we are left with a solid, mass-like SET and must decide on surveillance, sampling for histologic diagnosis, or en-bloc resection for diagnosis and cure [2, 3, 5, 6].

In the recent past, endoscopic and minimally invasive surgical resection of intramural tumors have made progress, so now most SET in the GI tract are safely resectable without ensuing GI dysfunction. But we must individualize strategies and make balanced decisions between surveillance or en-bloc resection for such SET, choosing the safest and least invasive technique [5–9].

F. Berr (✉)
Department of Internal Medicine I, Paracelsus Medical University, Salzburg, Austria
e-mail: frieder.berr@pmu.ac.at

J. Hochberger
Department of Gastroenterology, Vivantes Klinikum Berlin Friedrichshain, Berlin, Germany

T. Oyama
Department of Endoscopy, Saku Central Hospital Advanced Care Center, Saku, Nagano, Japan

F. Berr et al. (eds.), *Atlas of Early Neoplasias of the Gastrointestinal Tract*,
https://doi.org/10.1007/978-3-030-01114-7_4

4.2 Differential Diagnosis of Gastrointestinal Subepithelial Lesions

SEL are covered with normal mucosa and when quite protruded have bridging folds in the stomach (Fig. 4.1). Most of these lesions are asyptomatic and are overlooked when smaller than 5 mm. Considering the most common differential diagnoses for frequent and rare SELs in various organs (Table 4.1), we can exclude several non-neoplastic SEL with endoscopic and EUS findings.

Polypoid lesions are mainly hyperplastic or fibromatous polyps or hamartomas, such as in Peutz-Jeghers syndrome. Most polypoid lesions are easily removed with snaring for clearance and diagnosis. However, they have a wide differential diagnosis in the duodenum and small bowel; examination of the entire small bowel may be required, using capsule endoscopy or MRI enteroclysis, with double balloon enteroscopy for confirmation and resection when positive. (Compare Chap. 10.)

Sessile or elevated SET Endoscopic gross features, color, consistency on gentle forceps palpation, and morphology on high-resolution endoscopic ultrasound (hr-EUS) allow the clinical diagnosis of vascular tumor, lymphangioma, lipoma, aberrant pancreas, and duplication cyst [3, 4]. Distinguished by gross morphology are hemangioma ("blue rubber bleb sign") and soft SETs that are pliable with forceps ("cushion sign"), such as soft bulging SEL with white-grayish color (*lymphangioma*), yellowish color (*lipoma*), or isochrome color (*cyst*). Diagnosis is made with hr-EUS (20 MHz) for typical echostructure and intramural layer of origin, and with fine needle aspiration cytology or puncture histology of solid lesions using EUS (7.5 MHz) [3, 10] (Compare Chap. 5). None of these lesions, except intermittently bleeding hemangioma, is an indication for endoscopic ablation.

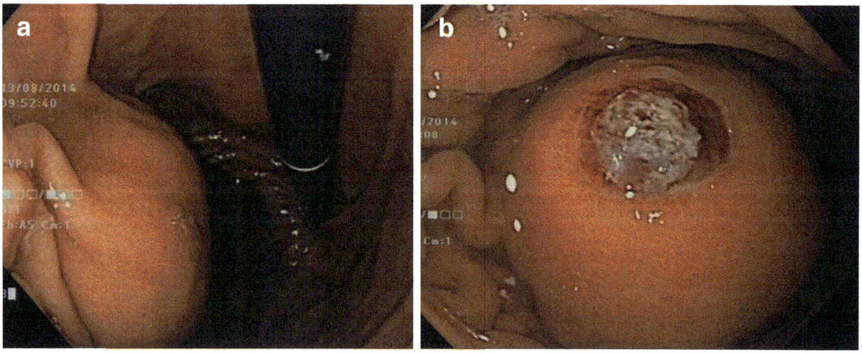

Fig. 4.1 Subepithelial tumor (d 3 cm, hard) in major curve of gastric body of a 75-year-old man with acute myocardial infarction and melena. (**a**) Typical bridging folds in normal gastric mucosa. (**b**) Central ulcer with fresh fibrin clot (after bleeding episode) Fine needle puncture (FNP) showed GIST with low mitosis rate 0/4 HPF; Ki-67 index 2%; cKIT and DOG1+

Table 4.1 Predilection for localization and relative prevalence of subepithelial lesions in GI tract

SEL	Esophagus	Stomach	Small Intestine	Colorectum
Prevailing SET	Leiomyoma[a] GCT Lipoma	GIST NET MALT lymphoma Lipoma Leiomyoma	NET GIST MALT lymphoma Lipoma Lymphangioma	NET (carcinoid) Lipoma MALT lymphoma
Rare SET	GIST Hemangioma Neurofibroma Schwannoma	GCT Schwannoma Metastasis Lymphangioma	Leiomyoma Hamartoma (Peutz-Jeghers) GCT	GCT GIST Lymphangioma
Non-neoplastic SEL	Fibromatous polyp Duplication cyst	Heterotopic pancreas Fundic gland polyp Duplication cyst	Brunner gland adenoma Aberrant pancreas Fibromatous polyp Duplication cyst	Inverted diverticulum

Modified from Nishida et al. [3] and Wiech et al. [4]

GCT granular cell tumor, *GIST* gastrointestinal stroma tumor, *MALT* mucosa-associated lymphoid tissue, *NET* neuroendocrine tumor

[a]Most frequent in esophagus; transformation to sarcoma very rare

Lymphomas Mucosa-associated lymphoid tissue (MALT) lymphoma in stomach (Fig. 9.5) and intestine, or other malignant B-cell or T-cell lymphoma in small or large bowel, tend to infiltrate the mucosa (LPM) and submucosa, causing edema and superficial submucosal lesions with alterations of surface and capillary architecture. High-grade malignant lymphomas often present bulky masses. Malignant lymphoma requires a particle biopsy (e.g., with cold snare) for detailed cytology and histochemistry to select the appropriate systemic therapy. If these SEL are excluded, a few solid SET remain for diagnostic evaluation.

4.3 Solid Gastrointestinal SET

Solid SET mainly comprise premalignant or malignant GIST (~50%), gastroentero-pancreatic neuroendocrine tumors (GEP-NET, 20–25%), benign leiomyomas (~15%), rare granular cell tumors (GCT), and very rare highly malignant leiomyosarcomas (LMS) [3, 4, 6, 11]. The mesenchymal tumors—GIST, leiomyoma, leiomyosarcoma—and the NET have been exactly diagnosed since the late 1990s, when immunohistochemical markers were identified. Since then, the incidence of these neoplasias has increased by twofold to fivefold. GIST arises from interstitial cells of Cajal regulating GI motility; leiomyosarcomas, from the smooth muscle layer and only very rarely from leiomyoma; GCT, from Schwann neuronal cells (<4% malignant transformation); and NET, from paracrine neuroendocrine cells. Clinical diagnosis may be presumed from prevalence at the organ location, endoscopic gross appearance, and EUS features including the contingent EUS layer of tumor origin. For special EUS features, including the typical echostructure and characteristic wall layer of origin (layer of EUS contingency), refer to Chap. 5, Sect. 5.4. Retention of ^{18}fluorodeoxy-glucose in FDG-positron emission tomography is a sign of malignant transformation (sarcoma, NE carcinoma). However, clinical diagnosis is uncertain and requires histologic confirmation by EUS-guided core needle puncture (EUS-FNP) for histology or aspiration cytology (EUS-FNA).

Note *En-bloc resection* is preferable for diagnosis of *mesenchymal SET,* except leiomyomas, because differential diagnosis and exclusion of malignancy of SET is unreliable by hr-EUS, according to NCCN clinical guidelines for soft tissue sarcoma [12].

Gastrointestinal stromal tumor (GIST) is the most frequent mesenchymal SET and the most common type of *soft tissue sarcoma.* GIST arises in the wall of the GIT or in the retroperitoneum; relapses and metastases affect the peritoneum and/or the liver [13]. The annual incidence is about 1–1.5 per 100,000, and the prevalence is 13 per 100,000 [13–15]. Major locations are the stomach (60%), small intestine (20–30%), and rarely, the colorectum, esophagus, mesentery, and retroperitoneum [5, 16]. GIST grows to protuberant lesions with central dimpling (subserosal or submucosal) and shows invasion and ulceration at larger size (~2 cm). GIST can present as a polyp (originating from MM), a sessile lesion (0-Is) (Fig. 4.1), an obtusely protruded SET (0-Is, central in PM layer), or can be inapparent from the lumenal aspect (protruded subserosal tumor). Some cause symptoms (pain, weight loss) or bleed. On EUS, the tumors appear homogenous and hypoechoic or with heterogenous structure and anechoic cystic foci; they are contingent with the fourth echo layer (proper muscle) or rarely with the second layer (MM) [3, 4, 17]. They originate from Cajal pacemaker cells or GI stem cells and are negative for pancytokeratin (PCK), but are positive for activated/mutated oncogens (~95% DOG1, 80% cKIT, 15% PDGFRα pos.) or 5% wild-type [SDH-B pos., succinate dehydrogenase subunit B] [15, 18].

The behavior of GIST is variable and not exactly predictable [8]. Therefore, the tumors are stratified for clinical risk of malignancy based on size, primary tumor site, and rate of mitosis [5, 13, 19] (Table 4.2). Small GIST (<2 cm size; <5 mitoses/5 mm^2) behaves as if benign. Risk for malignant behavior becomes substantial

Table 4.2 Modified NIH Risk Classification for Primary GIST[a]

Risk category	Tumor size, cm	Mitotic index (*n*/50 HPF)	Primary tumor site
Very low risk	<2.0	≤5	Any
Low risk	2.1–5.0	≤5	Any
Intermediate risk	2.1–5.0	>5	Gastric
	<5.0	6–10	Any
	5.1–10	≤5	Gastric
High risk	Any	Any	Tumor rupture
	>10	Any	Any
	>5.0	>5	Any
	2.1–5.0	>5	Non-gastric
	5.1–10	≤5	Non-gastric

HPF high-power field
[a]Modified acc. to [13, 19]

with larger size (>2 cm), inhomogenous structure and unclear margins on EUS, extragastic primary tumor location, and high mitosis rate (>5/5 mm^2; Ki-67 index >7%) [5, 11]. They spread by hematogenous/peritoneal metastases, not by lymph node metastases. Larger tumors may need neoadjuvant targeted therapy with imatinib, but only after mutational analysis of GIST for predicted response or non-response. Patients with GIST 1–2 cm (or larger) in size or suspicious for malignant transformation should be referred to specialized centers and treated there according to current guidelines [13, 15]. In East Asia, surgical oncologists often resect GIST of size <2 cm, some with minimally invasive endoscopic techniques [20–23], and with very good overall survival [18, 24]. In Western countries, resection is recommended for GIST <2 cm in the rectum, but endoscopic and EUS follow-up (first after 6 months, then 12 months) is recommended for gastric GIST <2 cm [13]. Asymptomatic "incidental" gastric GIST of size <1 cm is a frequent finding in 20–30% of the elderly ("seedling GIST" or "micro-GIST"), and resection of such a small GIST is not indicated [25]. Apart from cutaneous and neurological manifestations, neurofibromatosis type 1 (von Recklinghausen disease) may be associated with multiple endocrine neoplasias, neurofibromas, NETs (e.g. carcinoid) and even symptomatic GIST, mainly of the duodenum and small intestine [26].

Standard treatment for localized GIST (≥2 cm) is surgical excision with no dissection of clinically negative lymph nodes. Laparoscopic-endoscopic cooperative surgery (LECS)— particularly non-exposed wall inversion surgery (NEWS)—is the best minimally invasive approach for moderate-size GIST (2–4 cm) in specialized centers, but open surgery is preferred to the laparoscopic approach for larger-size GIST because of the risk of tumor rupture and peritoneal seeding [13, 15]. Resection en-bloc with an intact pseudocapsule is mandatory to avoid tumor cell seeding, to examine histologic evidence of malignancy (such as infiltration of the pseudocapsule and focal mitosis count >5 per 5 mm^2), and for mutational analysis for targeted therapy [13, 15, 27].

Leiomyoma (LM) is the most frequent SET in the esophagus (middle and lower third); it arises in the PM layer and is seldom found elsewhere in the GI tract. Transformation to leiomyosarcoma is rare (<4%); most of these are of larger size (>3 cm). Leiomyomas that are larger than 1–2 cm, are growing, or are symptomatic with dysphagia should be resected en-bloc, e.g. with subepithelial tunneling endoscopic resection (STER) [3, 11, 28]. Small (3–5 mm) "seedling" leiomyomas and GIST are very frequent and cluster in the esophagus and stomach around the esophagogastric junction (EGJ), with leiomyomas found in 47% of patients with esophageal carcinoma, and GIST in 10% [29] (Fig. 4.2).

Granular cell tumors (GCT, Abrikosoff tumors) are solitary submucosal neoplasms that originate from neuronal Schwann cells and have low malignant potential [4, 30, 31]. About 60% of GCT localize in the GI tract, mostly in the esophagus (prevalence 0.3%) and anal canal; very seldom in the stomach or elsewhere. They present on endoscopy as a nodular, pale-whitish lesion ("molar tooth-like") covered with normal mucosa, and on EUS as an isoechoic or hypoechoic lesion in the submucosa layer [3, 30]. Diagnosis is made by EUS-FNP showing typical lysosome-rich cells (PAS +) strongly positive for S-100 protein and negative for PCK [11, 30]. Malignant transformation is rare (~4%); risk depends on location (AR > EG), size

>3–4 cm, and increased rate of mitosis (>2 mitoses/10 HPF). Large (>1–2 cm), growing, or symptomatic GCT should be resected [11, 31]. (*See* Case 1, Fig. 4.4). By contrast, the very rare *schwannoma* is located in the PM layer, is homogenous-hypoechoic and encapsulated on hr-EUS; FNP also shows S-100 positive cells.

Neuroendocrine tumors (NET) of the foregut (GEP-NET) and hindgut (colorectal CR-NET) have risen in incidence by twofold to fivefold in the past 20 years, but less so for intestinal midgut NET (SI-NET), which escape incidental endoscopic detection. Gastrointestinal NET are located in esophagus (5%), stomach (G-NET, 50–60%), small intestine (SI-NET, 20–30%), and colorectum (CR-NET, 5–15%) [6] (Fig. 4.3). Next to colorectal cancer, these are the most prevalent GI tumors (35 per 100,000 in the United States). They have malignant potential and metastasize to regional lymph nodes and hematogenically to liver. Midgut and colonic NET have the poorest prognosis and the highest risk of metastatic disease: SI-NET at a size of 1 cm have in 30% positive LNM, and nearly 100% at a size of 2 cm [6, 32]. NET are stratified for risk of malignancy based on tumor site, size, and mitosis count (Table 4.3). The prognosis of NE carcinoma G3 (<5% of NET) is as poor as for advanced gastric cancer [6, 32, 33]. Except for SI-NET, however, the risk for metastasis is low for NET of size ≤1 cm (category T1), and such incidental NET should undergo endoscopic en-bloc resection when in clinical stage N0 (negative EUS or CT scan and negative FDG-PET or DOTATOC scintigraphy) [6]. Nevertheless, we recommend evaluating such NET in accordance with guidelines in a specialized center if it is hormone-active or larger than 1 cm in size [6, 32].

Gastric NET are mainly (~70%) G-NET type 1, reddish hemispherical subepithelial tumors (SET) with enterochromaffin-like cell hyperplasia of grading G1 on Table 4.4. They are often multiple and caused by hypergastrinemia in all forms of atrophic gastritis. Very rarely, they show invasive growth to the PM layer and LN

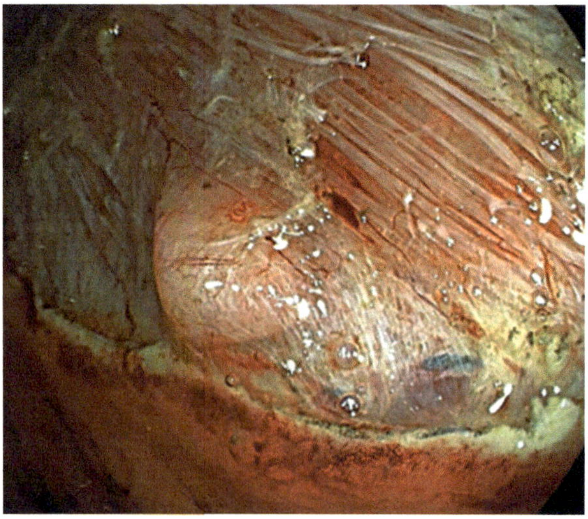

Fig. 4.2 Subepithelial tumor (d 8 mm, firm) in subcardial gastric wall of an 82-year-old woman, exposed at ESD of Barrett carcinoma, belonging to the "seedling-type" small, inapparent tumors (such as LM, GIST [29]) in EG junction area. Histology: leiomyoma

metastasis when exceeding 2 cm size. Annual surveillance endoscopy and cold snare resection (when ≤1 cm size) or ESD when slightly larger is recommended [6]. G-NET type 2 also arise from hypergastrinemia, in Zollinger-Ellison syndrome (ZES) or multiple endocrine neoplasia (MEN) type I. G-NET type 2 present as solitary and sporadic, usually showing grading G2 and moderate size (1–2 cm), but already with LN metastasis. They tend to seed LN more frequently than G-NET type 3, and need clinical staging, even when smaller (0.5–1 cm), prior to endoscopic

Table 4.3 Characteristics for malignant transformation of GI SET and resection strategy [2, 5, 11, 17, 30, 32]

	Signs of malignant transformation or behavior						Indication
SET type	SET location	Malignancy risk, %	Critical size, cm	EUS signs	Mitoses, *n*/*x* HPF	Ki67 index, %	Resection technique
GIST [5, 17]	R, D, I > G[a]	size <1 cm: 2–10%	>1[b]	Hypoechoic or echogenic & anechoic foci/invasive margin	>5/50	>7	STER (if 1–2 cm)[c] LECS (if >2 cm) Surg res (≥2 cm)[a]
		size <5 cm: 4–57%	>2[b]				
LM [11]	E, G, I	<1%	>4 or ↑ size[b]	Anechoic & echogenic foci/invasive margin	>2/10	n.g.	STER (sympt.) Surg res (≥2 cm)[c]
GCT [2, 30]	E, A	<4%	>3 or ↑ size	Anechoic & echogenic foci/invasive margin	>2/10	n.g.	ESD (<2 cm) STER[c], LECS
NET [6, 32]	G-NET types 2 & 3	*T1 < 1 cm* <5%	>1–2[d]	Anechoic & echogenic foci/invasive margin into PM/enlarged regional LN	2–20/10	3–20	EMR, EFTR (<1 cm)[e] ESD, STER (if cT1N0) Surg res & LND (if ≥2 cm)[f]
	D-NET	<5%					
	SI-NET	**<10%**					
	CR-NET	<2%					

A anus, *EFTR* endoscopic full-thickness resection, *EMR* endoscopic mucosal resection, *ESD* endoscopic submucosa dissection, *HPF* high power field (50 HPF = 5 mm^2), *LECS* laparoscopic-endoscopic cooperative surgery, *LND* lymph node dissection, *PM* proper muscle layer, *n.g.* not given, *STER* submucosal tunneling endoscopic resection, *TE* thoracoscopic enucleation

[a]Higher malignant potential in *rectum* and *intestine* (>10%, when size >1 cm). Consider for GIST >2 cm neoadjuvant therapy with imatinib before surgery (referral to specialized center)

[b]Avid ^{18}FDG retention in FDG-PET scan is sign of malignancy

[c]Resection (without LND) when growing, signs suspicious for malignant transformation or symptomatic

[d]Negative somatostatin-receptor scintigraphy with DOTATOC indicates endoscopic resection (only for T1 cN0)

[e]Resection for any size recommended, e.g. snare-PE for NF-NET ≤1 cm; ESD/STER for NF-NET ≤2 cm cLN 0; referral to specialized center (radioscintigraphic diagnostics), when >1 cm or hormonally active NET

[f]Surgical resection with lymphadenectomy when ≥2 cm or suspicion of malignant NET

Table 4.4 Histological Risk Grading of Gastroenteropancreatic Neuroendocrine Tumors (GEP-NET) [32]

ENETS Grade	Mitotic index, (×10 HPF)[a]	Ki-67 proliferation index, %[b]	WHO classification 2010
G1	<2	≤2	NET G1 (carcinoid)
G2	2–20	3–20	NET G2
G3	>20	>20	NEC G3, large cell or small cell type

ENETS European Neuroendocrine Tumor Society, *NEC* neuroendocrine carcinoma
[a]10 HPF (high power field) = 2 mm^2
[b]MiB1antibody: % pos of 2000 cells

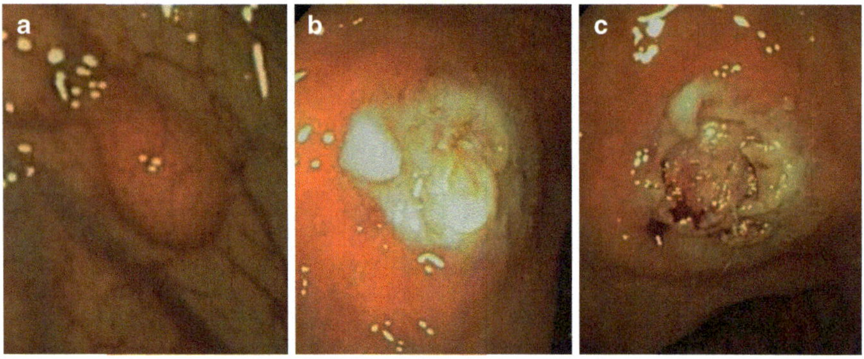

Fig. 4.3 Subepithelial tumor (SET, 8 mm) in anterior wall of the rectum in a 54-year-old man. (**a**) Firm SET with yellowish permeation, suspicious for neuroendocrine tumor (NET). (**b**) Snaring after sm-injection apparently was R2. (**c**) The resection bed was cleared down to the proper muscle layer with jumbo biopsy forceps. Histology: NET G1 T1 (Ki-67 index 1.3%). Follow-up was without recurrence at 2.5 years

Note: Better resect NET en-bloc (e.g. with band-ligation EMR).

en-bloc resection (when cT1 N0). G-NET type 3 are poorly differentiated NE carcinoma G3; most are larger (>3–5 cm) and have very poor prognosis, with about 50% first-year mortality [6, 32, 33].

Duodenal NET include gastrinomas (50–60%), somatostatin-secreting NET (10–15%), non-functional serotonin-producing NET (20%), and NE carcinomas G3 (<3%); they are mainly located in parts I and II of the duodenum.

Note Referral to a specialized center is recommended for management of

- NET of >1 cm size (except G-NET type 1)
- Hormone-active NET and G-NET types 2 and 3
- Gastric GIST of size >2 cm, or with size >1 cm in other locations

4.4 Minimally Invasive Resection Techniques for SET of the GI Tract

Gastrointestinal SET is a new indication for minimally invasive resection techniques and treatment is still investigational, without consensus guidelines. See Chap. 3, Sect. 3.5 for explanation of resection techniques.

4.4.1 Endoscopic Resection Techniques

Band-ligation EMR-L and ESD. SET of small size (≤1 cm) may undergo endoscopic surveillance, especially small gastric GIST (≤1 cm, contiguous with PM) in the elderly [25]. Resection for diagnostic and curative purpose is recommended for gastric small-size G-NET type 1 (often multiple) in atrophic gastritis, small-size G-NET type 2, and rectal NET. These submucosal NET can be resected en-bloc with band-ligation EMR-L (Chap. 3). Moderate-size (1–2 cm) SET situated in EUS layers 2 and 3 (MM and SM) in the esophagus and stomach may be resected with ESD, when a faint echo-band of layer 3 (echogenic sm layer) is preserved, such as with GCT, moderate-size gastric NET (cT1 N0), and superficial gastric GIST with only a narrow connection with the gastric PM layer on hr-EUS [8]. (See Case 4, Figs. 4.5 and 4.6).

Submucosal tunneling endoscopic resection (STER) is still investigational and is performed in highly specialized centers [20, 22, 23]. Moderate-size insuspect SET (1–2 cm) in the middle of the PM layer (near EUS band 4) may be amenable to STER in the lower esophagus and most locations of the stomach (except in the fundus or lesser curvature) [20, 23]. Ping-Hong Zhou and coworkers have reported a large retrospective series ($n \geq 180$) of esophageal and gastric SET (maximum longitudinal size up to 5 cm) with en-bloc resection rate ≥ 85%, without mortality, serious morbidity, or recurrent or metastatic disease within a median 10 to 24 months [21, 34]. When implemented in less specialized centers, however, a low complete resection rate and risk of perforation of the organ wall or pseudocapsule might cause morbidity or even peritoneal dissemination of GIST [8]. Therefore, guidelines recommend surgical resection for GIST larger than 2 cm [17, 18, 27].

4.4.2 Laparoscopic-Endoscopic Cooperative Surgery (LECS)

In general, gastric or esophageal SET larger than 2 cm and in wide contact with EUS layer 4 (PM) should be referred to specialized endoscopic-laparoscopic surgical centers. For proven GIST, pretreatment with imatinib and resection after partial remission may be an option in such a center. SET larger than 2 cm generally require laparoscopic surgery [17, 18, 27]. The best minimally invasive technique is LECS to guarantee complete and organ-sparing resection lines. But classic LECS opens the gastric lumen to the peritoneal space, allowing peritoneal transfer of luminal bacteria or tumor cells from ulcerated GIST [8, 35]. Non-exposed endoscopic wall-inversion surgery (NEWS) does not open the gastric wall and avoids peritoneal infection or tumor dissemination, but transoral harvesting of the specimen limits the NET size to about 3 cm [35, 36] (*see* Fig. 3.3). The alternative LECS non-exposure technique, wrapping the full-thickness wall and GIST specimen into peritoneum (CLEAN-NET), can remove larger NET by laparoscopic surgery when widening the access incision [7]. Nevertheless, guidelines recommend open surgery for large-sized GIST [13, 15, 27].

4.5 Cases of Subepithelial Tumors of the GI Tract

Case 1: NET in Part III of the Duodenum
In a 76-year-old man, a 1-cm SET was pointed out in the superior wall of duodenum part III during extraction of the common duct. On high-resolution EUS (20 MHz miniprobe), the small SET (9 × 9-mm) showed homogenous, hypoechoic structure with a clear border. In a second session, the lesion was snared en-bloc after sm-injection with good lifting, and the resection bed was closed with clips (Fig. 4.4).

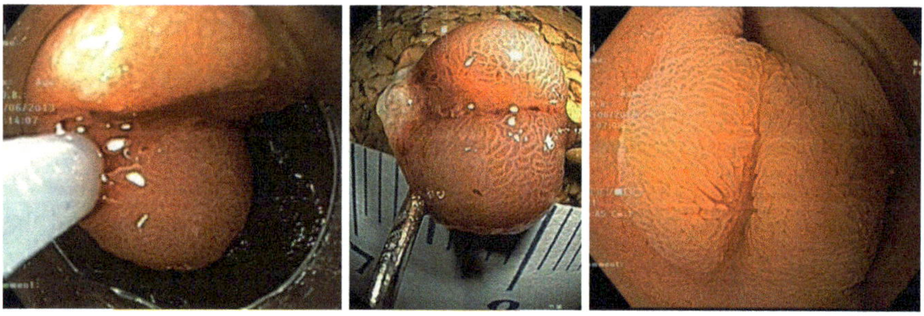

Fig. 4.4 Submucosal 9-mm tumor in the horizontal duodenum (part III), *Right pannel*, Normal villous surface epithelium is evident (WLI, magnification 40×). *Left pannel*, EMR en bloc. *Middle*, Specimen. Histology: NET G1 (Ki-67 <2%) pT1, R0. No recurrence at follow-up after 2 years

Case 2: Gastric GIST Located Below Esophagogastric Junction
A 56-year-old woman was referred for endoscopic resection of a GIST (diameter 2.5 cm) located in the posterior gastric wall towards the minor curvature. Two weeks previously, an attempt to snare the SET had been unsuccessful, only unroofing the GIST. ESD was curative (Fig. 4.5).

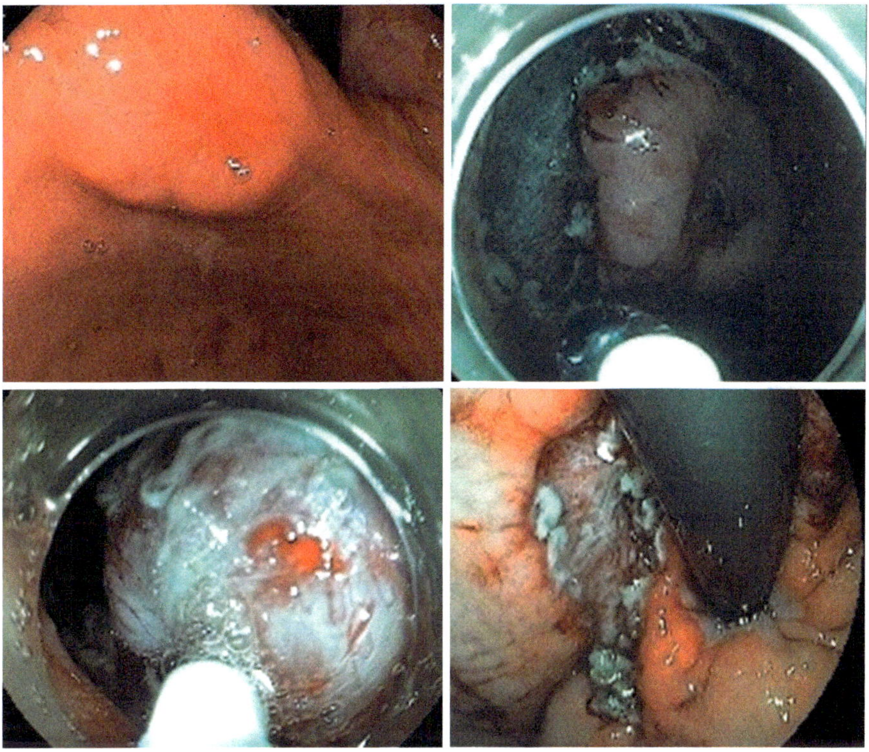

Fig. 4.5 Gastrointestinal stroma tumor (d 2 cm) located below EG junction in posterior gastric wall towards minor curve. ESD was performed with a hybrid knife (*upper right*). The GIST was in narrow contact with the PM layer (*upper left*), and was extracted with intact pseudocapsule in a harvesting net (*lower left*). Resection bed after prophylactic coagulation of vessel stumps (*lower right*). Histology: gastric GIST, maximum diameter 21 mm, cKIT+, mitoses 3.5/50 HPF. Resection en-bloc with intact pseudocapsule (probably curative)

Case 3: Esophageal SET of SM Layer with Intermittent Dysphagia

A 46-year-old otherwise healthy woman with intermittent dyspagia for solids was referred with a 1.5-cm, smoothly subepithelial, protuberant lesion in the midesophagus. On EUS, the lesion was solid, hypoechoic, and contingent with the third layer (SM), and was separated by a faint echoband from the fourth layer (proper muscle). FNA had shown PAS stain–positive cylindrical cells with positive IHC stain for S-100 protein. The Ki-67 index was 1%, consistent with benign granular cell tumor in the SM layer (Abrikossof tumor) (Fig. 4.6).

Note Esophageal SM tumor separated from PM on hr-EUS can be easily resected with ESD.

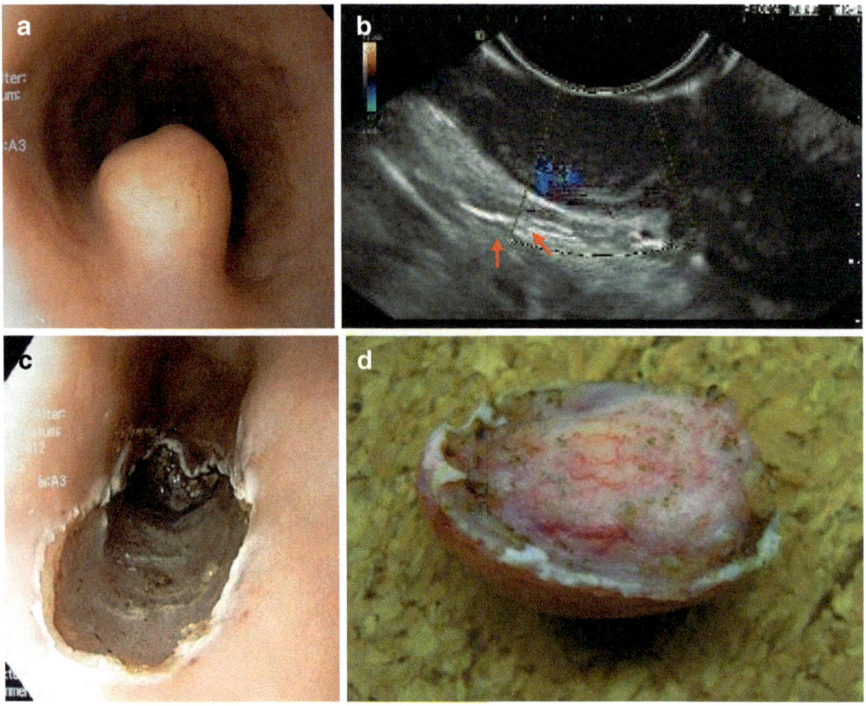

Fig. 4.6 Pale, "molar-tooth-like" SM tumor of 15 × 10 × 10-mm size in midesophagus (standard white light limaging [WLI]). (**a**) SM tumor of mid-esophagus. (**b**) EUS (7.5 MHz) shows a hypoechoic lesion contiguous with the SM layer (*arrow*), EUS FNP reveals S-100 expressing granular cell tumor (Abrikossof). (**c**) Resection bed after endoscopic submucosa dissection (ESD), on WLI. (Courtesy of G. Kleber, Aalen, Germany; and T. Oyama, Nagano, Japan.) (**d**) Specimen of granular cell tumor, ESD R0

Case 4: Symptomatic Esophageal SET Originating from the PM Layer

A 78-year-old man underwent UGI endoscopy for intermittent dysphagia of solids over about 6 months. In mid-esophagus, he presented a 15-mm elevated, bulging, sessile SET with smooth margins and firm consistency. The SET showed no malignant signs on EUS. FNA had inconclusive results. He was referred for endoscopic resection of this symptomatic, probably benign PM-SET (Fig. 4.7).

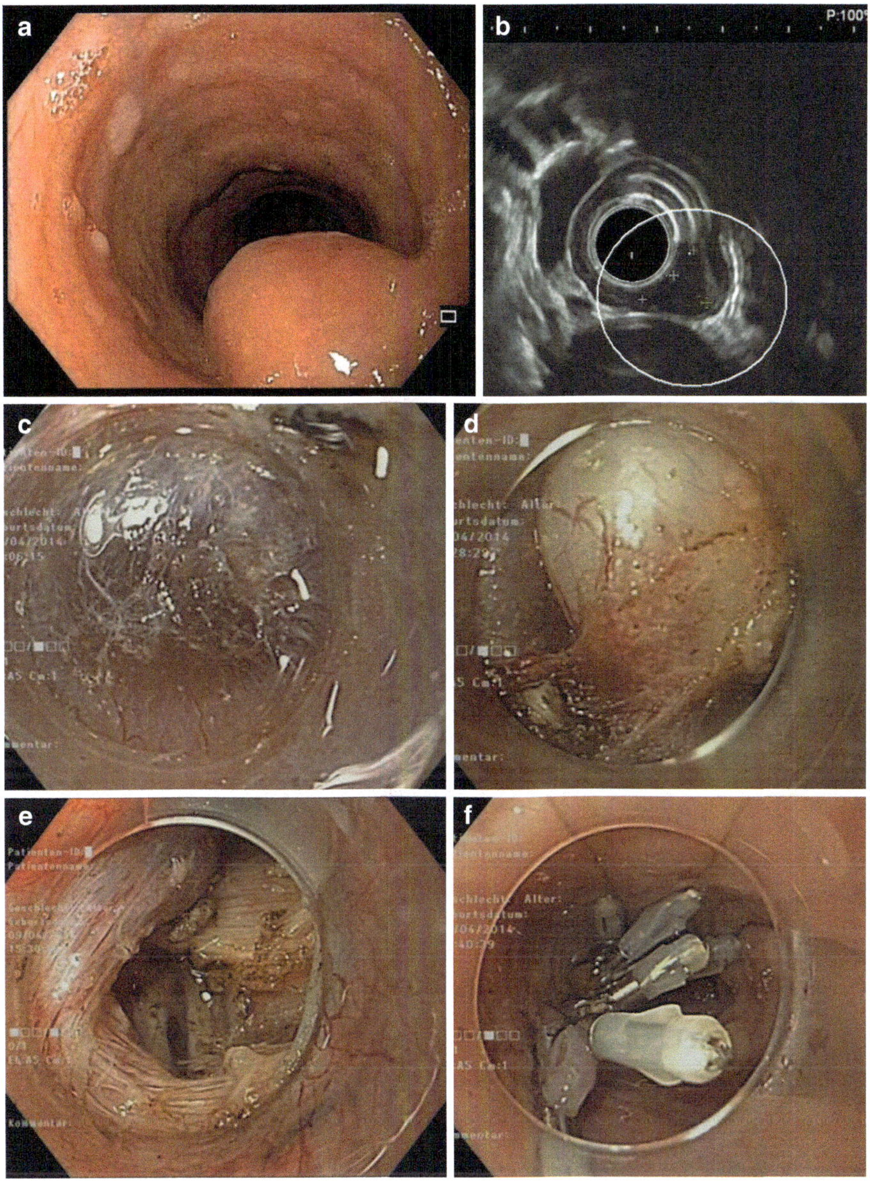

Fig. 4.7 Submucosal tunneling endoscopic resection of SET in PM layer. (**a**) 15-mm elevated bulging, obtusely sessile subepithelial tumor with firm consistency in mid-esophagus (25 cm p.i.), normal mucosa with a few glycogen acanthoses (WLI). (**b**) EUS shows a 15 × 12 × 17-mm homogenous, hypoechoic solid lesion with clear borders, contiguous with the fourth echo layer, PM. (**c**) Submucosal tunneling for 4 cm distance. (**d**) Dissection of encapsulated tumor in the sm space and resection with inner PM layer. (**e**) Gap of inner PM layer and small longitudinal transsection (5 mm) of outer PM layer. (**f**) Clip closure of the mucosal incision for SM access. (Courtesy of G. Kleber, Aalen, Germany; and T. Oyama, Nagano, Japan)

Case 5: Duodenal NET with Fibrosis of Submucosa Layer – Hybrid ESD

A 72-year-old man had a hemispherical SET (0-Is, 10 mm) under normal, reddish mucosa ín the inferior wall of the duodenal bulb, found on endoscopy for melena from NSAID-induced, right-sided colopathy. EUS showed a smooth, hyopoechoic tumor in SM layer. Fine-needle aspiration (FNA) identified epitheloid cells, synaptophysin ++. Enrichment of SET in octreotidscan. The diagnosis was NET of unknown grade – hormonal inactive. ESD was performed with curative intention (Fig. 4.8). DOTA-TOC scinti-scan remained negative, and endoscopy with EUS showed no evidence of recurrence during 2 years follow-up.

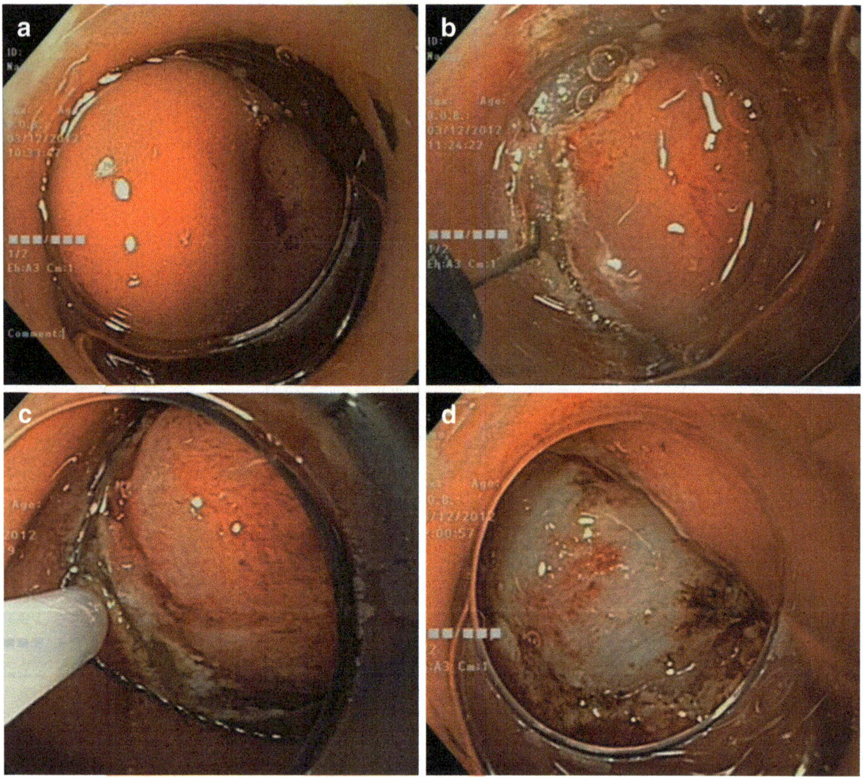

Fig. 4.8 (**a**) Duodenal bulb contained a 1.3-cm-sized, semispherical SET postpyloric in the anterior wall (WLI), difficult to access from the pylorus. (**b**) After circumferential incision (hook knife) no lifting of SET upon sm injection (severe sm fibrosis). (**c**) Snaring only of SET was feasible (hybrid ESD, no bleed). (**d**) Bland resection bed with PM layer. (**e**) Histology: *Well-differentiated neuroendocrine carcinoma NET G2* pNX L0 V0 Pn0 (HE); resection en-bloc, $R_{0.}$ Ki-67 index was 3.74%. (**f**) synaptophysin was positive (IHC). (Courtesy of H.P. Allgaier, Freiburg, Germany and T. Oyama, Nagano, Japan)

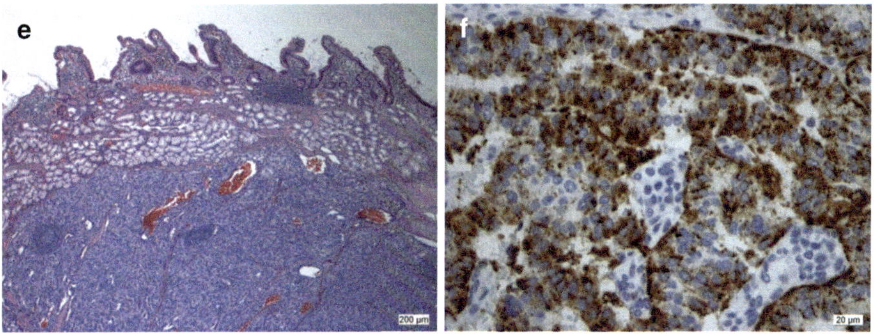

Fig. 4.8 (continued)

Acknowledgments The contribution of cases and histology by Drs. Tsuneo Oyama, Nagano, Takashi Toyonaga, Kobe, Japan, Hans P. Allgaier/Freiburg, Gerhard Kleber/Aalen, Germany, and Daniel Neureiter/Salzburg, Austria is gratefully acknowledged.

References

1. Hedenbro JL, et al. Endoscopic diagnosis of submucosal gastric lesions. The results after routine endoscopy. Surg Endosc. 1991;5:20–3.
2. Hwang JH, et al. American Gastroenterological Association Institute technical review on the management of gastric subepithelial masses. Gastroenterology. 2006;130:2217–28.
3. Nishida T, et al. Submucosal tumors: comprehensive guide for the diagnosis and therapy of gastrointestinal submucosal tumors. Dig Endosc. 2013;25:479–89.
4. Wiech T, et al. Histopathological classification of nonneoplastic and neoplastic gastrointestinal submucosal lesions. Endoscopy. 2005;37:630–4.
5. Miettinen M, Lasota J. Gastrointestinal stromal tumors: pathology and prognosis at different sites. Semin Diagn Pathol. 2006;23:70–83.
6. Sato Y, et al. Management of gastric and duodenal neuroendocrine tumors. World J Gastroenterol. 2016;22:6817–28.
7. Inoue H, et al. Endoscopic mucosal resection, endoscopic submucosal dissection and beyond: full-layer resection for gastric cancer with non-exposure technique (CLEAN-NET). Surg Oncol Clin N Am. 2012;21:129–40.
8. Kim HH. Endoscopic treatment for gastrointestinal stromal tumor: advantages and hurdles. World J Gastrointest Endosc. 2015;7:192–205.
9. Liu F, et al. The fourth space surgery: endoscopic subserosal dissection for upper gastrointestinal subepithelial tumors originating from the muscularis propria layer. Surg Endosc. 2018;32:2575–82.
10. Dumonceau JM, et al. Indications, results, and clinical impact of endoscopic ultrasound (EUS)-guided sampling in gastroenterology: European Society of Gastrointestinal Endoscopy (ESGE) Clinical Guideline – updated January 2017. Endoscopy. 2017;49:695–714.
11. Miettinen M, et al. Esophageal stromal tumors: a clinicopathologic, immunohistochemical, and molecular genetic study of 17 cases and comparison with esophageal leiomyomas and leiomyosarcomas. Am J Surg Pathol. 2000;24:211–22.
12. von Mehren M, et al. Soft tissue sarcoma, version 2.2018, NCCN clinical practice guidelines in oncology. J Natl Compr Cancer Netw. 2018;16:536–63.

13. Judson I, et al. UK clinical practice guidelines for the management of gastrointestinal stromal tumours (GIST). Clin Sarcoma Res. 2017;7:6.
14. Nilsson B, et al. Gastrointestinal stromal tumors: the incidence, prevalence, clinical course, and prognostication in the preimatinib mesylate era--a population-based study in western Sweden. Cancer. 2005;103:821–9.
15. Nishida T, et al. The standard diagnosis, treatment, and follow-up of gastrointestinal stromal tumors based on guidelines. Gastric Cancer. 2016;19:3–14.
16. Tran T, et al. The epidemiology of malignant gastrointestinal stromal tumors: an analysis of 1,458 cases from 1992 to 2000. Am J Gastroenterol. 2005;100:162–8.
17. Nishida T, et al. Clinical practice guideline for gastrointestinal stromal tumors (GIST) in Japan. Int J Clin Oncol. 2008;13:416–30.
18. Nishida T. Asian consensus guidelines for gastrointestinal stromal tumor: what is the same and what is different from global guidelines. Transl Gastroenterol Hepatol. 2018;3:11.
19. Joensuu H. Risk stratification of patients diagnosed with gastrointestinal stromal tumor. Hum Pathol. 2008;39:1411–9.
20. Cai MY, et al. Endoscopic full-thickness resection for gastrointestinal submucosal tumors. Dig Endosc. 2018;30(Suppl 1):17–24.
21. Chen T, et al. Long-term outcomes of submucosal tunneling endoscopic resection for upper gastrointestinal submucosal tumors. Ann Surg. 2017;265:363–9.
22. Inoue H, et al. Submucosal endoscopic tumor resection for subepithelial tumors in the esophagus and cardia. Endoscopy. 2012;44:225–30.
23. Lu J, et al. Heading toward the right direction--solution package for endoscopic submucosal tunneling resection in the stomach. PLoS One. 2015;10:e0119870.
24. Joensuu H, et al. Risk of recurrence of gastrointestinal stromal tumour after surgery: an analysis of pooled population-based cohorts. Lancet Oncol. 2012;13:265–74.
25. Scherubl H, et al. Management of early asymptomatic gastrointestinal stromal tumors of the stomach. World J Gastrointest Endosc. 2014;6:266–71.
26. Abdessayed N, et al. Rare triad of periampullary carcinoid, duodenal gastrointestinal stromal tumor and plexiform neurofibroma at hepatic hilum in neurofibromatosis type 1: a case report. BMC Cancer. 2017;17:579.
27. ESMO/European Sarcoma Network Working Group. Gastrointestinal stromal tumors: ESMO Clinical Practice Guidelines for diagnosis, treatment and follow-up. Ann Oncol. 2012;23(Suppl 7):vii49–55.
28. Maehata T, et al. Cutting edge of endoscopic full-thickness resection for gastric tumor. World J Gastrointest Endosc. 2015;7:1208–15.
29. Abraham SC, et al. "Seedling" mesenchymal tumors (gastrointestinal stromal tumors and leiomyomas) are common incidental tumors of the esophagogastric junction. Am J Surg Pathol. 2007;31:1629–35.
30. Iwamuro M, et al. Esophageal granular cell tumors can be differentiated from leiomyomas using endoscopic ultrasonography. Intern Med. 2018;57:1509–15.
31. Moten AS, et al. Granular cell tumor experience at a comprehensive cancer center. J Surg Res. 2018;226:1–7.
32. Rindi G, et al. TNM staging of foregut (neuro)endocrine tumors: a consensus proposal including a grading system. Virchows Arch. 2006;449:395–401.
33. Scheruebl H, et al. Neuroendocrine carcinomas of the bowel are on the rise: early aspects and management. World J Gastrointest Endosc. 2010;2:325–34.
34. Chen T, et al. Submucosal tunneling endoscopic resection vs thoracoscopic enucleation for large submucosal tumors in the esophagus and the esophagogastric junction. J Am Coll Surg. 2017;225:806–16.
35. Namikawa T, et al. Laparoscopic endoscopic cooperative surgery as a minimally invasive treatment for gastric submucosal tumor. World J Gastrointest Endosc. 2015;7:1150–6.
36. Goto O, et al. Laparoscopy-assisted endoscopic full-thickness resection of gastric subepithelial tumors using a nonexposure technique. Endoscopy. 2016;48:1010–5.

Chapter 5
High-Resolution Endoscopic Ultrasound: Clinical T-Staging of Superficial and Subepithelial Gastrointestinal Neoplasias

Hans Seifert, Daisuke Kikuchi, and Naohisa Yahagi

5.1 Introduction

High-resolution endoscopic ultrasound (hr-EUS) uses frequencies of 12–30 MHz, which in theory allows echo resolution of 0.18 to 0.07 mm. At these frequencies, penetration depth is reduced to about 2 cm. The miniprobe transducers (diameter $\leq$ 2.5 mm) are applied through the working channel, and hr-EUS imaging is made under endoscopic view. Hr-EUS examines the integrity of the echo layer structure of the organ wall mainly for two purposes: (1) detection of deep submucosal invasion of epithelial neoplasias (early cancer), and (2) delineation of the echo structure of *subepithelial lesions* (SEL) in regards to three features: the *echo structure*, the *wall layer of origin*, and the *margin*—that is, is there a clear margin with a capsule or pseudocapsule, or an unclear margin with signs of invasiveness? In addition, observing vessels of the lesion and adjacent structures will give safety information for any intended endoscopic resection.

H. Seifert (✉)
Department of Internal Medicine – Gastroenterology, University Hospital Oldenburg, Oldenburg, Germany
e-mail: hansseifert@web.de

D. Kikuchi
Department of Gastroenterology and Endoscopy Unit, Toranomon Hospital, Tokyo, Japan

N. Yahagi
Division of Research and Development for Minimally Invasive Treatment, Cancer Center, Keio University School of Medicine, Shinjuku-ku, Tokyo, Japan
e-mail: yahagi-tky@umin.ac.jp

F. Berr et al. (eds.), *Atlas of Early Neoplasias of the Gastrointestinal Tract*,
https://doi.org/10.1007/978-3-030-01114-7_5

5.2 Performance of High-Resolution EUS Examination

After cleaning any superficial neoplasia or overlying mucosa of SEL with a water-jet, the area of the lesion is submerged in degassed water filled in through the working channel. The subsequent EUS registration—after optimizing EUS frequency and image resolution with zoom and contrast—is performed under endoscopic control of the EUS-transducer position as well as real-time EUS imaging. Positioning of the transducer probe parallel to the surface of the lesion is essential to avoid artefacts and take optimum still images. The "pullthrough" over the neoplastic lesion is repeated a few times under close inspection and image documentation. Precautions must be taken during upper GI hr-EUS recordings to avoid aspiration of refluxed water.

Miniprobes for high-resolution ultrasound with a frequency of 20 MHz display the gastrointestinal wall in a five-layered structure or in a seven-layered echo structure; with a frequency of 30 MHz, up to seven or nine mural echo-layers may be identified (Fig. 5.1). The usual image of gastric or colonic wall is a *five-layered echo-structure* and this is referred to in textbooks as well as in this endoscopy atlas. However, when we use hr-EUS, we should be aware of faint additional echostructures that occasionally may be revealed, as well as of the most common technical artefacts, which may simulate wall structures. Three basic *types of echogenicity* are distinguished: *Anechoic* (*black* without internal echos) is water or clear fluid, and it typically shows a bright acoustic enhancement in the structure behind the fluid-filled structure such as a cyst. *Hypoechoic* is equivalent or lower than the echogenicity of the second or fourth wall layer (lpm or pm); typical examples are gastrointestinal stromal tumor (GIST), leiomyoma, or mucin-filled cyst. *Hyperechoic* is higher echogenicity than the first (ep) or third (sm) echo layers; a typical example is lipoma.

5.3 Endosonographic Anatomy of the Gastrointestinal Tract

Gastric wall. Normal echo-structure of gastric wall shows five echo layers corresponding to anatomic wall structures by 20 MHz EUS (Fig. 5.1a, b). The first *hyper*-echoic layer (1) is the reflected boundary echo of the epithelial surface and epithelial layer; the second *hypo*echoic layer (2) comes from lamina propria (lpm) of the mucosa (with glands); and the third *hyper*echoic layer (3), slightly wider, corresponds to the submucosa (sm) layer and includes upfront the echo from the muscularis mucosa (mm) layer. The broader fourth *hypo*echoic layer (4) corresponds to the proper muscle layer; and the fifth (5), to the subserosa and peritoneal serosa. Hr-EUS with 30 MHz separately resolves seven layers, adding the hyperechoic mm surface and hypoechoic mm layer, and the hyperechoic interstitial fascia between the circular and longitudinal pm layer [1] (Fig. 5.1a).

Colonic wall, like gastric wall, shows the same five echo layers, but the third layer (sm) more often contains three divided "ladder-like" echos (mm, sm, interface to pm) [1].

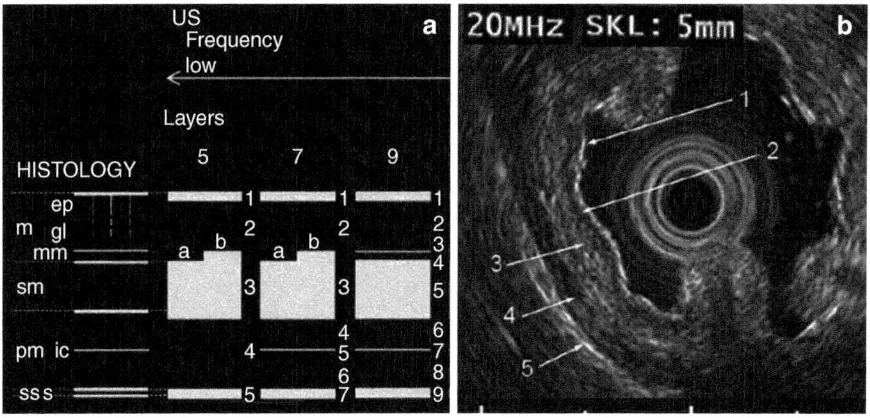

Fig. 5.1 (**a**, **b**) *Gastric wall*. (**a**) Schematic echo layers, (**b**) Five-layered echo-structure as in (a) (20 MHz)

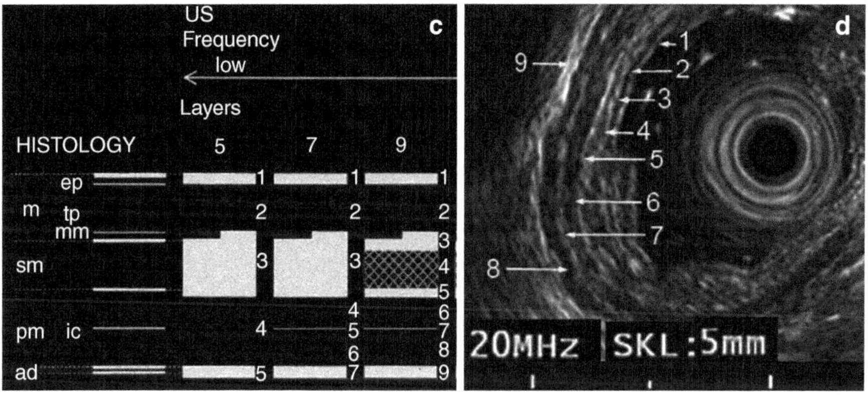

Fig. 5.1 (continued) (**c**, **d**) *Esophageal wall*. (**c**) Schematic echo layers. (**d**) Nine wall echo layers as in (c) (20 MHz). Multiple echo layering (below arrow #5) is a very short-lasting electronic artefact of the rotating echo probe. *1–9*—number of layers that can be identified; *ad*—adventitia; *ep*— epithelial layer; *gl*—glands; *ic*—intermuscular connective tissue; *m*—mucosa; *mm*—muscularis mucosae; *pm*—muscularis propria; *sm*—submucosa; *s/ss*—serosa/subserosa; *tp*— tunica/lamina propria (lpm). (**a**, **c**, Modified from Yamanaka [1], with permission of John Wiley & Sons Inc.)

Esophageal wall generally shows the same echo layers as the gastric wall, but differs in two aspects: layer 2 (*lpm*, hypoechoic) of squamous epithelium and layer 3 (*interface on sm*, hyperechoic) are broadly reflected and separately visualized, resulting in a nine-layered echo-structure (Fig. 5.1c, d). Sometimes even the boundary echoes at mm and the surface of sm may be divided into three hyperechoic layers [1].

Note Only *perpendicularly targeted* segments display exact echo layering (as in Fig. 5.1b)!

5.4 Staging by hr-EUS of Superficial Epithelial Neoplasias

Both T staging and N staging are important for differential indication of endoscopic versus surgical resection, and EUS appears to be more reliable than CT scans in detecting lymph nodes. Conventional EUS using frequencies of 7.5 (3.5–15) MHz offers good visualization of involved surrounding lymph nodes or major arteries. However, hr-EUS (20 MHz) clearly is more accurate than conventional EUS (7.5 MHz) for endosonographic uT staging of sm invasiveness, and it can distinguish T1a vs T1b-sm2 cancer with 88–93% accuracy for esophageal squamous cell cancer, and with 65–86% accuracy for differentiated gastric cancer [2].

5.4.1 Staging of Tumor Category (uT) by hr-EUS

T-staging by hr-EUS has a higher accuracy than conventional EUS (81% vs. 56%) in the upper gastrointestinal tract [3]. Pretherapeutic hr-EUS (for uT1a vs 1b) distinguished pT1a and pT1b of early esophageal cancer with 71–85% accuracy [3–6]. In general, the accuracy of miniprobe hr-EUS has been shown to be around 80% in the esophagus, the stomach, and the colon and rectum [7–9].

There are typical echo shape patterns signaling risk and depth of tumor invasion into hyperechoic submucosal wall layer. The risk of invasion of the submucosa layer was 60% when an "irregular narrowing" of the sm echo-layer was seen under the lesion, and it was 86% when the sm echo-layer showed a "*budding sign*" (a 2-mm-wide hypoechoic zone) under the lesion [10]. With 90% accuracy, tumor invasion of m3/sm1 layer was predicted in the presence of a "*hypoechoic fan shape*" in the sm-echolayer (Fig. 5.2a), and deep invasion of the sm2/sm3 layer in the presence of a "*hypoechoic arch*" in the sm-echolayer (Fig. 5.2b), as well as invasion of the pm layer (uT2) in presence of an *hypoechoic arch spreading from sm-layer into pm-layer* [11] (Fig. 5.2c). The presence of an unequivocal "hypoechoic arch sign" indicates that endoscopic resection is inappropriate.

Key Points

Depth of mural invasion by epithelial tumor on hr-EUS (uT category) is based on:

- Extension of ***hypoechoic lesion*** into wall echo layer (→ ***layer number***)
- Identification of ***uppermost intact*** wall echo layer
- Typical ***shape pattern*** of sm echo layer → risk/depth of sm invasion:
  - "*irregular* ***narrowing*** of sm-echo" → 60% risk of sm1 invasion
  - "**budding sign**" (2 mm wide) in sm → 86% risk of sm1 invasion
  - "*hypoechoic* ***fan shape***" in sm → m3/sm1 invasion (uT1a/b)
  - "*hypoechoic* ***arch shape***" in sm → sm2/sm3 invasion (uT1b)

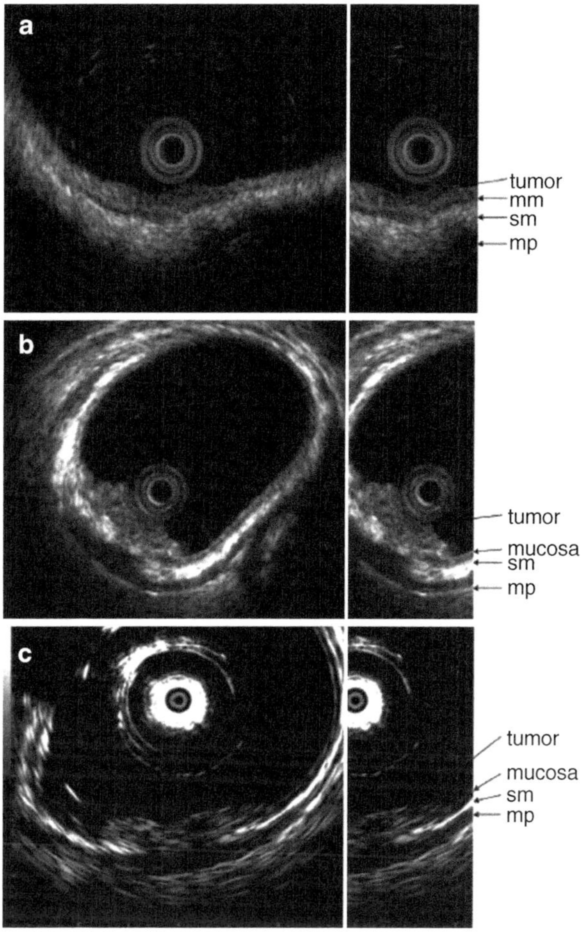

Fig. 5.2 (**a**) Lateral spreading tumor of the sigmoid, uT1-m in high-resolution endosonography. (**b**) Cancer lesion 0-Is of the rectum, uT1b-sm2 in high-resolution endosonography (arch into sm). (**c**) Cancer lesion 0-IIa + IIc at the rectum, uT2 in high-resolution endosonography (arch into mp). mp—muscularis propria

5.4.2 N Staging Using EUS

Conventional EUS (7.5 MHz) was more sensitive and accurate than CT for TN staging of early adenocarcinoma of the esophagus [12]. However, hr-EUS clearly was less sensitive (25–73%) and less accurate (56–87%) for N staging than conventional EUS with 7.5-MHz echoendoscopes [13–15]. Therefore, preoperative N staging for malignant neoplasias requires *conventional echoendoscopes* with 7.5 MHz.

5.4.3 Limitations of hr-EUS for Superficial uT Staging

High-resolution endosonographic imaging depends on good transmission of the acoustic signal, which easily is disturbed by microsludge and small air bubles in the water layer used for acoustic coupling to the organ wall, and by sludge adherent to the lesion. In addition, parallel alignment of the transducer probe to the lesion and perpendicular hr-EUS targeting of the lesion plane is essential for artefact-free hr-EUS imaging, and sometimes this alignment is not well maintained. Irregular shape of the lesion surface (e.g., polyp, large nodule, ulcer –/+ scars) and difficult anatomic locations such as the esophagogastric junction interfere with the anatomic echo planes and result in incontingent echo layers and poor resolution of echo structure [16–18]. The chances of error may rise to 29% for early esophageal cancer, and 19% of cases may be overstaged [19].

For detection of sm invasiveness of early cancer, magnifying endoscopic analysis of superficial vessel and surface structure was slightly more sensitive and accurate than hr-EUS imaging [17, 20], but both techniques combined seem to be most accurate. Image-enhanced endoscopy of an early cancer by itself is sufficient to decide on endoscopic versus surgical resection, especially in the esophagus. Supplementary hr-EUS analysis is even better, but not a standard requirement.

In a prospective study evaluating hr-EUS–based diagnosis of SET in 100 consecutive patients, only 48% of diagnoses were correct, and most misclassifications happened with hypoechoic tumors in the third and fourth layers (sm and pm), such as NET, GIST, and GCT [21]. Thus, *histologic diagnosis* is the gold standard for risk assessment of such SET.

5.5 Diagnosis and Staging of Subepithelial Tumors by hr-EUS

5.5.1 Differential Diagnosis of Subepithelial Lesions by hr-EUS

Subepithelial lesions (SEL) are seen as a bulge or elevation, and diagnosis may be evident by endoscopy, such as a typical varix. Or the bulge may show color permeation of underlying tissue, such as yellowish for lipoma or carcinoid-NET (both mainly in the colorectum) or whitish-greyish for lymphangioma. Consistency also is important for differential diagnosis, as softness favors lipoma, lymphangioma, cyst, or varix. On palpation with a biopsy forceps, such SEL plies like a pillow ("cushion sign"). On the other hand, a firm bulge is evidence of a solid submucosal tissue mass, most likely subepithelial tumor (SET). The predilection sites and characteristics of the most frequent differential diagnoses are listed in Table 5.1.

Differential diagnosis of SEL. Vascular tumors (Table 5.1) are often evident from their endoscopic aspect, e.g. dark-blue cavernous submucosal hemangioma; on hr-EUS, they present a hyperechoic vessel wall and anechoic vessel spaces, demonstrable when in doubt by intravenous injection of sonocontrast medium. On the other hand, *lypmphangioma* shows multiple anechoic lesions and similar wall echos, but without enhancement on sonocontrast examination. *Duplication*

Table 5.1 Characteristics of SET in the GI Tract

SE Mass	Predilection site, Endosc. signs	EUS signs	Contingent with Echo-nr. Layer		Diagnosis (by EUS-FNP)	
					[a]Benign	[b]Malignant
GIST	G > SI > CR > E 0-Is, central dimpling/ulcer	Clear/unclear margin (capsule), homogenous-hypoechoic or heterogenous	4 (2)	pm (mm)	DOG1 + [a] cKIT+ or [a] PDGFRA+ [b]	Size >2 cm Mitoses >5/5mm^2
NET	G > D > SI > R 0-Is, firm, yellowish	Clear capsule (+/−breaks?), homogenous-isoechoic or hypervascular-hypoechoic	2 (3)	lpm (sm)	ChromograninA & Synaptophysin positive	Size >1 cm Mitoses >2/10 HPF
GCT	E >> D > G > R 0-Is, firm, white-yellowish	Clear capsule, homogenous-isoechoic (echogenicity = sm layer)	3	sm	S100+ PAS+, PCK-	Size ≥4 cm Mitoses >2/10 HPF
Leiomyoma	E > G-EGJ > R; 0-Is/p, iso-chrome, firm	Clear capsule, homogenous-hypoechoic (echogenicity = pm layer)	4	pm	Benign, actin & desmin *positive*. *Leiomyosarcoma* very rare	
MALT lymphoma	G > CR > SI 0-II /-I, reddish, bulging or ulcer	Unclear margins, homogenous-hypoechoic	1, 3	m, sm	G-MALT-lymphoma → *Helicobacter pylori*-associated, histology for oncologic therapy	
Malignant lymphoma	SI > G > CR 0-II / 0-I, bulging or ulcer	Unclear margins, hypoechoic (multiple bulky masses)	1, 3	m, sm	Histology for oncologic therapy	
Vascular tumor	G-antrum >CR 0-IIa, 0-I-s, blue-purple	Varied echo pattern, enhanced by contrast-echo-bubbles	3, 4	sm, pm	−/−	(DD: Kaposi sarcoma)
Lipoma	G > right-side C 0-Is, yellowish, soft, cushion sign	Hyperechoic lesion, clear capsule	3	sm	Mature lipocytes	−/−
Fibroma	G > E 0-Ip cylindrical-polypoid	−/−	1, 3	m, sm	Fibrotic-inflammatory	
Lymphangioma	G > right-side C 0-Is/IIa, whitish, soft, cushion sign	Multiple anechoic lesions (few anechoic lesions → differential diagnosis: duplication cyst)	3	sm	Aspirated fluid: lymph vs. mucus	−/−

Modified from References [22–26]

C colon, *D* duodenum, *DD* differential diagnosis, *E* esophagus, *EUS* endoscopic ultrasound, *G* stomach, *GCT* granular cell tumor, *LM* leiomyoma, *MALT* mucosa-associated lymphoid tissue, *PCK* pancytokeratin, *R* rectum, *SE mass* subepithelial mass lesion, *SI* small intestine

[a]DOG1, discovered on GIST-1; cKIT = CD117

[b]PDGFRα = CD34

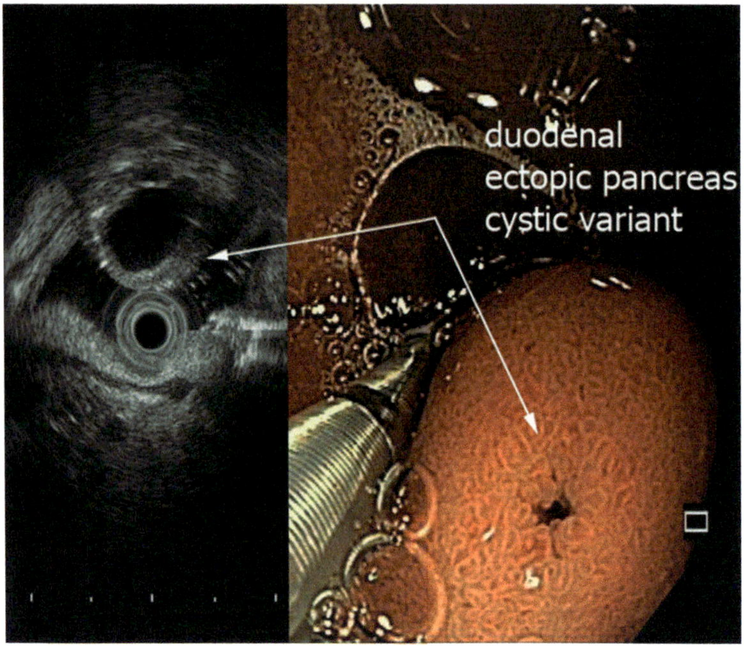

Fig. 5.3 Aberrant pancreas in duodenum pars II. *Right panel:* Porus of main duct of duodenal aberrant pancreas (M-WLI, 20×). *Left panel:* Hr-EUS showing slightly hypoechoic sm-lesion (*top*) with cyst-like dilated duct in sm layer, a thin underlying sm-layer, and hypoechoic pm layer

cyst—seen more often in proximal small intestine than in esophagus, stomach, or colon—is filled with anechoic mucoid fluid, which can be aspirated or drained by puncture or incision. These lesions usually are asymptomatic and do not need intervention. *Lipoma,* most common in the colorectum, rarely presents symptoms of intestinal obstruction. On hr-EUS, lipoma displays a homogenous-*hyper*echoic structure and clear capsule echo. The overlying mucosa can be lifted ("tenting sign"), and in about half of the cases, the "cushion sign" is positive and quite specific. *Aberrant pancreas* is usually observed at the major curve or posterior wall of the antrum or the inner curve of the duodenum as an elevated SEL, often depressed in the center, and on EUS as a a hyperechoic or isoechoic SET with central hypoechoic dilated duct [24, 27] (Fig. 5.3).

Diagnosis of solid SEL is made by typical echostructure and involvement of intramural layers on hr-EUS (20 MHz) and, when findings are ambiguous, with needle aspiration cytology or puncture histology using a 7.5 MHz echoendoscope [24, 28].

Lymphomas spread as infiltrating hypoechoic mases in the sm layer and in lpm of mucosa (Fig. 5.4). They usually cause visible edema and alterations in mucosal vascular structure; malignant lymphoma often produces protruded submucosal masses. Particle biopsy (e.g. with cold snaring) for histologic or immune histologic diagnosis is basic for the selection of oncologic therapy and is much more important than hr-EUS.

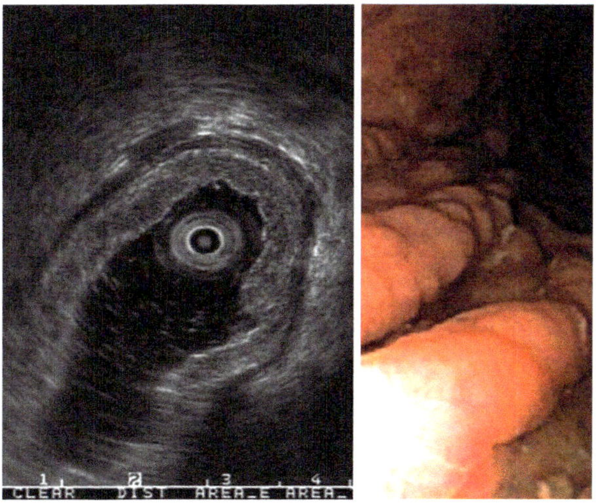

Fig. 5.4 Infiltration of lpm and sm of gastric corpus by slightly inhomogenous, hypoechoic infil-trates extending the diameter of sm. PM layer maintained (*left panel*). On WLI endoscopy, hypertrophic, slightly edematous gastric folds, i.e. solid infiltrates in sm layer (*right panel*). The diagnosis made by particle biopsy (cold snaring) is mucosa-associated lymphoid tissue (MALT) *B-cell lymphoma*

5.5.2 *Tumors Originating from SM or PM Layer*

The typical characteristics of original intramural SET are summarized in the first four rows of Table 5.1. SET in the sm layer with a clear pseudocapsule include rare gastrointestinal stromal tumors (GIST) originating from mm layer (or from pm layer with very narrow contact area on pm) and granular cell tumors (GCT).

Granular cell tumors (GCT), found mainly in the esophagus and anorectal canal, rarely in stomach, show clear capsule echo and homogenous *hyper*echoic structure, isoechoic to the sm layer, the layer of origin of GCT. This is different from leiomyoma [22] (Fig. 5.5a, b).

Leiomyomas, by contrast, present different, slightly *hypo*echoic homogenous echogenicity identical to that of the pm layer, which also is the contingent layer of origin of leiomyoma. There is a faint echo of fibrous capsule [22] (Fig. 5.5c, d).

Gastrointestinal stromal tumors (GIST) with benign behavior typically exhibit homogenous hypoechoic lesions with well-defined margins and moderate size (≤3 cm). GIST are in contact with or located in the *pm layer*, which is the layer of origin (Figs. 5.6 and 5.7). Predilection sites are stomach (~65%), small intestine (~25%), colorectum (5%), and esophagus (<5%). Gastric GIST of size <20 mm without high-risk features may undergo EUS surveillance at intervals of 6–12 months when the size is 10–19 mm, or 2 years if the size is <10 mm [29, 30]. High-risk EUS signs of malignant behavior of GIST or other mesenchymal tumors are growth in size, irregular borders (invasiveness), cystic spaces ≥5 mm (liquid necrosis), echogenic foci, heterogeneity on hr-EUS, ulceration, and extragastric location [31, 32]. Contrast-enhanced EUS provides irregular hypervascularization as an additional criterion suspicious for malignant behavior of GIST [32, 33]. However, GIST basically are soft-tissue sarcomas and have malignant potential regardless of size. The risk of malignant behavior requires histology of the entire primary tumor (invasion of pseudocapsule, foci with high mitosis count) as well as molecular genetic mutation analysis predictive of response to targeted therapy. (See Chap. 4.)

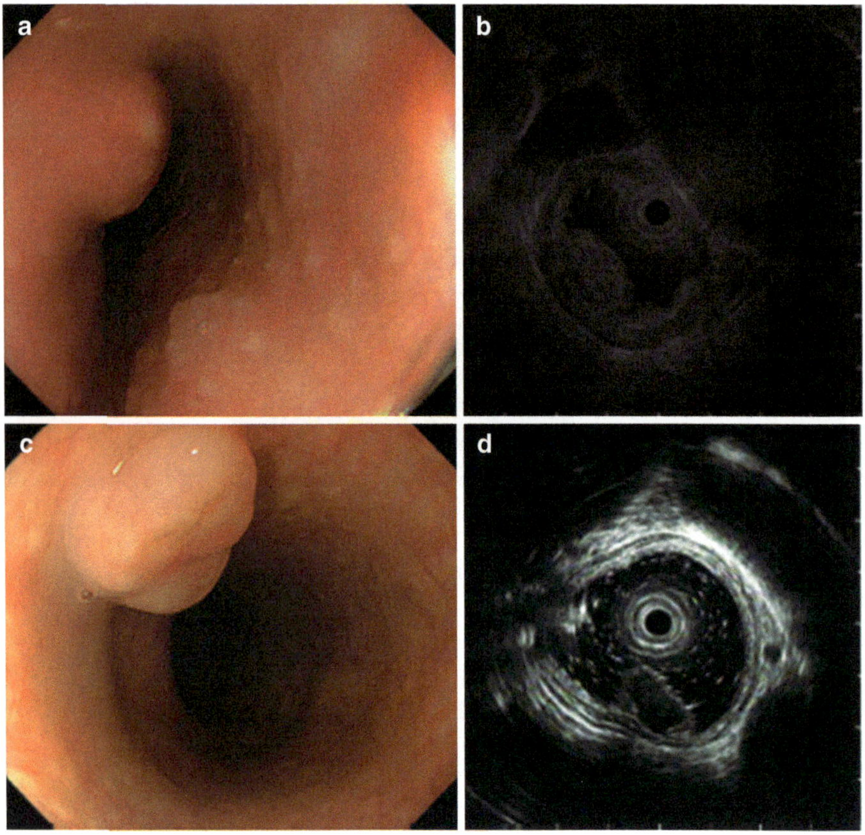

Fig. 5.5 Superficial SET in esophagus may show a steep-bulging, molar tooth-like appearance. (**a**) Endoscopic aspect (WLI) of GCT in normal, partly whitish SC mucosa. (**b**) Hr-EUS (20 MHz) exhibits slightly hyperechoic homogenous SET (isoechoic to sm layer) with clear margins in continuity with sm echo band. (**c**) Endoscopic view (WLI) of a superficial leiomyoma with normal, partly whitish SC mucosa. (**d**) On hr-EUS, the SET is homogenous hypoechoic (isoechoic to pm layer) and separated by the sm-echo band from the pm layer. The layer of origin presumably was MM. (From Iwamuro et al. [22], under the terms of the Attribution-NonCommercial-NoDerivatives 4.0 International (CC BY-NC-ND 4.0) License https://creativecommons.org/licenses/by-nc-nd/4.0/)

Note The guidelines of the National Comprehensive Cancer Network recommend en-bloc resection of intramural mesenchymal tumors (SET) of size >2 cm or SET of any size with high-risk features, for cure and diagnosis of malignancy risk [34].

Neuroendocrine tumors (NET) arise from lamina propria mucosae (lpm, second echo layer) and can extend into the sm layer on hr-EUS. They show homogenous *hypo*echoic or *iso*echoic lesions (vs. lpm) with regular capsule echo (Fig. 5.8). Duodenal and especially small intestinal NET, often carcinoids, and rectal carcinoids may have adjacent sentinel lymph node metastasis at a moderate NET size of 1–2 cm. An enlarged, inhomogenous lymph node may show up within the extramu-

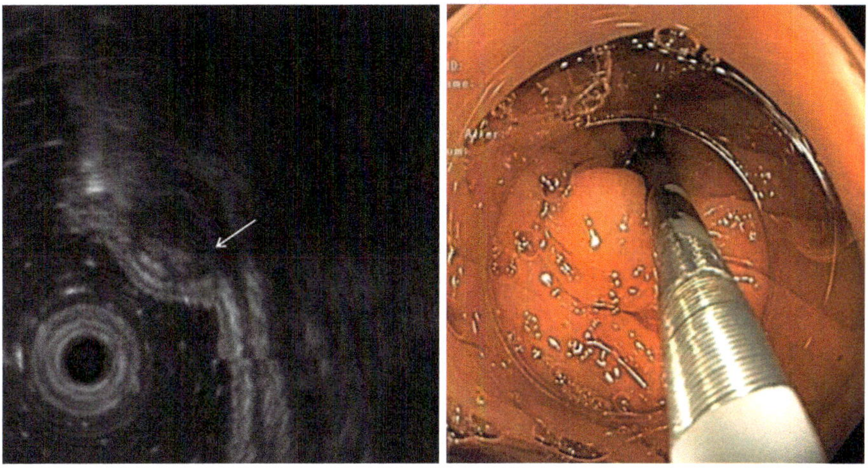

Fig. 5.6 Firm SET in descending colon covered with normal mucosa (WLI, *right panel*). Hr-EUS imaging (20 MHz) (*left panel*) reveals a SET (7.3 × 6 mm) with inhomogenous hypoechoic structure and central anechoic area. The SET is in continuity (↓) with fourth layer (pm); the pm echo band is preserved. There is a clear capsule margin. GIST is suspected. Endoscopic resection en-bloc is performed using a hook knife. Diagnosis: GIST, low-risk (Ki-67, 4%)

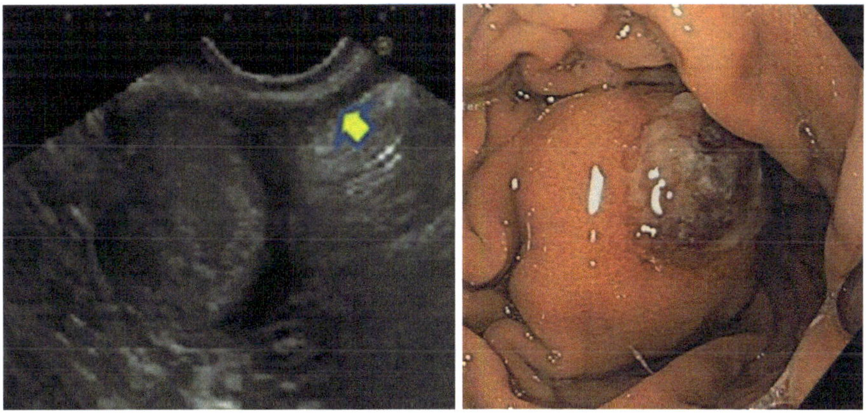

Fig. 5.7 WLI endoscopy 2 hours after melena shows a ball-like SET approximately 2.5 cm in size, with central ulcer and fibrin thrombus, located in the major curvature of the gastric body (*right panel*). EUS imaging (7.5 MHz) of a similar case displays an SET (18.3 × 18 mm) with inhomogenous hypoechoic (compared to sm) structure arising from the fourth layer (*arrow*, pm), suggesting GIST. Pseudocapsule is intact (*left panel*). Later EUS-guided fine needle aspiration (FNA) revealed GIST (*right panel).* Resection is recommended for symptomatic GIST with nearly 2-cm size and heterogenous echo structure. (EUS from Yegin et al. [30] with permission of Springer under Creative Commons Attribution-NonCommercial-ShareAlike 3.0 License)

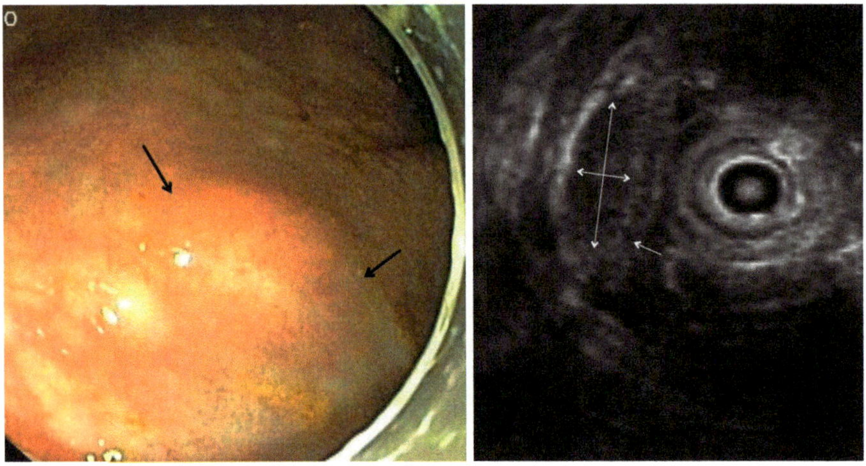

Fig. 5.8 Rectal SET (~10 mm), pale and translucent under normal epithelium, standard WLI (*left*). Hr-EUS demonstrates fairly homogenous hypoechoic SET above the intact echo bands of sm and pm. The SET is isoechoic and in continuity (↓) with second layer (lpm) (*right*). The clinical diagnosis is suspected small-size NET. Resection using band-ligation EMR was recommended. Histology: CR-NET, G1 (Ki-67, 2%), low risk

ral imaging distance (~2 cm) of hr-EUS. In these cases, conventional EUS (7.5 MHz), octreotidscan scintigraphy, and CT or MRI (for lymph node and/or liver metastases) are required, as well as examination for functional NET. Patients are best referred to a specialized center. NET are most frequent in the stomach, and there are three types of G-NET. Type 1 is caused by hypergastrinemia in any type of chronic atrophic gastritis and has often multiple NET of size ≤1 cm, and very rarely lymph node metastasis when NET are larger. Annual follow-up with endoscopic resection of all G-NET type 1 is indicated. All other gastrointestinal NET are sporadic and solitary; they show malignant behavior, at least when >1 cm in size, and should be referred to a specialized center [25, 35]. (See Chap. 4.)

Rare malignant neoplasias include *malignant melanoma* as a primary tumor in esophagus or anorectum and *mucosal metastases* of extragastrointestinal cancer (e.g. breast cancer, extraintestinal lymphoma, or malignant melanoma). These lesions are mostly located in the sm and lpm layer and show some superficial mucosal involvement. Diagnosis is made by biopsy.

5.6 Cases: High-Resolution EUS and Endoscopic Analysis of Superficial and Subepithelial Neoplasms

Case 1: Small Rectal Lesion 0-Is

On screening endoscopy, a small 10-mm polyp 0-Is with an irregular, partially depressed surface was found in the mid-rectum. Analyis by magnifying chromoendoscopy and hr-EUS allowed decision-making on resective strategy (Fig. 5.9).

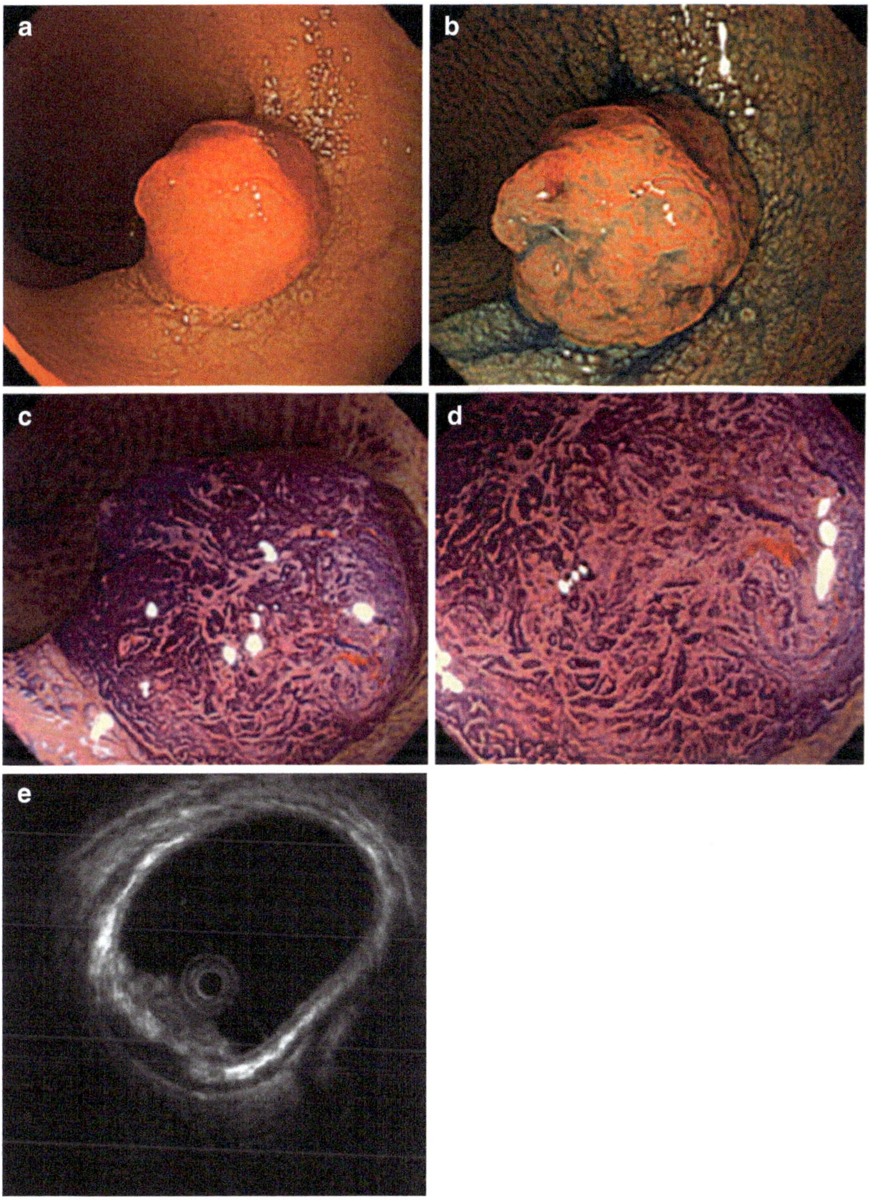

Fig. 5.9 (**a**) Small 10-mm rectal polyp 0-Is, (**b**) Irregular surface shown on indigo carmine spraying. (**c**, **d**) Crystal violet CE revealed pit pattern (**c**) type Vi and (**d**) type V_N, typical of a submucosa-invasive cancer. (**e**) Hr-EUS showed massively sm-invasive cancer with a break in the hyperechoic sm echoband and a hypoechoic arch reaching the proper muscular layer: eusT1sm3/T2. Surgical resection: adenocarcinoma G2, *psm3* (3500 μm), ly0, *v1*, pPM0, pDM0, pRM0

Case 2: Lesion 0-IIc Located at the Upper Gastric Body
In a 70-year-old male, a reddish lesion 0-IIc was found at the upper gastric body. Deeper submucosa-invasive cancer was suspected on conventional endoscopy but not on hrEUS (Fig. 5.10). The patient underwent gastrectomy.

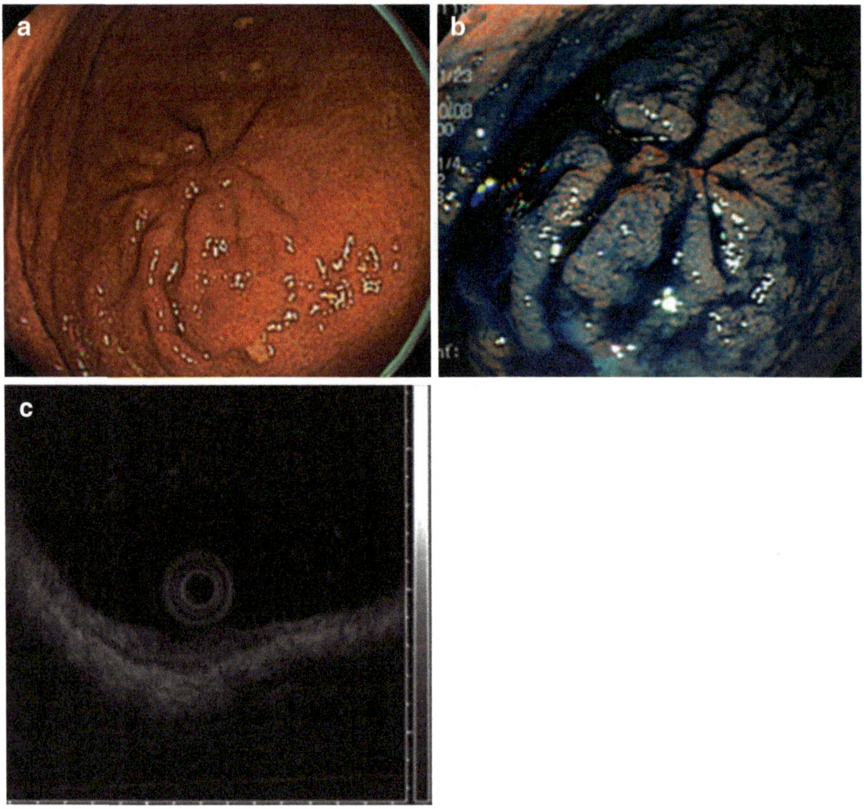

Fig. 5.10 Reddish lesion 0-IIc in the upper gastric corpus. (**a**) Mucosal folds converging at the lesion showed irregular tapering at the depression. (**b**) Indigo carmine spraying enhanced the irregularities, tapering and break of folds at the depression. Deeper submucosa-invasive cancer was suspected at this lesion with conventional endoscopy. (**c**) Radial EUS image by a miniprobe (20 MHz) demonstrated a continuous hyperechoic submucosal echo layer. On hrEUS examination, an intramucosal cancer was suspected, but based on macroscopic analysis, gastrectomy was performed. *Histopathology* confirmed intramucosal adenocarcinoma (tub2 > tub1), pT1(M), ly0, v0, pPM0, pDM0, 0-IIc, 35 × 30 mm

Note
When endoscopic analysis stages a lesion as sm2-invasive, albeit hrEUS would endorse endoscopic resectability (suspected understaging), usually surgery is favoured to ascertain curative resection of cancer. And overstaging with hrEUS (and combined macroscopic type of lesion) also is possible.

Case 3: Neoplasia Type 0-IIc Located at the Upper Gastric Body

On conventional gastroscopy a small, pale depressed lesion with break and some fusion of folds was pointed out at the upper gastric body. Analysis using conventional WLI, chromoendoscopy and hrEUS favoured gastrectomy (Fig. 5.11).

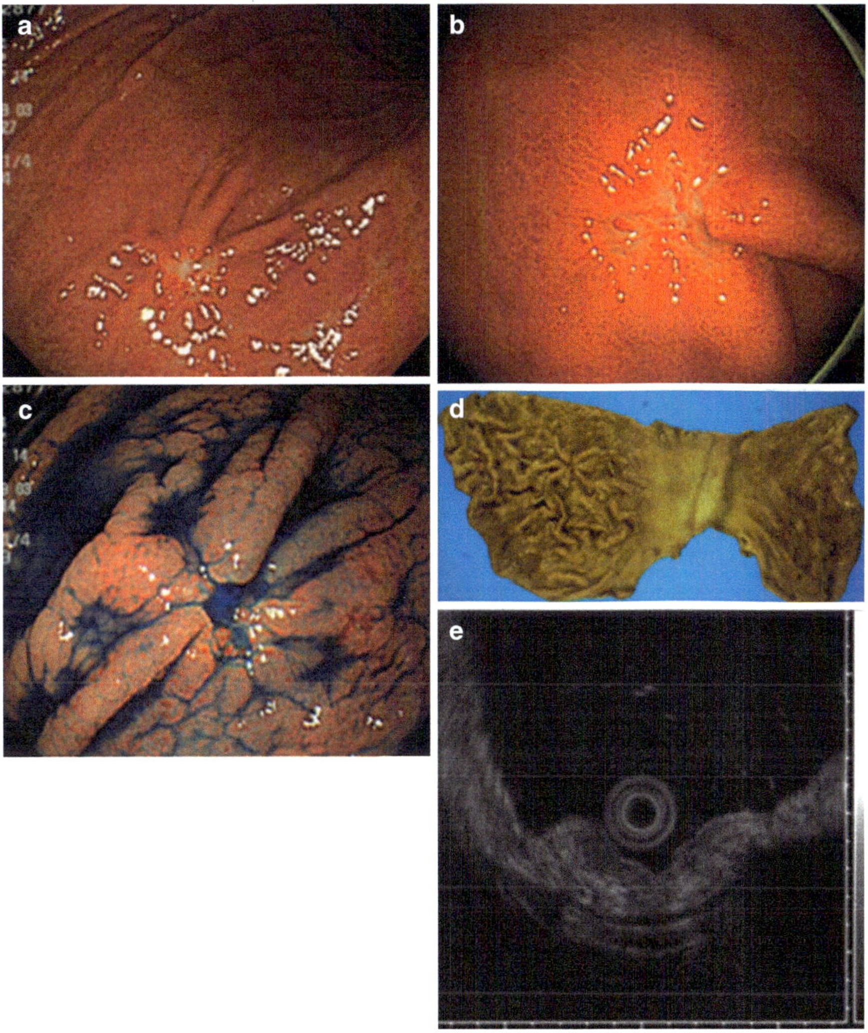

Fig. 5.11 (**a, b**) Small, pale depressed lesion with break and some fusion of folds at the upper gastric body, WLI. (**c**) Irregularity of folds was enhanced after indigo carmine spraying suggesting deep sm invasion. (**d**) Radial EUS image (20 MHz) demonstrated breaks in the hyperechoic sm echo layer. Clinical diagnosis: eusT1b,sm2–3, suspicious for poorly differentiated cancer (on WLI). (**e**) Gastrectomy confirmed *pathological diagnosis*: adenocarcinoma, in part signet ring cell cancer (sig > tub2), pT1b(sm2), ly0, v0 pPN0

Case 4: Gastric Lesion 0-IIc

In a 42-year-old man, a gastric lesion 0-IIc (d 20 mm) was pointed out at the posterior of the middle gastric body. According to EUS finding, SM2 invasion was suspected, and we recommended surgical operation. Histopathology of surgical specimen showed sm invasion and lymph node metastasis (Fig. 5.12).

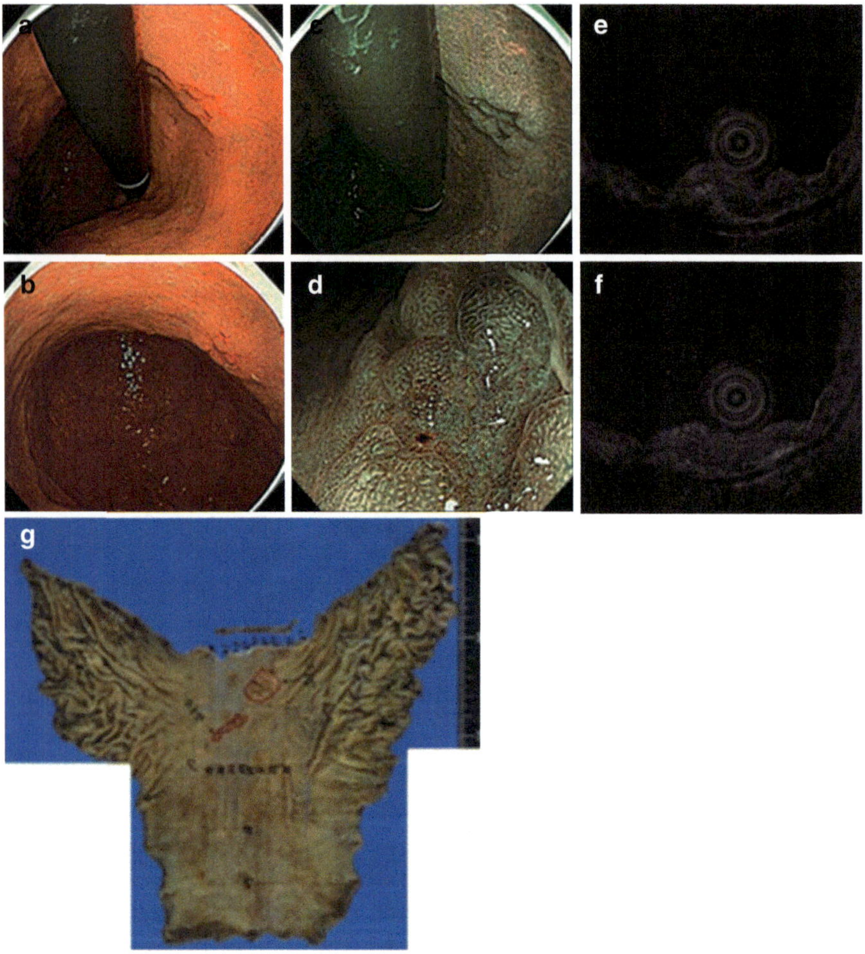

Fig. 5.12 Lesion 0-IIc in posterior wall of middle gastric body. (**a**, **b**) WLI: Reddish and depressed lesion was detected in posterior wall of middle gastric body. (**c**, **d**) Narrow band imaging (NBI) and NBI magnification: Lesion was detected as brownish area on NBI. By NBI magnification, microstructure was completely destructive, and irregular microvascularity was detected. Using VS classification proposed by Yao et al., the tumor border could be diagnosed precisely. (**e**, **f**) EUS: Radial EUS image (20 Mhz) showed diffuse invasion of hyperechoic sm layer by a hypoechoic mass. According to EUS finding, the invasion depth of this lesion was diagnosed as SM2 with high confidence. (**g**) Gastrectomy: Adenocarcinoma (tub2 > por2 > tub1) with lymphoid stroma, T1(SM2, 1500 μm), 15 × 14 mm, ly0, v0, N1

Case 5: SET in distal Esophagus

On WLI, a bulging tumor was observed under regular SC mucosa in lower esophagus. Based on WLI and EUS findings, this lesion was diagnosed as SET in sm layer and treated by EMR (Fig. 5.13).

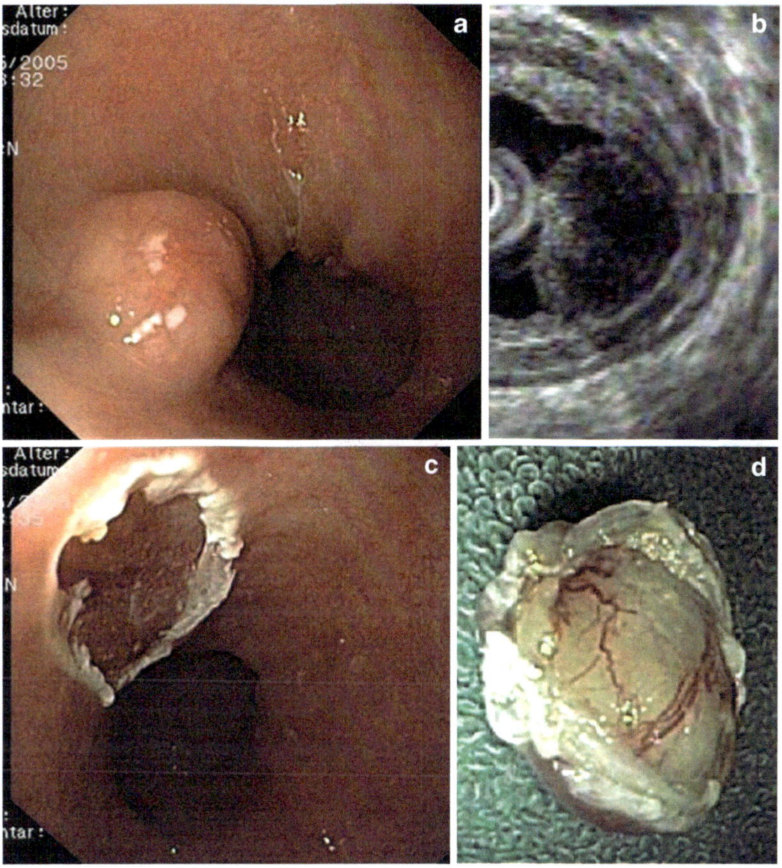

Fig. 5.13 (**a**) Bulging SET with with regular SC-mucosa in lower esophagus (WLI). (**b**) Hr-EUS (20 MHz) shows homogenous hypoechoic, ~1 cm sized SET with distinct margins in sm layer, with preserved sm-echo layer beneath the SET (→ leiomyoma from mm, or less likely GIST). (**c**) Resecection bed after snaring. (**b**) Specimen: intact encapsulated SET. Histology: Leiomyoma

Note Most *leiomyomas*, however, reside within pm layer and require *STER* for indicated resection (Fig. 4.7)!

Case 6: Early Neoplasia 0-IIc at the Gastric Body

On WLI, a reddish depressed lesion was pointed out at posterior wall of gastric body. Tumor border was clearly detected by chromoendoscopy with indigocarmine and acetic acid and NBI magnification. Based on EUS finding, this lesion was diagnosed as intramucosal cancer and treated by ESD (Fig. 5.14).

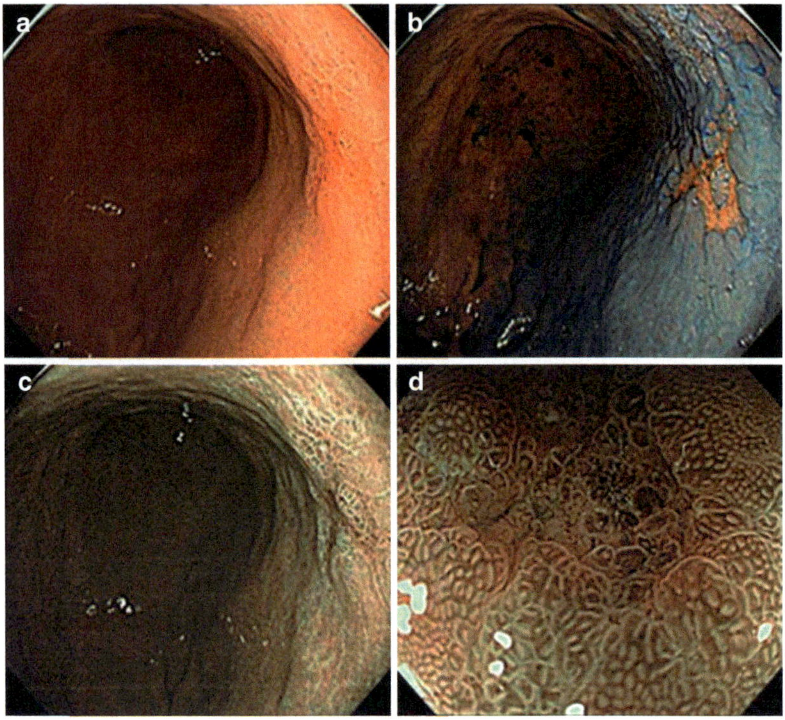

Fig. 5.14 (**a**) Reddish lesion 0-IIc on minor curve of gastric corpus (**a**) standard WLI and (**b**) acetic acid indigocarmine CE, and (**c**) NBI. (**d**) Pit-shape fundic mucosa with clear demarcation and encroachment of the lesion with irregular VP (network) and irregular pit-like SP (M-NBI ~50-fold). (**e, f**) Hr-EUS (20 MHz) showed irregular mass in second layer (Lpm) and irreg. Surface (first echo), but no break nor narrowing of third layer (sm). (**g**) ESD bed (WLI). (**h**) Specimen (3.5 × 4 cm): WDAC T1a –Lpm, L(−)V(−), R0 – curative

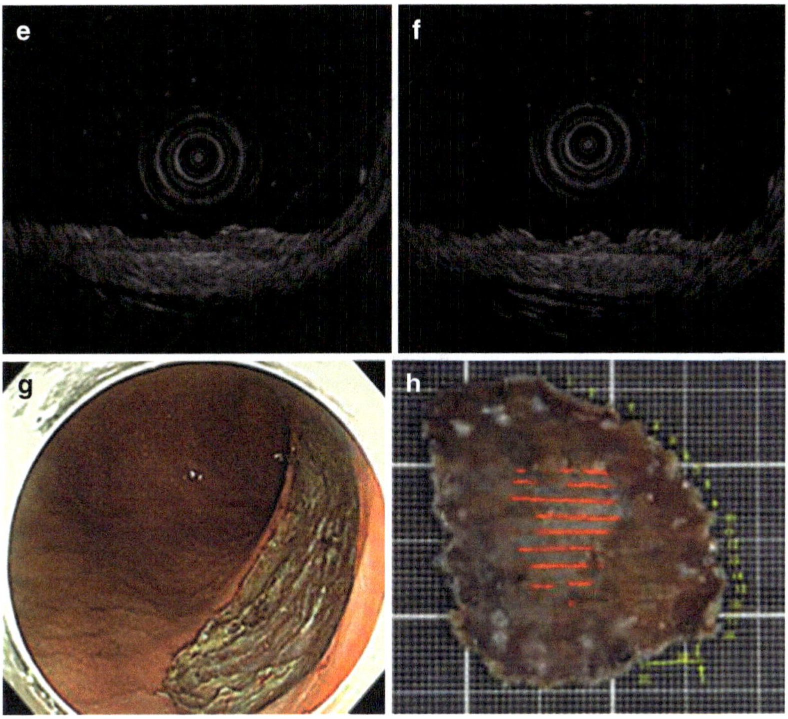

Fig. 5.14 (continued)

Note Preoperative diagnosis should be made in a comprehensive manner with WLI, magnifying NBI & Chromoendoscopy, and hr-EUS.

References

1. Yamanaka T. JGES consensus meeting report in DDW-Japan 2000, Kobe: interpretation of the layered structure of gastrointestinal wall with endoscopic ultrasonography. Dig Endosc. 2002;14:39–40.
2. Yoshinaga S, et al. Endoscopic ultrasound using ultrasound probes for the diagnosis of early esophageal and gastric cancers. World J Gastrointest Endosc. 2012;4:218–26.
3. Goda K, et al. Magnifying endoscopy with narrow band imaging for predicting the invasion depth of superficial esophageal squamous cell carcinoma. Dis Esophagus. 2009;22:453–60.
4. He LJ, et al. Endoscopic ultrasonography for staging of T1a and T1b esophageal squamous cell carcinoma. World J Gastroenterol. 2014;20:1340–7.
5. Jung JI, et al. Clinicopathologic factors influencing the accuracy of EUS for superficial esophageal carcinoma. World J Gastroenterol. 2014;20:6322–8.
6. Lee MW, et al. Predicting the invasion depth of esophageal squamous cell carcinoma: comparison of endoscopic ultrasonography and magnifying endoscopy. Scand J Gastroenterol. 2014;49:853–61.

7. Kim GH, et al. Accuracy of high-frequency catheter-based endoscopic ultrasonography according to the indications for endoscopic treatment of early gastric cancer. J Gastroenterol Hepatol. 2010;25:506–11.
8. Yoshida M, et al. Endoscopic assessment of invasion of colorectal tumors with a new high-frequency ultrasound probe. Gastrointest Endosc. 1995;41:587–92.
9. Yoshinaga S, et al. Current status of endoscopic ultrasound for the upper gastrointestinal tract in Asia. Dig Endosc. 2015;27(Suppl 1):2–10.
10. Matsumoto Y, et al. Endoscopic ultrasonography for diagnosis of submucosal invasion in early gastric cancer. J Gastroenterol. 2000;35:326–31.
11. Yoshida S, et al. Diagnostic ability of high-frequency ultrasound probe sonography in staging early gastric cancer, especially for submucosal invasion. Abdom Imaging. 2005;30:518–23.
12. Pech O, et al. The impact of endoscopic ultrasound and computed tomography on the TNM staging of early cancer in Barrett's esophagus. Am J Gastroenterol. 2006;101:2223–9.
13. Hasegawa N, et al. Preoperative staging of superficial esophageal carcinoma: comparison of an ultrasound probe and standard endoscopic ultrasonography. Gastrointest Endosc. 1996;44:388–93.
14. Hunerbein M, et al. Endosonography of upper gastrointestinal tract cancer on demand using miniprobes or endoscopic ultrasound. Surg Endosc. 2003;17:615–9.
15. Menzel J, et al. Preoperative staging of esophageal carcinoma: miniprobe sonography versus conventional endoscopic ultrasound in a prospective histopathologically verified study. Endoscopy. 1999;31:291–7.
16. Akashi K, et al. Ulcerous change decreases the accuracy of endoscopic ultrasonography diagnosis for the invasive depth of early gastric cancer. Int J Gastrointest Cancer. 2006;37:133–8.
17. May A, et al. Accuracy of staging in early oesophageal cancer using high resolution endoscopy and high resolution endosonography: a comparative, prospective, and blinded trial. Gut. 2004;53:634–40.
18. Tsung PC, et al. Miniprobe endoscopic ultrasonography has limitations in determining the T stage in early colorectal cancer. Gut Liver. 2013;7:163–8.
19. Chemaly M, et al. Miniprobe EUS in the pretherapeutic assessment of early esophageal neoplasia. Endoscopy. 2008;40:2–6.
20. Arima M, et al. Diagnostic accuracy of tumor staging and treatment outcomes in patients with superficial esophageal cancer. Dig Endosc. 2007;4:145–53.
21. Hwang JH, et al. A prospective study comparing endoscopy and EUS in the evaluation of GI subepithelial masses. Gastrointest Endosc. 2005;62:202–8.
22. Iwamuro M, et al. Esophageal granular cell tumors can be differentiated from leiomyomas using endoscopic ultrasonography. Intern Med. 2018;57:1509–15.
23. Nishida T, et al. The standard diagnosis, treatment, and follow-up of gastrointestinal stromal tumors based on guidelines. Gastric Cancer. 2016;19:3–14.
24. Nishida T, et al. Submucosal tumors: comprehensive guide for the diagnosis and therapy of gastrointestinal submucosal tumors. Dig Endosc. 2013;25:479–89.
25. Sato Y, et al. Management of gastric and duodenal neuroendocrine tumors. World J Gastroenterol. 2016;22:6817–28.
26. Wiech T, et al. Histopathological classification of nonneoplastic and neoplastic gastrointestinal submucosal lesions. Endoscopy. 2005;37:630–4.
27. Hwang JH, et al. American Gastroenterological Association Institute technical review on the management of gastric subepithelial masses. Gastroenterology. 2006;130:2217–28.
28. Dumonceau JM, et al. Indications, results, and clinical impact of endoscopic ultrasound (EUS)-guided sampling in gastroenterology: European Society of Gastrointestinal Endoscopy (ESGE) Clinical Guideline - Updated January 2017. Endoscopy. 2017;49:695–714.
29. Gao Z, et al. The cut-off value of tumor size and appropriate timing of follow-up for management of minimal EUS-suspected gastric gastrointestinal stromal tumors. BMC Gastroenterol. 2017;17:8.

30. Yegin EG, et al. Small EUS-suspected gastrointestinal stromal tumors of the stomach: An overview for the current state of management. Endosc Ultrasound. 2016;5:69–77.
31. Soweid AM. Endosonographic features predictive of benign and malignant gastrointestinal stromal cell tumors. Gastrointest Endosc. 2001;53:836–8.
32. Zhao Y, et al. The diagnostic value of endoscopic ultrasonography and contrast-enhanced harmonic endoscopic ultrasonography in gastrointestinal stromal tumors. Endosc Ultrasound. 2016;5:111–7.
33. Ignee A, et al. Contrast-enhanced (endoscopic) ultrasound and endoscopic ultrasound elastography in gastrointestinal stromal tumors. Endosc Ultrasound. 2017;6:55–60.
34. von Mehren M, et al. Soft Tissue Sarcoma, Version 2.2018, NCCN Clinical Practice Guidelines in Oncology. J Natl Compr Canc Netw JNCCN. 2018;16:536–63.
35. Rindi G, et al. TNM staging of foregut (neuro)endocrine tumors: a consensus proposal including a grading system. Virchows Arch. 2006;449:395–401.

Chapter 6 Endoscopic Screening and Surveillance: Indications and Standards

Thierry Ponchon, Frieder Berr, and Tsuneo Oyama

6.1 Introduction

The gastrointestinal (GI) tract is the organ system with the highest cancer burden (incidence 1.0–1.4 × 10^3) and cancer mortality (700–900 per 10^5 and year). The annual mortality-to-incidence ratio ranges from 43% for colorectal to 75% for gastric, and 84% for esophageal cancer, but has fallen for gastric cancer below 40% in Japan, where now more than 70% of cases are detected as early gastric cancer [1–3]. Curative radical surgery with complete removal of first- and second-tier lymph nodes for early gastric cancer (EGC ≤ pT1) achieved 5-year overall survival rates (OS) exceeding 90% [4, 5]. Overall survival was as good after endoscopic en-bloc resection of EGC (93% / 5 years, no recurrence of GC) for patients selected according to criteria of the Japanese Gastric Cancer Association or expanded criteria of National Cancer Centre (NCC) Tokyo [6, 7].

Early GI cancers show differentiated grading in most cases (>95%), except for gastric cancer in low-incidence regions (only ~60%). Early cancer, when differentiated (HGIN, G1, G2) progresses more slowly to systemic disease (e.g. within 3 years) than undifferentiated cancer [4, 8]. This slow progress allows detection at an early stage, as necessary for screening and surveillance programs.

T. Ponchon (✉)
Department of Digestive Diseases, Hôpital Eduard Herriot, Lyon, France
e-mail: thierry.ponchon@chu-lyon.fr

F. Berr
Department of Internal Medicine I, Paracelsus Medical University, Salzburg, Austria

T. Oyama
Department of Endoscopy, Saku Central Hospital Advanced Care Center, Saku, Nagano, Japan

F. Berr et al. (eds.), *Atlas of Early Neoplasias of the Gastrointestinal Tract*,
https://doi.org/10.1007/978-3-030-01114-7_6

6.2 Rationale for Endoscopic Screening and Surveillance

Endoscopic screening of the population aims to reduce mortality from frequent GI cancers. Beyond the average risk of GI cancers in the general population, there are many individuals with a high risk profile depending on environmental factors (e.g. carcinogen exposure, smoking, alcohol abuse) and/or individual disposition (familial inheritance, chronic GI inflammatory diseases). Such individuals require opportunistic screening endoscopy earlier in life and more frequent surveillance [9–11]. However, even in specialty practice, up to 39% of patients had colorectal cancer (CRC) screening without taking the risk profile and family history. Therefore, 55% of patients with strong family history had received inappropriate surveillance [12].

Note Taking the history of family and carcinogenic risk factors is a prerequisite for any screening endoscopy and for scheduling endoscopic surveillance.

CRC is the third most common cause of cancer-related death worldwide, ranking second in Western countries and third in Japan [1, 2, 13], with similar yearly incidence rates (cases per 100,000 per year) in the United States (range 28–38), Western Europe (33–50), and Japan (22–58) [1, 2, 13]. In the US National Polyp Study, the incidence rate of CRC was much lower after clearing colonoscopy (with resection of all neoplasias) than predicted from the US population [14]. This finding delivered the rationale for nationwide colonoscopy screening programs in many countries, to reduce mortality from CRC.

Gastric cancer (GC) is frequent in Japan (incidence ~25 per 100,000 per year), justifying screening of the general population [3, 13, 15]. Screening endoscopy is recommended to start at the age of 40 years and has decreased cancer-related mortality [13, 15]. In most Western countries, however, GC is too rare (e.g. ≤5/100,000/year in USA) to start an endoscopic screening program [2, 3, 9, 16]. In Western countries, evidence can be claimed for endoscopic surveillance of Barrett's esophagus [9]. Clinicians should refer to their own national guidelines for the appropriate screening and surveillance recommendations.

6.2.1 Screening Colonoscopy for Prevention of CRC

Colonoscopy is the best diagnostic standard for detection of neoplasias in the colon [10, 17], and combined with polypectomy of all detected adenomas (clearing colonoscopy), it reduces the risk of colon cancer by 66–71% for 10 years [14]. Annual fecal occult blood test (FOBT) screening (followed when positive by colonoscopy and polypectomy) reduced this risk by 23% [18, 19]. The risk of complications is low (diagnostic, 0.39%; therapeutic, 1.02%; mortality, 1:150,000) [10, 20].

Note Recommendations for asymptomatic, average-risk individuals [10, 17]:

- Age ≥ 50 years [≥40 years in Japan] → screening colonoscopy (every 10 years).
  - [Aim: prevention and early detection of CRC]
- If not → annual FOBT→ colonoscopy, if FOBT is positive
  - [Aim: (early) detection of asymptomatic colon cancer]

6.2.2 Individuals with Increased Risk for Colorectal Cancer

Approximately 75% of CRC cases occur sporadically in average-risk individuals, and up to 25% occur in persons with positive family history for colon adenomas or cancer, i.e. increased risk profile [10, 21]. Monogeneic autosomal dominant inherited familial cancer syndromes account for less than 10% of all CRC, including 1% with familial adenomatous polyposis coli (FAP) and 5% with hereditary non-polyposis colon cancer (HNPCC). Another 15–20% of all CRC cases report colon cancer or adenomas in the family history [10, 11]. The lifetime risk for CRC ranges from 60% to 80% with HNPCC, and is up to nearly 100% with classic FAP (>100 colon adenomas) by age 40–50 years, with onset at a young age [11] (Fig. 6.1). Attenuated FAP (with fewer adenomas [10–99] and later onset) is suggested by the following criteria: (1) At least two first-degree relatives (FDRs) with 10–99 adenomas at age > 30 years (none under age 30 years), or (2) One FDR with 10–99 adenomas and one FDR with CRC and few adenomas. There is a 25% chance of identifying an *APC* mutation in this attenuated FAP syndrome [11].

A very rare form of adenomatosis coli (10–100 adenomas) manifested *before* the age of 30 years is MAP (*MUTYH*-associated adenomatous polyposis), an autosomal recessive disorder due to biallelic *MUTYH* mutations. MAP persons show a

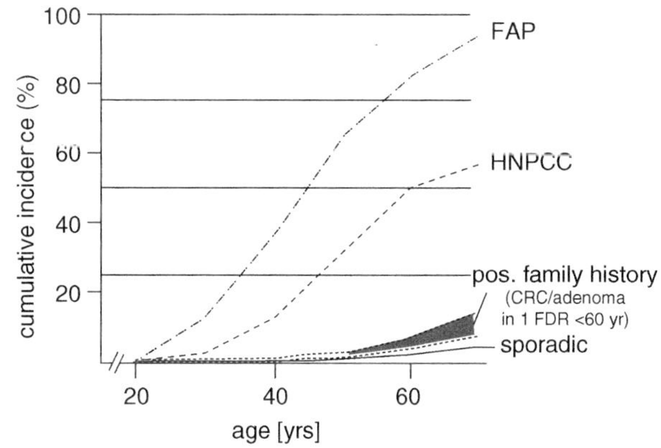

Fig. 6.1 Cumulative incidence of CRC by age in different risk groups. FAP familial adenomatous polyposis coli, FDR first-degree relative, HNPCC hereditary non-polyposis colon cancer. (Modified acc. to Winawer et al. [21]; permission granted by AGA Institute, W.B. Saunders Co.)

Table 6.1 Individuals with increased risk for colorectal cancer

Condition	References
Family history of colon adenoma or carcinoma	[18, 21]
Hereditary colorectal carcinomas (rapid progression, adenoma → carcinoma)	
Hereditary non-polyposis colon cancer (HNPCC), autosomal dominant	[18, 21]
Familial adenomatous polyposis coli (FAP), autosomal dominant	[11, 18]
MAP (*MUTYH*-associated adenomatous polyposis), autosomal recessive	[11]
Peutz-Jeghers syndrome (PJS)	[22]
Familial juvenile (hamartomatous) polyposis (FJP)	[22]
Chronic inflammatory bowel disease (ulcerative colitis, colitis Crohn)	[24–26]
Surveillance after polypectomy or surgery for CRC	[27, 28]

predilection for CRC in the right colon, as well as adenomas and cancer in the duodenum [11]. Peutz-Jeghers syndrome (PJS) has a lifetime risk of CRC up to 39%, and familial juvenile polyposis (FJP), 20% [22]. Chronic inflammation also increases the probability of cancer: the risk for ulcerative colitis is 7–15% after 20 years (even higher when combined with primary sclerosing cholangitis), and the risk is similar for colitis Crohn [23–25]. Table 6.1 lists increased risk conditions for CRC.

Screening with positive family history. The lifetime risk for colon cancer is about 1% in individuals without increased risk factors, and 2% in individuals with first-degree relatives (FDRs) with colonic adenoma or carcinoma at age < 60 years (i.e. positive family history). It is 3.5–4% when one FDR had colon cancer at age < 50 years or more than one FDR had colon cancer, or when two or more second-degree relatives (SDR) had colon cancer [11] (Fig. 6.1). The risk for colon cancer is only marginally increased (~1.5–1.8-fold) when one FDR at age > 60 years or one SDR had colon adenoma or cancer [11]. In cases of positive family history (and more so in cases with a strong hereditary risk for CRC, such as positive Amsterdam criteria, Table 6.2), the risk rises earlier in life and becomes very high in the cancer syndromes: about 60% in HNPCC and 80–90% in FAP at age of 60 years (*see* Fig. 6.1) [10, 11, 21]. Table 6.3 lists recommendations for surveillance.

Genetic testing for mutations (*APC*, mismatch repair (MMR) genes) is recommended for

- FAP of the colon (→ sequencing of *APC* gene).
- Presence of criteria compatible with HNPCC (Table 6.2).

Patients with *very high-risk family history* require genetic testing of the carcinoma (if MSI positive) of the index patient, first by immunohistochemistry for MMR proteins, followed by sequencing the gene of an unexpressed MMR protein to detect the specific MMR gene mutation. Consecutively, family members at risk

Table 6.2 Criteria for Microsatellite Instability (MSI) Genetic Testing (for HNPCC) [11]

Amsterdam Criteria II
At least three relatives with CRC or a Lynch syndrome–associated cancer[a] occurring in the following combinations: One is first-degree relative to others In at least two successive generations At least one diagnosed at age < 50 years Familial adenomatous polyposis coli (FAP) excluded in the CRC cases Tumors verified by histopathology
Revised Bethesda guidelines
one CRC diagnosed at age < 50 years, *or* MSI-H pos. CRC at age < 60 years, *and* Synchronous or metachronous Lynch syndrome–associated tumors,[a] or 1 CRC and 1 first-degree relative with Lynch syndrome–associated tumor,[a] 1 at age < 50 years 1 CRC with two or more first-degree or second-degree relatives with a Lynch syndrome–associated tumor[a]

[a]These include colorectal, endometrial, stomach, ovarian, pancreas, ureter, renal pelvis, biliary tract, and brain tumors; sebaceous gland adenomas; keratoacanthomas; and carcinoma of the small bowel

Table 6.3 Screening colonoscopy recommendations for high risk of CRC[a] [10, 11, 22, 24, 26]

	Screening colonoscopies	
Risk factors	Age to begin	Intervals, *y*
Positive family history only		
One SDR or 3[rd]DR (cousin) with CRC	50 years	10
One FDR with CRC/adenoma at age > 60 years, or more than two SDR with CRC	40 years	10
One FDR with CRC/adenoma at age < 60 years	40 years, or 10 years before manifestation in FDR	5
Monogenic hereditary syndromes		
FAP (classic form)	12 years	1 or 2
Attenuated FAP (10–100 adenomas)	25 years, or 10 years before CRC in FDR	1 or 2
HNPCC [panchromocolonoscopy, PCC]	20 or 25 years, or 10 years before earliest CRC in FDR	1 or 2
Peutz-Jeghers syndrome (PJS)	18 years	2
Familial juvenile polyposis (>10 polyps)	12 years	3–5
Chronic inflammation		
Ulcerative colitis, Crohn's colitis [PCC]	Pan-/Colitis for 8–10 years	2 (−1)

CRC colorectal cancer, *FDR* first-degree relative, *SDR* second-degree relative
[a]See Chap. 12 for surveillance of ulcerative colitis and colitis Crohn

must be screened for this MMR gene mutation by a center for genetic studies [11]. Carriers of the mutation need surveillance for CRC and related cancers.

Note Up to 20% of FAP cases have *negative family history* (probably new germline FAP mutations or biallelic autosomal recessive *MUTYH* gene mutations). Likely hereditary cancer syndromes must be evaluated at a center for genetic diseases. Subtotal or total colectomy with ileorectal anastomosis or even ileo-anal pouch may be indicated for FAP, HNPCC, and rarely for ulcerative colitis [10, 11, 22, 24, 26].

6.3 Gastric Cancer

Gastric cancer (GC) is the second leading cause of cancer-related death worldwide, and the fourth in the United States and Western Europe. The incidence rates for GC have decreased by 75–85% during the past 60 years to 3–5 per 100,000 per year in the USA and Western Europe, but they remain higher in Japan (five-fold), China, Chile, and Eastern Europe [1–3, 13]. Radiographic and endoscopic screening has decreased GC-specific mortality in Japan [13, 15, 16]. In Western countries, opportunistic screening and surveillance endoscopy is common [9, 16].

The two main types are *intestinal type*, forming gland-like tubular structures, and *diffuse type*, lacking cell cohesion and infiltrating the wall by spreading of single cells. The intestinal type is easier to detect at endoscopy and spreads more slowly. Table 6.4 outlines the disorders considered for surveillance gastroscopy in individuals at increased risk for GC.

Table 6.4 Individuals with increased risk for gastric cancer [8, 9, 16, 29, 30]

	Surveillance endoscopy[a] [9]	
Type of GC at high risk	Onset	Intervals
Intestinal type GC		
Atrophic gastritis type B with intestinal metaplasia (*Helicobacter pylori* positive)	Index endoscopy	→ *H. pylori* eradication, 2–3 years
Polypoid type chronic gastritis with IM	Individualize	1–3 years
Chronic. autoimmune gastritis type A with IM	Index endoscopy	1–3 years
Gastric IM		
IM and low-grade IEN	Check at 3 months with mapping and biopsies	3 months–1 year
IM and high-grade IEN	Confirm → ESD or surgery	6 months–1 year
Partial Billroth-II gastrectomy (PGE) (chronic bile reflux gastritis)	Index endoscopy 15 years after PGE	→ *H. pylori* eradication
		2–3 years
Gastric adenoma (35% malignant foci, [29])	EMR or ESD	1–3 years
FAP (gastro-/duodenoscopy) and HNPCC [9]	Index endoscopy and individualize	6 months–3 years
Diffuse type GC		
Hereditary diffuse GC (30% *CDH1* mutation)	Genetic diagnosis [31]	Prophylactic gastrectomy

EMR endoscopic mucosal resection, *ESD* endoscopic submucosal dissection, *IEN* intraepithelial neoplasia, *IM* intestinal metaplasia

[a]Recommendations of the American Society for Gastrointestinal Endoscopy (ASGE) [9, 16]

The precursor lesions for intestinal type GC are severe chronic atrophic gastritis (autoimmune type A or *Helicobacter pylori*-induced type B) with intestinal metaplasia (IM), or biliary reflux–induced chronic remnant gastritis after partial gastrectomy [8, 9, 16, 29, 30]. Intestinal metaplasia with HGIN has a 33–85% chance of GC [9]. Families with autosomal dominant diffuse-type GC require genetic diagnosis and prophylactic gastrectomy [31], because the efficiency of surveillance is unproven for diffuse-type GC, which is poorly detectable.

6.3.1 Esophageal and Pharyngeal Squamous Cell Cancer (SCC)

Cancer of the squamous cell epithelium of the esophagus is relatively rare, with incidence rates of 1.5–5 per 100,000 per year in most countries, except for a few high-prevalence areas such as Hunyuan County in China, Singapore, and Iran (incidence rates up to $140/10^5$/year) [1, 9, 32]. Therefore, endoscopic screening is not generally indicated, but index endoscopy and surveillance is recommended for some groups with high risk for SCC in the esophagus and head and neck region [9, 32, 33].

Evidence for inheritance of esophageal cancer is lacking, although familial clustering has rarely been reported for SCC and for Barrett's esophagus [32].

The risk of esophageal SCC is increased four-fold in men versus women, in particular with chronic heavy smoking and alcohol abuse (approximately 25-fold) [32–34]. The latter group may undergo surveillance endoscopy starting at the age of 50 years without proven evidence [9]. In addition, some cancers of the upper GI tract are strongly associated. Head-and-neck SCC exhibits about a 20% risk of synchronous or metachronous esophageal SCC [34], and the latter presents about a 10% risk of metachronous intestinal-type GC. About 10% of cases of oropharyngeal SCC show synchronous or metachronous SCC in the esophagus [34]. Patients treated for these carcinomas need surveillance endoscopies of the oropharynx, hypopharynx, esophagus, and stomach.

Diseases with increased risk of esophageal SCC include prolonged esophageal mucosal damage caused by achalasia, lye injury, or chronic caustic injury such as caused by hot beverages [35, 36]. Some hereditary diseases of squamous epithelium have a high risk of esophageal cancer, such as tylosis with palmar and plantar hyperkeratosis [37]. Endemic human papillomavirus (HPV) infection of the esophagus may increase the risk of esophageal SCC [34]. Table 6.5 lists groups at high risk for SCC, in which surveillance endoscopies every 1 to 3 years may be justified.

Table 6.5 Individuals with high risk of esophageal cancer [9, 33, 34, 37–39]

Type of esophageal cancer at high risk	Surveillance endoscopy [9, 33, 38] Recommended onset	Intervals, years)
Esophageal squamous cell carcinoma (SCC)		
Aerodigestive tract SCC (head and neck ~, lung ~)	One index endoscopy	Unknown
Synchronous or metachronous esophageal SCC (in 10% of patients)	Individualize	Unknown
Gastric cancer (risk of double cancer)	One index endoscopy	Unknown
Achalasia (16-fold↑ risk after ~14 years)	15 years after onset	Unknown
Strictures from lye, radiation, or caustic injury	10–15 years after injury	1–3 years
Partial gastrectomy (PGE) (chronic bile reflux esophagitis)	15 years after PGE	2–3 years
Hereditary diseases of squamous epithelium (e.g. tylosis)	At age 30 years	1–3 years
Papillomavirus infection	(High-risk immigrant)	Unknown
Adenocarcinoma of esophagus or GEJ		
Barrett's esophagus in GERD	See Chap. 8	
Alcohol and smoking	Index endoscopy	See Table. 6.6
Obesity (abdominal type)	–	Unknown

GEJ gastroesophageal junction, *GERD* gastroesophageal reflux disease

6.3.2 Adenocarcinoma of Esophagus or Gastroesophageal Junction

In the past 40 years, the incidence of adenocarcinoma (AC) of the esophagus and the gastroesophageal junction (GEJ), which was previously rare, has rapidly increased, so this AC is now the prevailing type of esophageal cancer in the United States and Western Europe [1, 38, 40]. Nearly all of these cases of AC arise from intestinal metaplastic epithelium in *Barrett's esophagus* (BE), i.e. columnar epithelium (without or with goblet cells), which has replaced esophageal squamous epithelium [40–42]. The cause for transformation to BE is chronic gastroesophageal reflux disease (GERD) [40–42]. Risk factors for malignant transformation (metaplasia → dysplasia → AC) are uncontrolled GERD, extent of BE (long-segment vs. short-segment), older age, male sex, smoking, and family history of BE or AC [38, 40, 43]. Persons with GERD-suspect symptoms should receive an index endoscopy (opportunistic screening).

Endoscopic diagnosis of BE must be confirmed by biopsies. BE is an indication for *endoscopic cancer surveillance*, because on surveillance BE-AC is detected at an early, curable stage ($pT \leq 1$), in contrast to sporadic esophageal AC [44]. Endoscopists from community centers detected lesions only in 60% of dysplastic BE, whereas 40% of diagnoses were made by protocol random biopsies. However, the BE expert centers detected visible lesions in 87% of dysplastic BE, and in 76% of referred random biopsy-positive BE on re-endoscopy [45]. Hence, we endorse random biopsies and referral to BE centers for therapy of dysplastic BE. Guidelines

Table 6.6 Recommendations of European Society of Gastrointestinal Endoscopy (ESGE) for Barrett's Esophagus Surveillance

Intraepithelial Neoplasia	Management and Surveillance Intervals
Non-dysplastic BE (NDBE)	Surveillance 3–5 years for short-segment BE
Low-grade dysplastic BE (LGDBE)	Visible lesion,[a, b] refer to BE expert center 6 months, then 12 months when LGD pos. → LGD confirmed → BE ablation[a, c] Like NDBE after 2× remission (without LGD)
High-grade dysplastic BE (HGDBE)	Patient referral to BE expert center
Visible HGD lesion	Endoscopic resection (en-bloc) & BE ablation
Invisible HGD	Re-endoscopy with random biopsies → HGD confirmed → BE ablation[c] → Negative for HGD → 3 months surveillance
Indefinite for dysplasia	Confirmation by second GI pathologist; PPI therapy Re-endoscopy at 6 months in BE expert center
Superficial BE-AC (T1a)	Endoscopic resection en-bloc[a] Subsequently, BE ablation[a, c]
Long-segment BE of length > 10 cm	Surveillance in BE expert center

Modified from Weusten et al. [46]
BE Barrett's esophagus, *PPI* proton pump inhibitor
[a]Any endoscopic therapy (resection; ablation) should be done in BE expert center
[b]Endoscopic resection of visible lesion according American College of Gastroenterology (ACG) [47]
[c]Preferably with radiofrequency ablation (RFA)

(Table 6.6) do not yet require magnifying or NBI endoscopy [38, 46–48]. However in Japan, BE is examined with WLI & NBI endoscopy. Lesions are analysed with M-NBI and acetic acid CE, and targeted biopsies [49].

Note *Guidelines* recommend for BE surveillance endoscopy after proton pump inhibitor therapy [38, 46–48]:

- high definition (HD-WLI) endoscopy and acetic acid chromoendoscopy,
- targeted biopsy of any visible lesion *and*
- protocol random biopsies (4-quadrant biopsies every 2 cm; Seattle protocol)
- histologic examination by GI pathologist (& reference pathologist for dysplasia +)
- referral for resection of high grade dysplasia (HGD) or BE-AC to specialized center (see Chap. 8)

Beyond actual guidelines, we strongly recommend

- analysis of visible lesion first with M-NBI (V, vessels), then M-CE (S, surface).

6.4 Standards for Screening and Surveillance Endoscopy

Detection of small (<10 mm) and minute (<5 mm) neoplastic lesions during screening or surveillance endoscopy depends on proper cleaning and preparation of the organs, examination technique and endoscopic equipment, and the experience and

Table 6.7 General aspects to document for endoscopy [50]

I. Preprocedure
(a) Proper indication, including justification of non-standard indications
(b) Proper consent (with risks, e.g. in Table 6.8), documentation of anticoagulation
(c) Pre-procedure history and physical examination for risk stratification
(d) Level of desired sedation.
II. Intra-Procedure
(a) Patient monitoring with documentation of vital parameters and medications
(b) Image documentation of endoscopic landmarks and abnormalities
III. Postprocedure
(a) Discharge letter (endoscopy procedure report) and documentation
(b) Patient instructions (for sedation and potential postprocedure complications)
(c) Pathology follow-up and report
(d) Record-keeping of adverse events and complications in the endoscopy unit
(e) Communication with patient (patient satisfaction) and referring physician
(f) Anticoagulation plan

alertness of the examiner. To ensure the outcome quality of these diagnostic procedures, benchmark criteria known as key performance indicators (KPI) should be monitored, evaluated, and achieved in every endoscopy unit, along with procedural documentation (Table 6.7).

The *Endoscopic Procedure Report* includes the *conclusive diagnosis of any neoplasia*, recommendation for staging (EUS/MRI/CT) and resection technique; it is the legally binding document. Complex or malignant lesions must be documented by several pictures showing location, size, and structural detail on magnification in white light endoscopy (WLI), narrow-band imaging (NBI), or chromoendoscopy (CE).

Note The *Endoscopic Procedure Report* on any neoplastic lesion must contain several elements:

- Macroscopic type and characteristics (e.g. air-induced alteration of shape)
- Microsurface and microvascular structure
- Conclusive endoscopic diagnosis of predicted tumor category

6.4.1 Colonoscopy

Approximately 8% of patients with newly diagnosed colorectal carcinoma had a negative colonoscopy within the past 3 years (i.e. interval cancer) [51, 53, 54]. Endoscopists with higher rates of interval cancer have a lower adenoma detection rate (ADR) [51]. Hence, ADR is a key performance indicator for quality of diagnostic colonoscopy [20]. Likely causes for missed detection are a miss rate for detectable adenomas (~11% for 5–10 mm size) and overlooked tiny flat adenomas or carcinomas of <5 mm size [53].

Bowel preparation is essential for diagnostic outcome. Oral intake of iron medications (causing discoloration of mucosa) and fruits or bread with small seeds should be discontinued for a few days. Standard preparation is intake of sodium picosulfate solution (10 mL) to empty the rectum, followed by intake of 2 to 3 liters of polyethylene glycol–sodium sulfate solution (PEG-ELS) within 60 to 90 min the evening before the examination and/or early in the morning 3–4 h before the examination. We recommend adding 5 mL of dimethicone solution (Gascon) per litre of PEG solution to remove mucus from the colonic mucosa. The interval between last oral fluid intake and colonoscopy should be 3 h, to ensure gastric emptying before sedation. The quality of preparation (i.e. discharge of yellowish stool fluids without solids) should be checked before settling the patient. Cleanliness should be achieved for >95% of examinations and documented with Boston Bowel Preparation Score ≥ 7 (BBPS range 1 to 9) [55].

Examination. Magnifying (≥50-fold) colonoscopes should be used and colonoscopy performed as one-examiner method with loop-less insertion technique. Sedation (e.g. midazolam 0.7 mg/kg body weight) or propofol intravenous anesthesia can be used according to national guidelines. Completeness of the colonoscopy must be documented by images of the cecal end and mound of the appendix and ileum. Prior to withdrawal of the scope, an antispasmodic is given intravenously (butylscopolamine 10–20 mg, or glucagon 1 mg in cases of glaucoma or frank prostatic hypertrophy). To scrutinize the entire mucosal surface including the proximal sides of the haustral folds, withdrawal time will last at least 6 min. Complications and quality indicators for screening colonoscopy should be recorded for all examinations per examiner and per endoscopy unit, and should meet benchmark indicators [52] (Tables 6.8 and 6.9). For endoscopic detection of neoplasias see Chap. 11.

Table 6.8 Risks of diagnostic colonoscopy [10, 51, 52]

Complication	Risk
Bleeding	0.01% (after snare polypectomy, 0.8%)
Perforation	0.01% (after snare polypectomy, 0.06%)
Mortality	2 / >300,000 colonoscopies

Table 6.9 Key Performance Indicators (KPI, Benchmarks) for Colonoscopy [10, 20]

Quality Indicator	Parameter (% of colonoscopies)
Bowel preparation	>90% clean (Boston Scale score > 6; target >95%, >7)
Cecal intubation rate	>95% for screening of healthy adults (target >97%) >90% of all cases (photodocumentation)
Adenoma detection rate	>25% of colonoscopies in >50 y.o. men >15% of colonoscopies in >50 y.o. women
Adequate polypectomy	% fraction (snare polypectomies / lesions > 3mm)
Complication rate	No benchmark yet (e.g. 7-day re-admission rate)

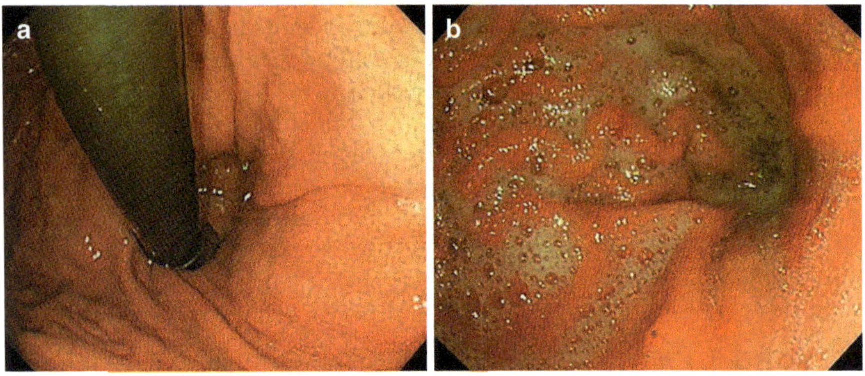

Fig. 6.2 (**a**) Gastric body cleaned with proteinase pretreatment and washing using a water jet. (**b**) Gastric body without proteinase pretreatment. In spite of water-jet rinsing of the mucosa, adherent mucin forms a foamy gel on gastric mucosal folds, severely impairing assessment of the epithelial surface structure. (Reprinted from Oyama [56], permission granted by Nankodo Co., Ltd., Tokyo, Japan)

6.4.2 Upper Gastrointestinal Endoscopy

Upper GI endoscopy for detection of neoplasias should be performed 10–20 min after oral intake of a glass of water with proteinase or acetylcysteine (see below), to clean mucus from the mucosa (Fig. 6.2), using conscious or deep intravenous sedation complying with national guidelines. High-definition video endoscopes with magnifying virtual chromoendoscopy (NBI, blue laser imaging [BLI], i-scan) must become standard equipment that supports accurate diagnosis of mucosal lesions.

Note Upper GI diagnostic endoscopy has a number of general requirements [57]:

- Mucolytic and defoaming preparation (0.25 g Pronase®/25 mL water, Kaken Seiyaku Corp., Tokyo; *or* 400 mg N-acetylcysteine and 20 mg activated dimethicone/25 mL water) 15 min before, and a glass of water right before, endoscopy
- Anticholinergics to reduce secretion and peristalsis (Buscopan® 10–20 mg i.v. or, if contraindicated, glucagon 1 mg i.v.)
- Lignocain spray for pharyngeal anesthesia (and hypopharyngeal inspection)

- Intravenous sedation in most cases (midazolam 2–5 mg or pethidine 20–30 mg for conscious sedation, or propofol 5–10 mg for unconscious sedation)
- Copious rinsing of mucosa with a water jet is essential for endoscopic assessment of mucus-devoid gastric surface and capillary pattern.
- Avoiding blind spots during the procedure, in particular using
  - distension of the gastric wall by insufflation
  - irrigation (water with dimethicone) to clean the gastric mucosa
  - systematic WLI inspection of all areas of the organs (hypo−/pharynx, esophagus, stomach, duodenum parts 1 to 3) to detect any lesions

Examination

Sensitive detection of small and minute neoplastic lesions on conventional WLI endoscopy depends on examiner capability—examination technique, knowledge, and diagnostic experience—and a standardized screening procedure [58].

Insertion of scope: Pharyngeal and laryngeal regions are inspected during insertion of the endoscope, taking care to avoid direct contact with the mucosa of the soft palate, the pharynx, and the base of the tongue. For detection of early SCC, NBI mode (with adequate illumination) is superior and preferable to WLI mode while slowly advancing in view of the hard and soft palate and the posterior wall of the hypopharynx. Complete endoscopic inspection of the oropharynx and hypopharynx is detailed in a recent atlas by Muto et al. [57]. First advance the scope into the apex of the right piriform sinus during inspiration, while inspecting the larynx, and empty any saliva collection there (particularly in case of Zenker's diverticulum). The piriform sinus and oropharynx are wider and better seen when the scope is withdrawn during expiration. Then observe the arytenoid and laryngeal area above the vocal cords, and the left piriform sinus, before inserting the scope into the esophageal orifice from the base of the right piriform sinus. The cranial entrance part of the esophagus (15–18 cm post incisors) will better be seen during scope withdrawal. Observe the insufflated, fully distended esophagus on WLI during insertion and in NBI mode to scrutinize for tiny brownish lesions during withdrawal at the end.

For precise description of the localization of any lesion in the esophagus, straighten the shaft of the endoscope and look for the notch of the left main bronchus (25–28 cm from incisor teeth and between 10 and 12 on a clockface) corresponding to the ventral side. For endoscopy of Barrett's esophagus, see Sect. 6.3.2.

Stomach. After washing off all mucus and debris from the gastric mucosa, first identify high-risk conditions for early cancer (Tables 6.4 and 6.5), fully distend the stomach by insufflation to avoid blind spots, map the entire stomach with a standardized screening protocol (Fig. 6.3), and take additional pictures of any suspicious lesion and its location. Targeted biopsy specimens are taken from gastric ulcers and any lesion suspicious for neoplasia [9, 29]. Protocols of esophagogastroduodenoscopy for early cancer screening are more explicit in Japan than in Western countries. For basic technique, systematic observation, and judgment of suspicious lesions in WLI, we recommend the e-learning program by Kenshi Yao [58].

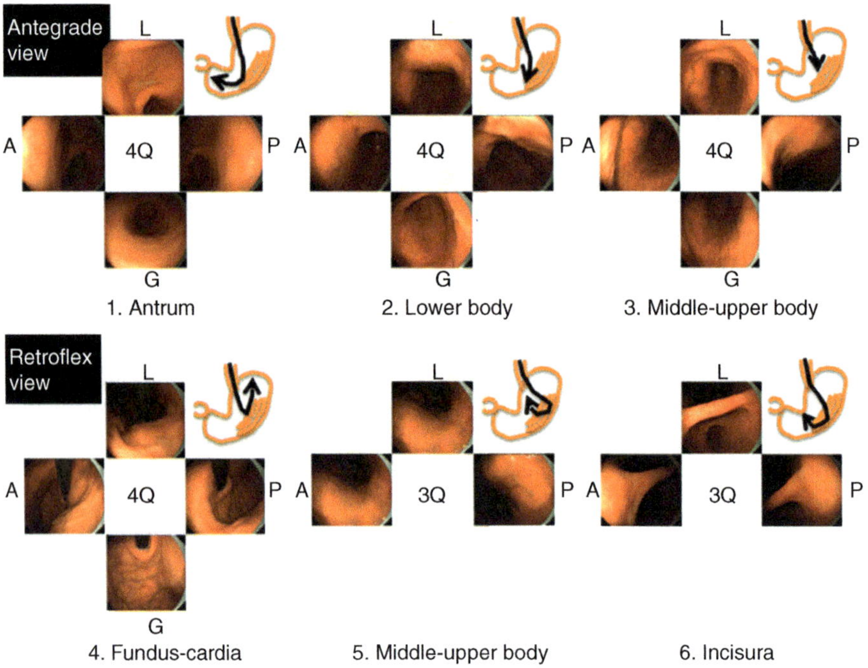

Fig. 6.3 Systematic screening protocol for the stomach (SSS). The SSS should be started as soon as the endoscope is introduced into the gastric antrum. In the antegrade view, endoscopic images of four quadrants of the gastric antrum, body and middle-upper body are obtained; then, in the retroflex view, images of the four quadrants of the gastric fundus and cardia and three quadrants of the gastric middle-upper body and incisura are taken. Overall, the SSS comprises 22 endoscopic images. *A* anterior wall, *G* greater curvature, *L* lesser curvature, *P* posterior wall, *Q* quadrant. (Reprinted from Yao [58], under the terms of the Creative Commons Attribution 4.0 International License (http://creativecommons.org/licenses/by/4.0/)

Recommendations for detection and magnifying endoscopic analysis of neoplasias are given in Chap. 1 and Chaps. 7, 8, 9, and 10.

Duodenum is examined with the same processor settings as the stomach (*see* Table 1.2). Any biliary fluid is washed off and aspirated. Normal mucosa shows a carpet of mobile villi, particularly well seen on water immersion. Villous atrophy in celiac disease presents loss of mobile villi. Neoplasias exhibit well-demarcated margins. (See Chap. 10.)

Complications and quality measures should be recorded in upper GI endoscopy (UGE) reports (Table 6.10).

6.4.3 Periprocedural Precautions

Antibiotic prophylaxis is not required for upper or lower GI endoscopy, unless the patient is severely immune compromised, has cardiac valvular replacement or disease, or undergoes a procedure with high infective risk (e.g. placement of

Table 6.10 Key Performance Measures (KPM) for Upper GI Endoscopy (UGE) [59]

Documentation of KPM	Parameter fulfilled (in % UGE reports)
Fasting ≥6 h/solids, 2 h/liquids	≥95% (instructed, in consent form)
Procedure duration	≥90% of reports (UGE ≥ 7 min for screening)
Photodocumentation	≥90% (for landmarks n = 10 & lesions)
Standard terminology	≥95% of reports [59]
Seattle protocol for BE	≥90% of BE (BE inspection 1 min / C = 1 cm)
Complications of therapeutic UGE	≥95% documented in all therapeutic UGE reports (benchmark for UGE-EMR <2% perforations)

BE Barrett's esophagus, *C* circular extent of BE, *EMR* endoscopic mucosal resection

Table 6.11 Anticoagulant agents and washout period before biopsy

Drug	Washout period
Platelet aggregation inhibitor	
Aspirin	7 days
Ticlopidine hydrochloride	7 days
Ticagrelor	7 days
Ethyl eicosapentate	7 days or more
Cilostazol	4 days
Argatroban	1 day
Thrombolytic	
Urokinase	1 day
Anticoagulant	
Warfarin potassium	7 days
Enoxaparin, Paroxaparin	1/2 day
Rivaroxaban (anti-factor Xa)	1 day
Dabigatran (anti-factor IIa)	2 days[a]

Modified from Anderson et al. [61]

[a]24 h if glomerular filtration rate (GFR) is >80 mL/min; 4 days if GFR is 30–50 mL/min

percutaneous endoscopic gastrostomy (PEG), EUS-FNA of cystic GI lesions, or ligation of esophageal varices). In these situations, a single intravenous dose 30–60 min prior to endoscopy is recommended (depending on patient drug tolerance): amoxicillin 2 g, cefazolin 1 g, or ciprofloxacin 500 mg [60]. There are no such recommendations for endoscopic submucosal dissection (ESD), but high-risk individuals should receive antibiotic prophylaxis before esophagogastric or colonic ESD. Table 6.11 lists the washout period of anticoagulants prior to biopsy.

References

1. GLOBOCAN database, International Agency for Research on Cancer, WHO, http://globocan.iarc.fr/.
2. Ferlay J, et al. Cancer incidence and mortality worldwide: sources, methods and major patterns in GLOBOCAN 2012. Int J Cancer. 2015;136:E359–86.

3. Inoue M, et al. Epidemiology of gastric cancer in Japan. Postgrad Med J. 2005;81:419–24.
4. Everett SM, et al. Early gastric cancer in Europe. Gut. 1997;41:142–50.
5. Morita S, et al. Outcome of pylorus-preserving gastrectomy for early gastric cancer. Br J Surg. 2008;95:1131–5.
6. Abe S, et al. Short- and long-term outcomes of endoscopic submucosal dissection for undifferentiated early gastric cancer. Endoscopy. 2013;45:703–7.
7. Gotoda T, et al. Endoscopic resection of early gastric cancer treated by guideline and expanded National Cancer Centre criteria. Br J Surg. 2010;97:868–71.
8. Hamashima C, et al. Optimal interval of endoscopic screening based on stage distributions of detected gastric cancers. BMC Cancer. 2017;17:740.
9. Hirota WK, et al. ASGE guideline: the role of endoscopy in the surveillance of premalignant conditions of the upper GI tract. Gastrointest Endosc. 2006;63:570–80.
10. Rex DK, et al. Colorectal cancer screening: recommendations for physicians and patients from the U.S. Multi-Society Task Force on Colorectal Cancer. Gastroenterology. 2017;153:307–23.
11. Vasen HF, et al. Familial colorectal cancer risk: ESMO clinical recommendations. Ann Oncol. 2009;20(Suppl 4):51–3.
12. Fletcher RH, et al. Screening patients with a family history of colorectal cancer. J Gen Intern Med. 2007;22:508–13.
13. Torre LA, et al. Global cancer incidence and mortality rates and trends – an update. Cancer Epidemiol Biomark Prev. 2016;25:16–27.
14. Zauber AG, et al. Colonoscopic polypectomy and long-term prevention of colorectal-cancer deaths. N Engl J Med. 2012;366:687–96.
15. Hamashima C, et al. Mortality reduction from gastric cancer by endoscopic and radiographic screening. Cancer Sci. 2015;106:1744–9.
16. Evans JA, et al. ASGE guideline. The role of endoscopy in the management of premalignant and malignant conditons of the stomach. Gastrointest Endosc. 2015;82:1–8.
17. Ebell MH, et al. Cancer screening recommendations: an international comparison of high income countries. Public Health Rev. 2018;39:7.
18. Bevan R, Rutter RD. Colorectal cancer screening – who, how, and when? Clin Endosc. 2018;51:37–49.
19. Towler B, et al. A systematic review of the effects of screening for colorectal cancer using the faecal occult blood test, Hemoccult. BMJ. 1998;317:559–65.
20. Kaminski MF, et al. Performance measures for lower gastrointestinal endoscopy: a European Society of Gastrointestinal Endoscopy (ESGE) quality improvement initiative. United European Gastroenterol J. 2017;5:309–34.
21. Winawer SJ, et al. Colorectal cancer screening: clinical guidelines and rationale. Gastroenterology. 1997;112:594–642.
22. Dunlop MG. Guidance on gastrointestinal surveillance for hereditary non-polyposis colorectal cancer, familial adenomatous polyposis, juvenile polyposis, and Peutz-Jeghers syndrome. Gut. 2002;51(Suppl 5):V21–7.
23. Beaugerie L, et al. Cancers complicating inflammatory bowel disease. N Engl J Med. 2015;373:195.
24. Farraye FA, et al. AGA technical review on the diagnosis and management of colorectal neoplasia in inflammatory bowel disease. Gastroenterology. 2010;138:746–774, 774 e741–744; quiz e712-743.
25. Soetikno R, et al. Paradigm shift in the surveillance and management of dysplasia in inflammatory bowel disease (West). Dig Endosc. 2016;28:266–73.
26. Laine L, et al. SCENIC international consensus statement on surveillance and management of dysplasia in inflammatory bowel disease. Gastrointest Endosc. 2015;81:489–501.
27. Lieberman DA, et al. Guidelines for colonoscopy surveillance after screening and polypectomy: a consensus update by the US Multi-Society Task Force on Colorectal Cancer. Gastroenterology. 2012;143:844–57.

28. Watanabe T, et al. Japanese Society for Cancer of the Colon and Rectum (JSCCR) guidelines 2016 for the treatment of colorectal cancer. Int J Clin Oncol. 2018;23:1–34.
29. Hamashima C, et al. The Japanese guidelines for gastric cancer screening. Jpn J Clin Oncol. 2008;38:259–67.
30. Leung WK, et al. Screening for gastric cancer in Asia: current evidence and practice. Lancet Oncol. 2008;9:279–87.
31. Huntsman DG, et al. Early gastric cancer in young, asymptomatic carriers of germ-line E-cadherin mutations. N Engl J Med. 2001;344:1904–9.
32. Engel LS, et al. Population attributable risks of esophageal and gastric cancers. J Natl Cancer Inst. 2003;95:1404–13.
33. Kuwano H, et al. Guidelines for diagnosis and treatment of carcinoma of the esophagus April 2012 edited by the Japan Esophageal Society. Esophagus. 2015;12:1–30.
34. Muto M, et al. Early detection of superficial squamous cell carcinoma in the head and neck region and esophagus by narrow band imaging: a multicenter randomized controlled trial. J Clin Oncol. 2010;28:1566–72.
35. Appelqvist P, et al. Lye corrosion carcinoma of the esophagus: a review of 63 cases. Cancer. 1980;45:2655–8.
36. Sandler RS, et al. The risk of esophageal cancer in patients with achalasia. A population-based study. JAMA. 1995;274:1359–62.
37. Stevens HP, et al. Linkage of an American pedigree with palmoplantar keratoderma and malignancy (palmoplantar ectodermal dysplasia type III) to 17q24. Literature survey and proposed updated classification of the keratodermas. Arch Dermatol. 1996;132:640–51.
38. Spechler SJ, et al. American Gastroenterological Association medical position statement on the management of Barrett's esophagus. Gastroenterology. 2011;140:1084–91.
39. Shuyama K, et al. Human papillomavirus in high- and low-risk areas of oesophageal squamous cell carcinoma in China. Br J Cancer. 2007;96:1554–9.
40. El-Serag HB, et al. Epidemiological differences between adenocarcinoma of the oesophagus and adenocarcinoma of the gastric cardia in the USA. Gut. 2002;50:368–72.
41. Hvid-Jensen F, et al. Incidence of adenocarcinoma among patients with Barrett's esophagus. N Engl J Med. 2011;365:1375–83.
42. Kelty CJ, et al. Barrett's oesophagus: intestinal metaplasia is not essential for cancer risk. Scand J Gastroenterol. 2007;42:1271–4.
43. Gray MR, et al. The role of smoking and alcohol in metaplasia and cancer risk in Barrett's columnar lined oesophagus. Gut. 1993;34:727–31.
44. Kastelein F, et al. Impact of surveillance for Barrett's oesophagus on tumor stage and survival of patients with neoplastic progression. Gut. 2016;65:548–54.
45. Schölvinck DW, et al. Detection of lesions in dysplastic Barrett's esophhagus by community and expert endoscpists. Endoscopy. 2017;49:113–20.
46. Weusten B, et al. Endoscopic management of Barrett's esophagus: European Society of Gastrointestinal Endoscopy (ESGE) position statement. Endoscopy. 2017;49:191–8.
47. Shaheen NJ, et al. ACG clinical guideline: diagnosis and management of Barrett's esophagus. Am J Gastroenterol. 2016;111:30–50.
48. Fitzgerald RC, et al. British Society of Gastroenterology guidelines on diagnosis and management of Barrett's esophagus. Gut. 2014:7–42.
49. Oyama T. Diagnostic strategies of superficial Barrett's esophageal cancer for endoscopic submucosal dissection. Dig Endosc. 2013;25(Suppl 1):7–12.
50. Faigel DO, et al. Quality indicators for gastrointestinal endoscopic procedures: an introduction. Am J Gastroenterol. 2006;101:866–72.
51. Kaminski MF, et al. Quality indicators for colonoscopy and the risk of interval cancer. N Engl J Med. 2010;362:1795–803.
52. Lee TJ, et al. Colonoscopy quality measure experience from the NHS bowel cancer screening programme. Gut. 2012;61:1050–7.
53. Kudo S, et al. The problem of de novo colorectal carcinoma. Eur J Cancer. 1995;31A:1118–20.

54. Morris EJ, et al. Post-colonoscopy colorectal cancer (PCCRC) rates vary considerably depending on the method used to calculate them: a retrospective observational population-based study of PCCRC in the English National Health Service. Gut. 2015;64:1248–56.
55. Calderwood AH, et al. Boston Bowel Preparation Scale scores provide a standardized definition of adequate for describing bowel cleanliness. Gastrointest Endosc. 2014;80:269–76.
56. Oyama T. Endoscopic diagnosis of gastric adenocarcinoma for ESD. Tokyo: Nankodo Co., Ltd; 2010.
57. Muto M, Yao K, Sano Y. Atlas of endoscopy with narrow band imaging. Tokyo: SPRINGER Japan; 2015. p. 11–30.
58. Yao K, et al. Development of an e-learning system for teaching endoscopists how to diagnose early gastric cancer: basic principles for improving early detection. Gastric Cancer. 2017;20:28–38.
59. Bisschops R, et al. Performance measures for upper gastrointestinal endoscopy: a European Society of Gastrointestinal Endoscopy quality improvement initiative. United European Gastroenterol J. 2016;4:629–56.
60. Banerjee S, et al. Antibiotic prophylaxis for GI endoscopy. Gastrointest Endosc. 2008;67:791–8.
61. Anderson MA, et al. Management of antithrombotic agents for endoscopic procedures. Gastrointest Endosc. 2009;70:1060–70.

Part II
Organ-Specific Endoscopic Analysis of Early Neoplasias

Chapter 7
Squamous Cell-Lined Esophagus and Hypopharynx: Mucosal Neoplasias

Tsuneo Oyama

7.1 Introduction

Opportunistic screening of high-risk individuals and surveillance of high-risk conditions with upper GI endoscopy have led to more frequent diagnosis of early cancers or high-grade intraepithelial neoplasia (HGIN) of the head and neck region and the esophagus [1, 2]. Early squamous cell cancer (SCC, pT1m-sm1) of the esophagus has an almost 100% chance of permanent cure after radical esophagectomy [3]. Analysis of pT category in a large cohort of patients revealed that the risk of lymph node metastasis is 1–3% when the carcinoma is confined to the lamina propria mucosae (m2), 9% when it involves the muscularis mucosae (m3), and 20% with microinvasion of the upper third of the submucosa (sm1) (<200 μm below muscularis mucosae) [3–5], but only 4.2% for sm1 carcinoma with low-risk criteria (sm <200 μm, G1 or G2, L0, V0) [5, 6]. Endoscopic diagnosis of esophageal cancer in very early stages (HGIN, T0m1, T1m2) is essential for curative endoscopic resection [7].

7.2 Endoscopic Surveillance for SCC in the Esophagus and Hypopharynx

For optimal visibility, upper GIendoscopy should be performed with intravenous sedation, 10 min after intake of a glass of water containing dimethicone and proteinase or acetylcysteine. Systematically inspect the entire pharynx. Including the view onto the vocal cords (see Sect. 6.4.2).

T. Oyama (✉)
Department of Endoscopy, Saku Central Hospital Advanced Care Center, Saku, Nagano, Japan
e-mail: oyama@coral.ocn.ne.jp

F. Berr et al. (eds.), *Atlas of Early Neoplasias of the Gastrointestinal Tract*,
https://doi.org/10.1007/978-3-030-01114-7_7

Detection of neoplastic lesions requires a standardized approach. Insert the endoscope with close inspection in white light (WL) mode, but use narrow-band imaging (NBI) mode for analysis of lesions (with magnification) and during scope withdrawal in the esophagus and hypopharynx, in order to achieve these objectives:

- Focus on *mucosal color changes* (red or pale, WLI; brown, NBI), and *disappearance* of the branched submucosal vascular network.
- Watch for *bleeding* lesions or surface *irregularities* in WLI.
- Perform total NBI mapping of the esophagus.
- Detect on NBI mapping any *brownish spot with irregular microvessels* (on magnification ≥ 40-fold)—a pattern highly specific for dysplasia or carcinoma [8].
- Use chromoendoscopy (CE) with 0.75% *Lugol* solution for any flat lesion of squamous epithelium in high-risk individuals (in hypopharynx only after tracheal intubation!).

7.3 Endoscopic Signs of Neoplastic Lesions on WLI Observation

Squamous epithelium-lined esophagus shows pale-orange or whitish color, smooth surface with light reflex, no glandular pattern on WLI endoscopy, and on magnification (m-WLI 60×), a blank microsurface with tiny perforating gland holes, and brownish coloring with Lugol-CE. The submucosal vascular pattern is clearly visible on WLI and NBI observation (Fig. 7.1).

Note *Signs of mucosal neoplasias* on standard WLI endoscopy:

- Slightly reddish appearance (as compared with regular mucosa)
- *Or* tiny whitish coating (keratinizing-type SCC)
- Uneven, velvety to granular-appearing surface structure
- Disappearance of normal mucosal light reflex
- Disappearance of dendritic vascular network of submucosal veins

Macroscopic types of early SC neoplasias in the earliest stages (HGIN, SCC pT1a), confined to EP (m1) or LPM (m2), exhibit types 0–IIb by macroscopic classification of neoplasias (*see* Table 1.2). The likelihood of sm2 invasion is about 30% in slightly depressed neoplasias (0-IIc) and increases to about 50% with the elevated type (0-IIa or 0-IIa + IIc), paralleled by diagnostic alterations in IPCL pattern. Protuberant (0-Is) or ulcerated SCC (0-III) usually are deeply sm invasive. Table 7.1 presents the prevalence and risk of sm invasiveness of early SCC types diagnosed before the introduction of magnifying NBI analysis [4], a fact that explains why the relative prevalence of 0-IIb and 0-IIa types was low among early esophageal SCC. Very early detection using NBI yields a high prevalence of 0-IIb and 0-IIa types.

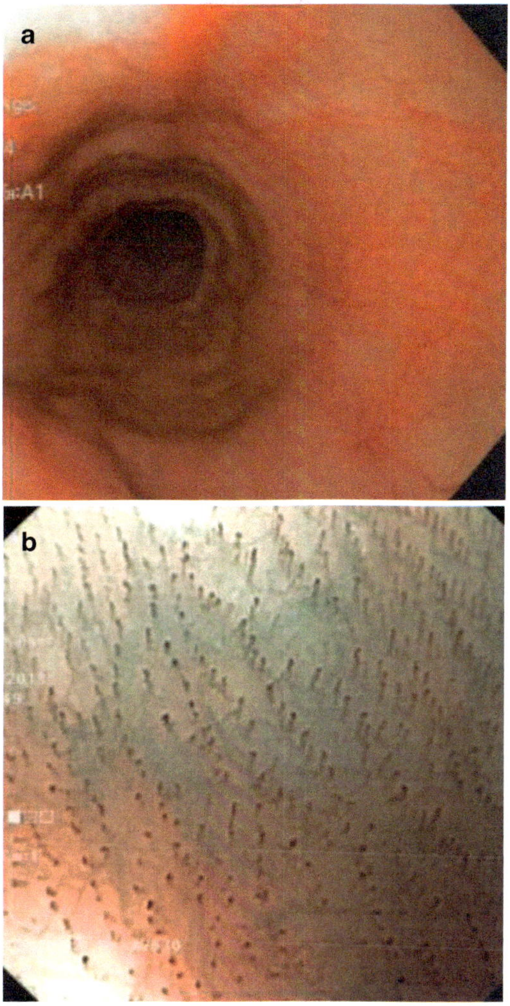

Fig. 7.1 Normal squamous epithelial esophagus. (**a**) Standard white light endoscopy (WLI) showing dendritic submucosal vascular pattern and very faint intrapapillary capillary loops (IPCLs), (**b**) Squamous epithelial esophagus with regular straight IPCL pattern of normal loop *type A JES*; (type I, Inoue), M-NBI (60×). (**c**) IPCL pattern *normal loop type A, JES* (*type II, Inoue*, with elongation of IPCL). M-NBI 40×. Mild post-esophagitic changes of SC mucosa (left, lower esophagus) in 70-year-old woman with axial hernia and chronic GERD on treatment with omeprazole (*insert*: cardia in retroflex view, WLI). (**d**) IPCL mildly abnormal *loop type A, JES* (*types II and III, Inoue*), with elongation, some variation of shape. M-NBI 60×, same patient as in (**c**). (**e**) Early squamous cell cancer type 0-IIa + b. Note partly reddish, partly whitish lesion (*arrows*) on WLI, and whitish, smooth glycogen acanthosis in upper right corner, (**f**) Lugol-CE shows unstained SCC with mild "pink color sign" and coloring of glycogen acanthosis

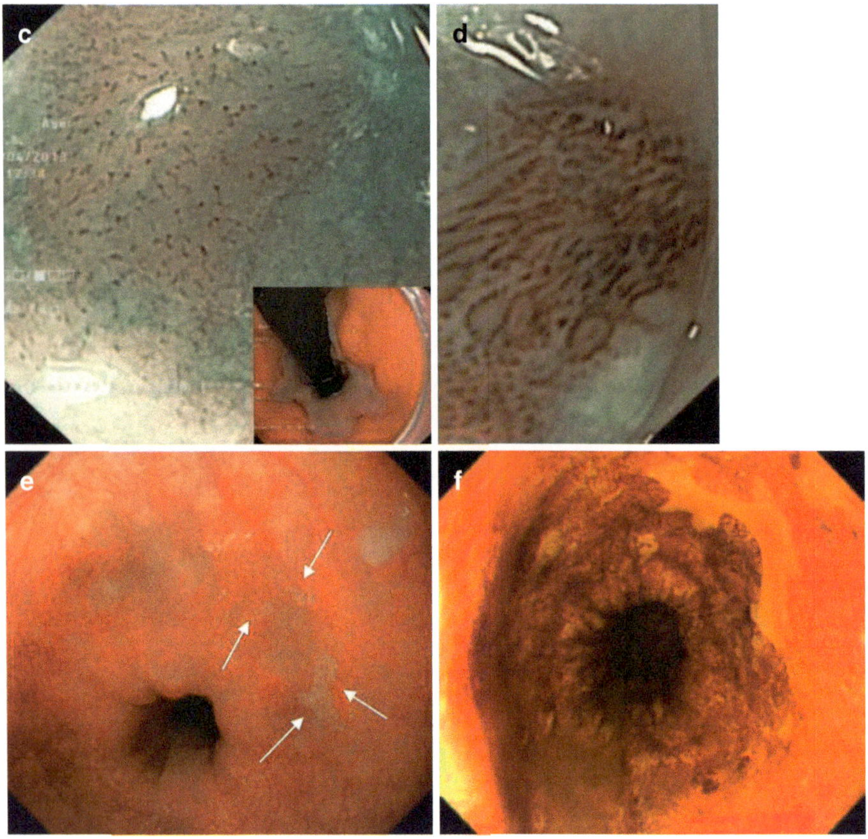

Fig. 7.1 (continued)

Chromoendoscopy with 0.75–1% iodine solution is useful for detection and analysis of lateral margins of superficial squamous cell cancer:

- *Lugol-unstained areas* signify SCC (or rarely inflammation) [9].
- A "*pink color sign*" on WLI ("silver sign" on NBI) appearing after 2–3 min in a Lugol-unstained area is typical for SCC [10].

The problem is inflammation caused by Lugol; sometimes the patient feels heartburn, and rarely, it causes shock.

Table 7.1 Early esophageal SCC: distribution of Paris types and relationship with depth of tumor invasion

	Type	Prevalence (% of ESCC[a])	Depth of tumor invasion (% of Type)		
			M1 & M2	M3 & sm1	≥sm2
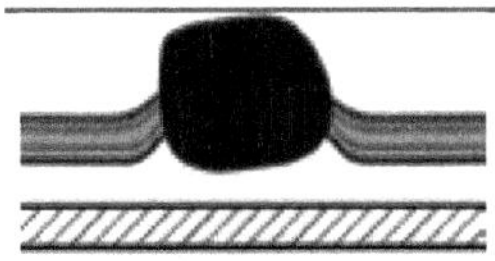	0-I (s, p)	14	4	**17**	**79**
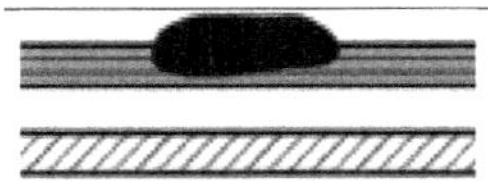	0-IIa	16	20	31	**49**
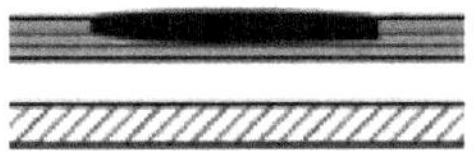	0-IIb	12	69	16	15
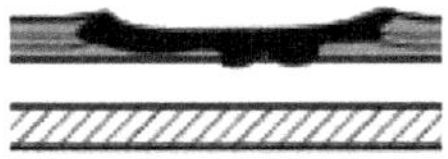	0-IIc	38	36	35	29
	0-IIa + IIc	8	10	**37**	**53**
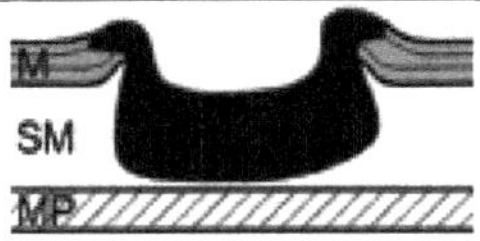	0-III	4	3	13	**83**

ESCC esophageal squamous cell cancer

[a]Multicenter analysis of 1853 specimens ESCC resected either surgically or endoscopically (between 1990 and 1994) in Japan [4]. Graphics modified from [3]

[b]**Bold** numbers indicate high probability of deep submucosal invasion, a contraindication for curative endoscopic submucosal dissection (ESD)

7.4 Endoscopic Diagnosis of Mucosal Lesions Based on Magnifying NBI Endoscopy: Basic Microvascular Patterns

Normal epithelium in squamous esophagus shows a regular pattern of intrapapillary capillary loops *(IPCL)*, which is well enhanced on magnifying NBI observation. Magnifying NBI (>60-fold) reveals a striking microvessel pattern (VP) that consists of a longitudinal array of fine, parallel, straight IPCLs in the lamina propria mucosae (VP type A, JES, i.e. type I, Inoue) and a branching pattern of thicker arterioles and oblique venules in the submucosa (*see* Fig. 7.1a, b). Alterations of mucosal VP are the key to accurate endoscopic diagnosis of mucosal lesions. VP types are defined by alterations in four IPCL characteristics—length (elongation), tortuosity, caliber (thickness), and shape (distortion of loop)—and reflect changes in anatomy of epithelial papillae, which are destroyed by vertical tumor invasion and neoangiogenesis. The recent consensus classification of the Japan Esophageal Society (JES) showed highly accurate (overall ~90%) prediction of malignant or invasive neoplasms [11] (Table 7.2a, b; Fig. 7.2). For comparison with the previously accepted classification of Inoue, see Table 7.3 and Fig. 7.3 [12]. *Non-neoplastic lesions* present variants of normal *JES type A pattern* that are typical of mild acute or severe chronic esophagitis (*see* Fig. 7.1c,d).

Table 7.2a M-NBI vessel classification of esophageal squamous epithelium and neoplasias by the Japan Esophageal Society (JES)

Scheme	Diameter, μm	Vessel type	Description	Invasion depth	Histology
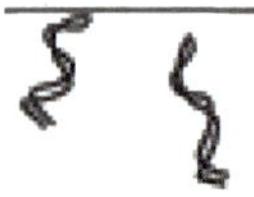		A	Normal IPCL vs. elongation and tortuosity	No invasion	Normal epithelium
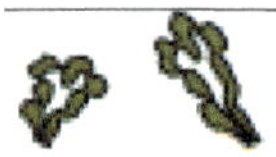	~7–10	B1	Abnormal VP, loop-like	T1a-EP, T1a-LPM	HGIN, SCC-Tis
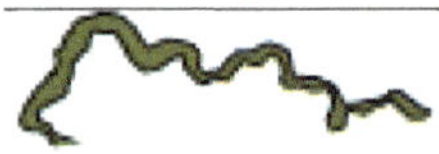	~20	B2	Non-loop formations	T1a-MM, T1b-SM1	SCC ~sm invasive
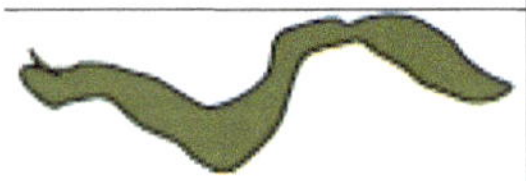	Most >60	B3	Thick vessel (neoangiogenesis)	T1b- ≥ SM2	SCC deep sm invasive

Table 7.2b M-NBI Vessel classification in squamous cell-lined esophagus—minor criteria: Avascular areas (AVA) according to diameter

	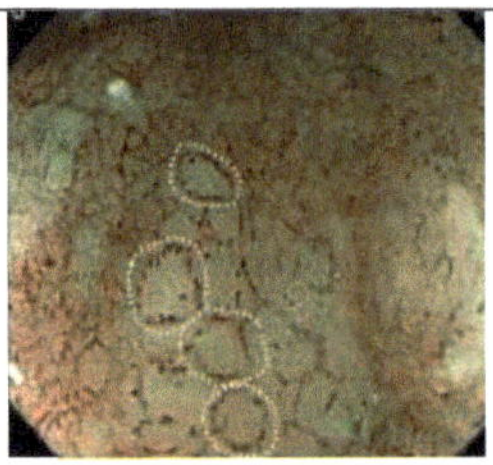	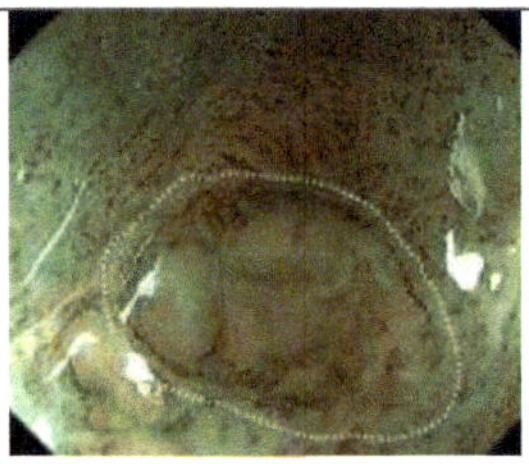	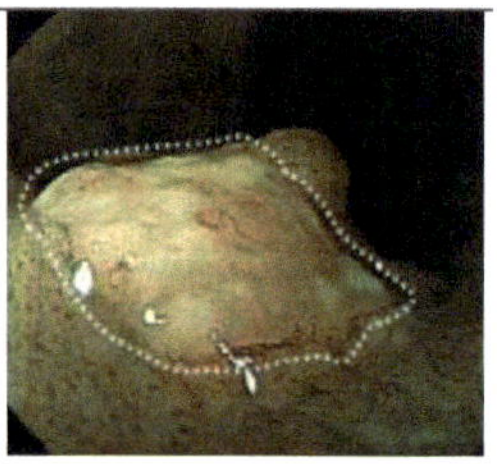
Size	AVA-small (<0.5 mm)	AVA-middle (0.5–3.0 mm)	AVA-large (>3.0 mm)
Invas.	T1a-EP or T1-LPM	T1a-MM or T1b-SM1	T1b- ≥SM2

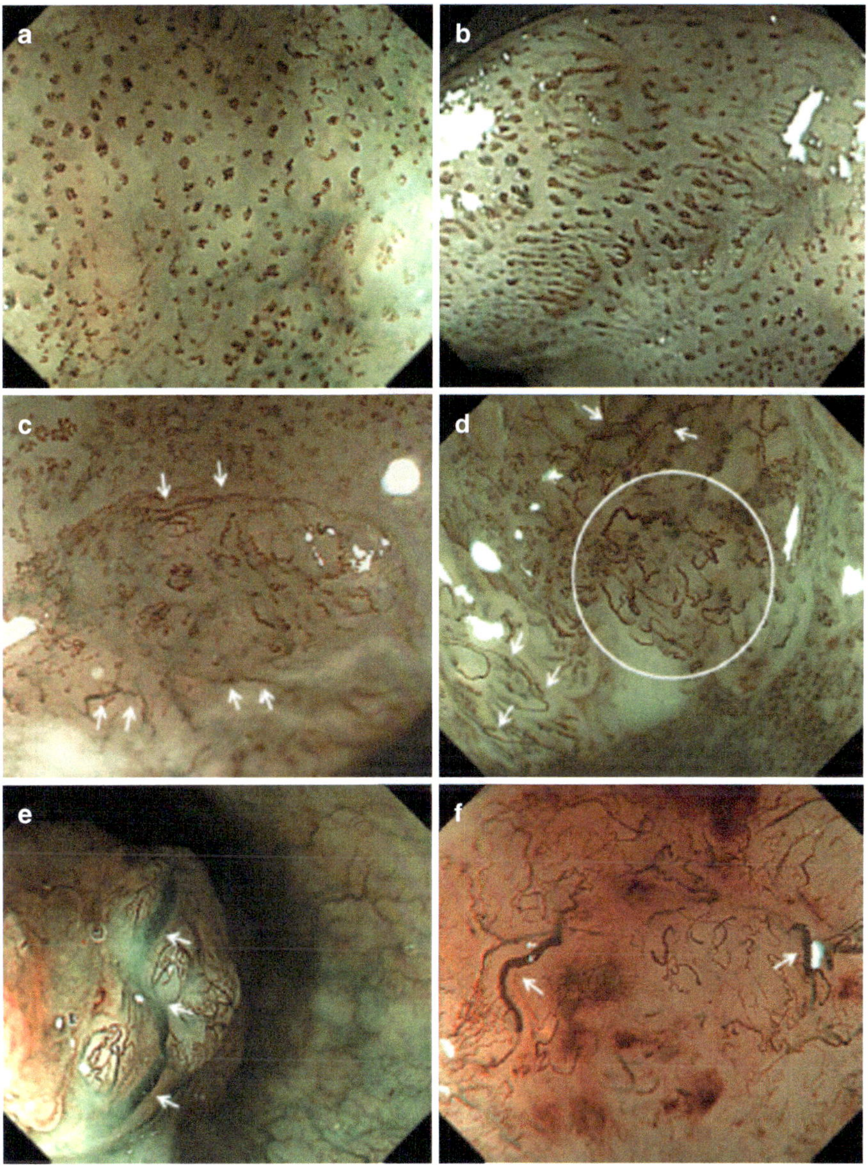

Fig. 7.2 M-NBI (~80×) classification of VP in esophageal squamous epithelium and neoplasms, consensus of Japan Esophageal Society (JES). (**a**) Type **B1** vessels, loop-like. (**b**) Type B1, loop-like. (**c**, **d**) Type **B2** vessels without a loop-like formation (*white arrows* and *inside white circle*). (**e**, **f**) Type **B3** of highly dilated abnormal vessels (*white arrows*); diameter is more than three times that of the B2 vessels. (Reproduced from Oyama et al. [11], under the terms of the Creative Commons Attribution 4.0 International License (http://creativecommons.org/licenses/by/4.0/))

Table 7.3 Comparison of VP classifications of squamous cell-lined esophagus (on M-NBI)

Inoue classification (modified)[a]		Histopathology		Japan Esophageal Society (JES). classification[b]	
VP type	IPCL	Invasion	LN+	IPCL pattern	VP type
I	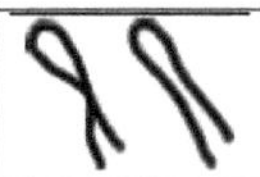	Nonneoplastic		Normal IPCL pattern	A
II	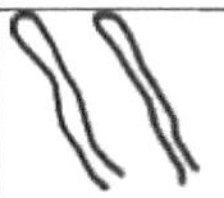				
III	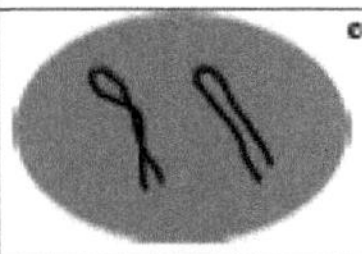 [c]				
IV	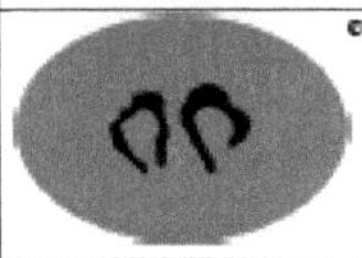 [c]	EP	0–1%	Abnormal loop pattern	B_1
V-1	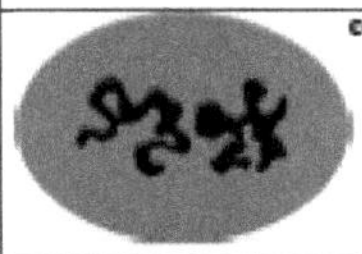 [c]	m1	2% (1–9%)		
V-2	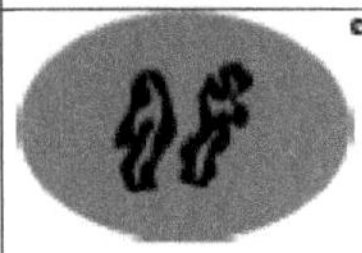 [c]	m2			
V-3	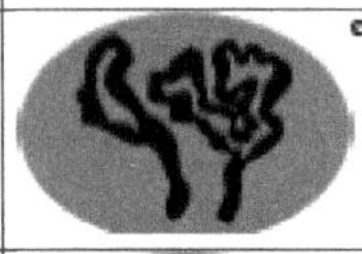 [c]	m3 (mm)/sm1	10–20%	Non-loop pattern	B_2
Vn	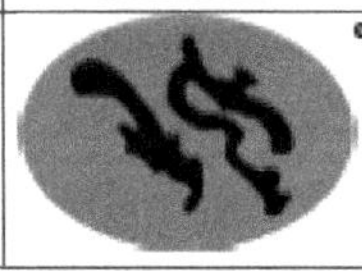 [c]	sm2 (massive invasion)	~50%	Very thick (tumor) vessel	B_3

[a]Modified according to [8, 12] (Compare Fig. 7.3a–f)
[b]Japan Esophageal Society Classification (JES) for Esophageal SCC [11]
[c]Un-/stained with Lugol

Neoplasias, when flat, appear as slightly reddish or whitish (keratinizing) areas that remain unstained on Lugol-CE and often show a "pink-color sign" a few minutes after Lugol spraying (*see* Fig. 7.1e, f). They are readily apparent on NBI as brownish areas that display (on magnifying NBI) augmented and *irregular VP and loss of normal dendritic sm vascular pattern* (Figs. 7.2 and 7.3). The brownish aspect on NBI is due to increased vascularity and brownish background coloration [11]. Rare small squamous cell cancer (SCC) lesions (<5%) show an entirely whitish aspect, easy to miss on WLI and NBI. *Inoue's VP classification* of squamous esophagus has been

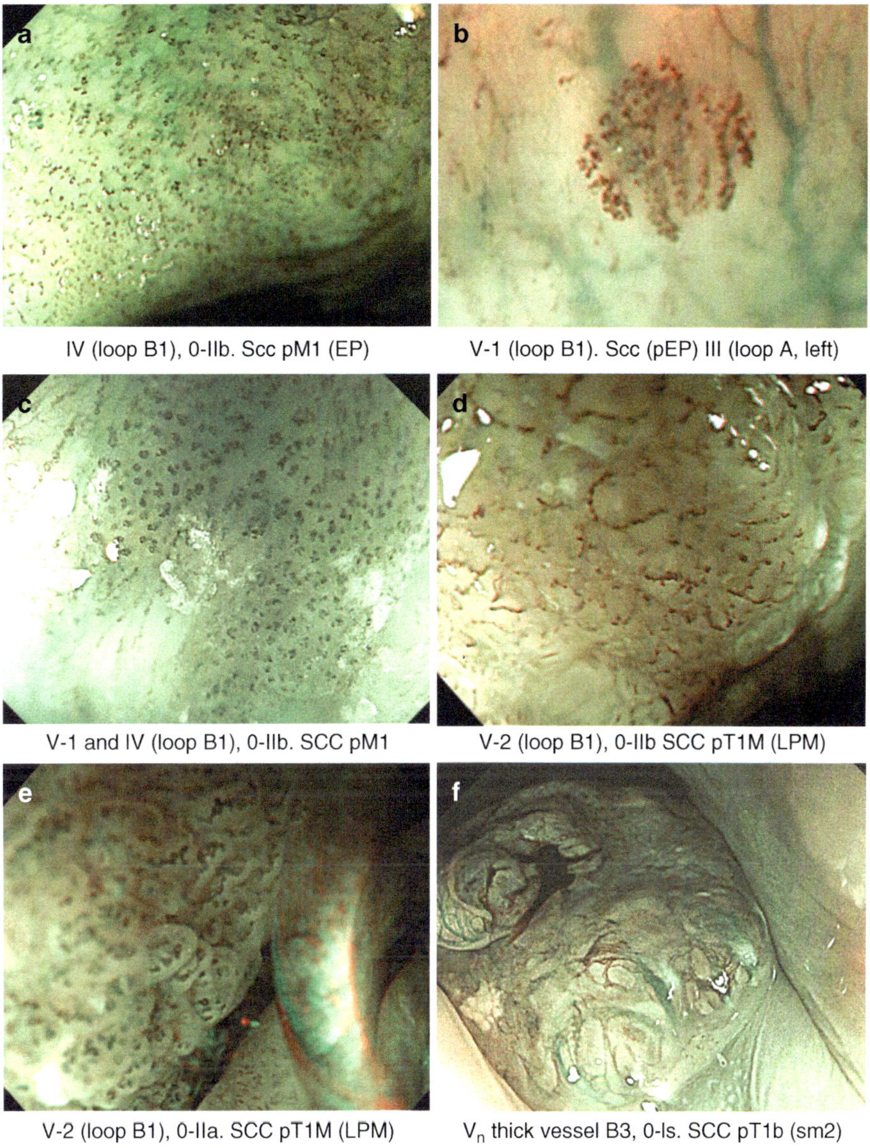

Fig. 7.3 (**a–f**) VP classification by Inoue (by JES in parentheses) of microvascular pattern types of squamous cell neoplasias, magnifying NBI (60–100-fold), and corresponding histology obtained after ESD. (Compare Table 7.3: Inoue VP, JES VP.)

most widely applied (Table 7.3) [12], but has now been simplified by consensus of the Japan Esophageal Society (JES) to the principal IPCL patterns A, B_1, B_2, and B_3 [11] (*see* Table 7.2a and Figs. 7.2 and 7.3). *Neoplastic changes* in caliber and shape of IPCL, with preserved IPCL loop configuration, progressive curling, and slight dilatation of IPCL tops, and elongation of IPCL, are typical for dysplasia (LGIN or HGIN) or intramucosal carcinoma (m1, m2), classified as *VP abnormal loop B_1, JES.*

SCC extending to the muscularis mucosae (m3) or minimally into submucosa (sm1) typically show some vanishing IPCL (due to destruction of epithelial papillae) and/or marked elongation of IPCL and connection of adjacent IPCL yielding *non-loop type* B_2, *JES* (*Inoue type V-3*). Distinctly nonstructured VP exhibits all four abnormalities (*Inoue type* V_N) including *disrupted thick vessel type* B_3, *JES* and is characteristic of SCC with deep sm invasion (*see* Figs. 7.2e, f and 7.3e, f) [11, 12].

Avascular area (AVA) is defined as an area of low or no vascularity surrounded by stretched, irregular vessels (type B1, B2, or B3). The size of AVA on m-NBI bears direct correlation with lack or degree of submucosal invasion of SCC in the esophagus [13] (Table 7.2b), but this correlation has not yet been proven in a prospective multicenter study [11].

Note In squamous cell-lined esophagus, M-NBI reveals changes in VP of IPCL, which permit to distinguish with high accuracy [11, 12, 14]:

- Nonneoplastic (*type A, JES*) *vs*. neoplastic lesions (*types B, JES*)
- Intramucosal HGIN/sm-microinvasive carcinoma (*types* B_1 / B_2 *-/+ AVA-small/-middle*) *vs*. carcinoma with deep submucosal invasion (*type* B_3 *-/+ AVA-large, JES*)

7.5 Endoscopic Diagnosis of Nonneoplastic and Neoplastic Lesions

Reddish flat lesions in squamous cell-lined esophagus cover a variety of *inflammatory and nonneoplastic lesions* as well as *neoplastic lesions*. For classification of macroscopic type of lesions, compare Fig. 1.2a. Most are *esophagitic lesions* (erosions, flat ulcerations, inflammatory hyperplasia) of different etiology (e.g., Fig. 7.4a). All these show inflammatory IPCL pattern type II or III (Inoue), i.e., mildly abnormal loop type A (JES), and unclear margins. Mechanical damage may cause IPCL hematomas (Fig. 7.4c–e). Severe ischemic damage may present *dark, livid areas*, the so-called *black esophagus* (with IPCL type A). This differs from *pigmented melanosis* (Fig. 7.4f), a sign of past toxic exposure with risk of SCC [2, 15]. Similar pigmented submucosal lesions may show *pigmented nevi* or *malignant melanoma* on biopsy.

Whitish flat lesions frequently reveal *Candida* esophagitis (Fig. 7.4b), *glycogenic acanthosis*, a smooth whitish spot with concealed dendritic sm vessel pattern (Fig.7.1e, f), rarely *foam cell nests* with yellowish lipid deposits, or flat *papillomas*. All these alterations exhibit nearly regular IPCL pattern JES loop type A (Inoue type I or II). Papillomas look like lesions type 0-IIa or type 0-Is, but the surface pattern is completely different from SCC. Papilloma shows a sea anemone–like shape with scanty IPCL pattern loop type A (Inoue type II or III) and surface light reflex (Fig. 7.4g–k). About 80% of papillomas are solitary; 20% are multiple and may be virus-induced.

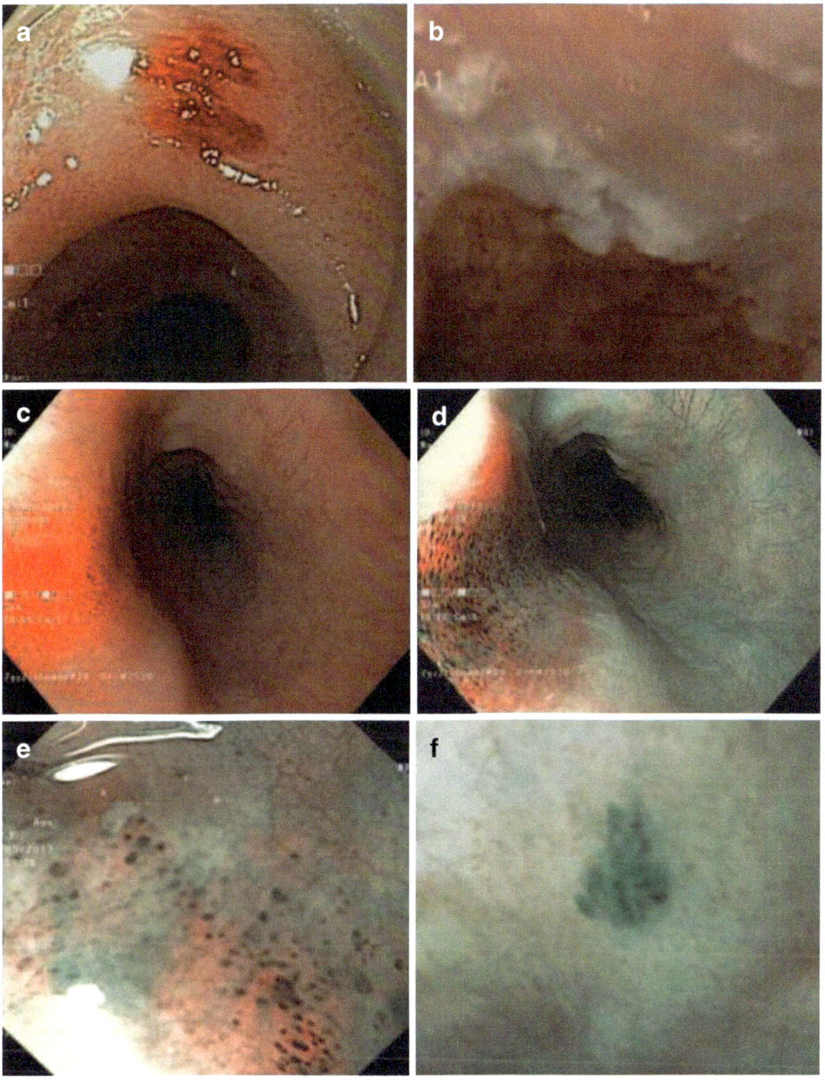

Fig. 7.4 (**a**) Acute inflammatory lesion in lower esophagus caused by pancreatobiliary reflux after removal of an enteric drainage tube, in a patient with Billroth-II partial gastrectomy. (**b**) *Candida* esophagitis at GE junction, white fungal plaques, on WLI. Note the epithelial lesion with white fungus plaque, without neovascularization. (**c**–**e**) Lesion 0-IIa (14–16 cm p.i., anterior wall) in a 59-year-old healthy woman with cricopharyngeal dysphagia. (**c**) Squamous epithelial damage (IPCL microhematomas) caused by mechanical shear stress within upper esophageal sphincter area, seen on WLI; (**d**) NBI; (**e**) M-NBI (60-fold). Histology: regular epithelial papillas and squamous epithelial layer with loss of superficial epithelial cell layers. (**f**) Pigmented melanosis in normal squamous mid-esophagus NBI (20×) in a 65-year-old healthy woman

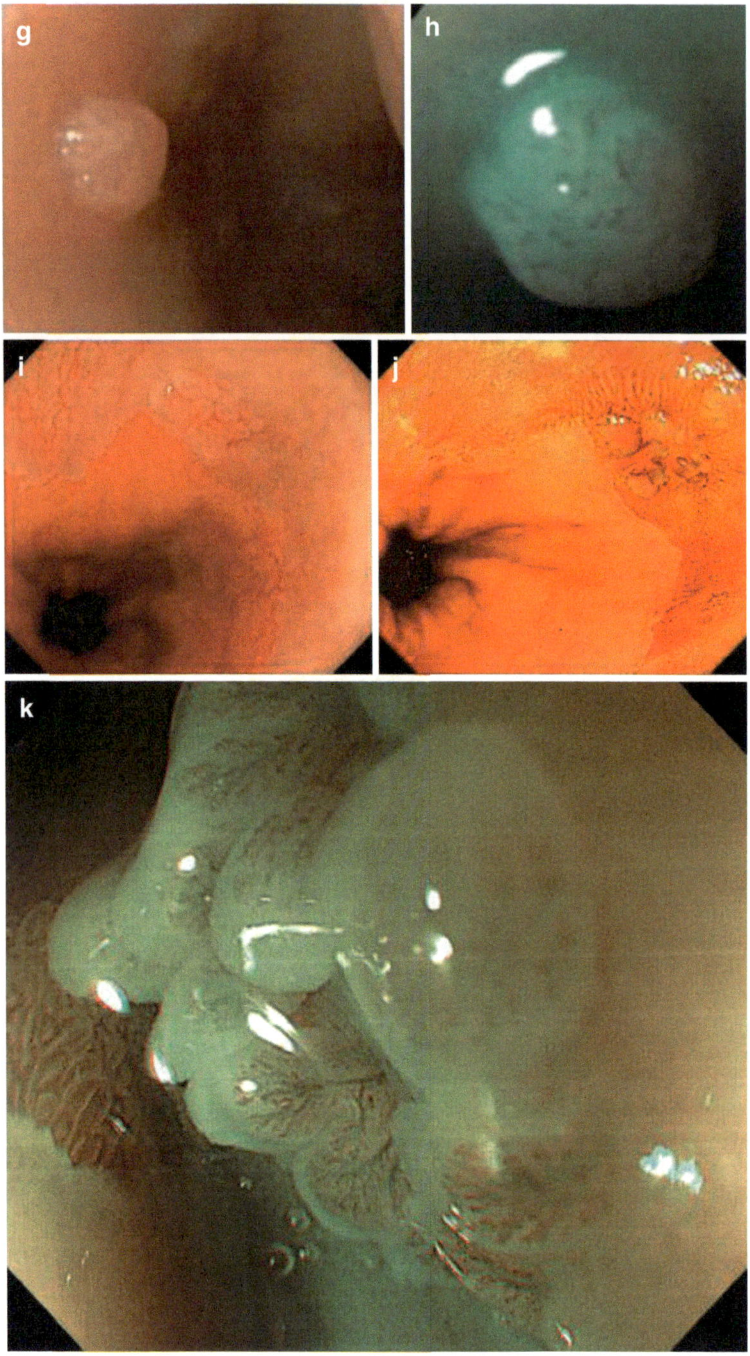

Fig. 7.4 (continued) (**g–k**) Papillomas in squamous esophagus. (**g**) WLI: whitish, 0-IIa-like; (**h**) M-NBI (40×): with IPCL pattern II; (**i**) WLI: papilloma in squamous cell-lined esophagus next to hiatal hernia; (**j**) Lugol stain: mild Lugol staining to Lugol-voiding lesion (WLI, four-fold zoom). (**k**) Sea anemone–like appearance (IPCL loop type A, JES) by M-NBI (100-fold)

Note *Permeation* of submucosal dendritic vascular pattern in the lesion indicates lack of neoplastic infiltration of LPM (*see* Fig. 7.4e).

Rarely, a white flat lesion (0-IIb, IIa) shows no or little permeation of VP type B_1–B_3 identifying *keratinizing squamous cell carcinoma* (Fig. 7.5).

Reddish protruding lesions comprise well-differentiated cancer (non-keratinizing type), inflammatory polyp, some submucosal tumors (e.g., NET, GIST, granular cell tumor), and rarely, intramucosal metastasis (e.g., from breast cancer).

Inflammatory polyps (0-Is or Isp) are covered with typical squamous cell epithelium and present unclear mucosal margins and often inflammatory erosions or ulcerations; the stroma shows fibrosis and chronic inflammatory or granulomatous mononuclear cell infiltrations without or with eosinophils. In non-eroded parts, squamous cell epithelium is smooth with normal IPCL loop type A, JES. Larger, symptomatic inflammatory polyps are removed with polypectomy, and precautions must be taken for vigorous bleeding from feeding vessels [16].

Neoplastic lesions of esophageal squamous epithelium are mostly flat (0-II, 79%); fewer are protruded (0-I, 16%) or excavated (0-III, 5%) (Table 7.1). In general, *protruded neoplasias* (0-I) and combined elevated and depressed types (0-IIa + c or 0-IIa + III) are easily detectable. Well-differentiated *SCC* as a protruding lesion (Fig. 7.5e–h) in general is deeply sm invasive (>200 μm) and shows VP type B_3, JES (Inoue type V_N) on M-NBI. However, some rare 0-Ip lesions, often with a narrow base showing AID (Fig. 1.2b) and softness and mobility on manipulation, may only be m3 (MM) or sm1-invasive, when without thick vessels type B3, JES. Staging including endoscopic ultrasound (EUS) clarifies resectability. Chromoendoscopy with *0.75–1% iodine solution* is useful for detection and analysis of lateral margins of superficial SCC [10, 12].

Note *For detection* of less-obvious *flat-type neoplasias* (*0-IIa*, *b*, *c*) in esophagus and hypopharynx, focus on:

- Mucosal color changes to *red* or pale on WLI examination
- Surface irregularities and loss of surface reflex and of dendritic sm vascular pattern
- Brown spots on NBI mapping of squamous epithelium (except whitish-keratotic ones)

You *must analyze* any such brown spot on *magnifying NBI* (±*Lugol-CE*) for:

- Atypias of microvascular pattern type, *type* B_1–B_2 (Inoue *IV–V3*), which indicate HGIN or mucosal cancer [8, 11]
- *Unstained lesion* −/+ *pink-color* sign on Lugol stain

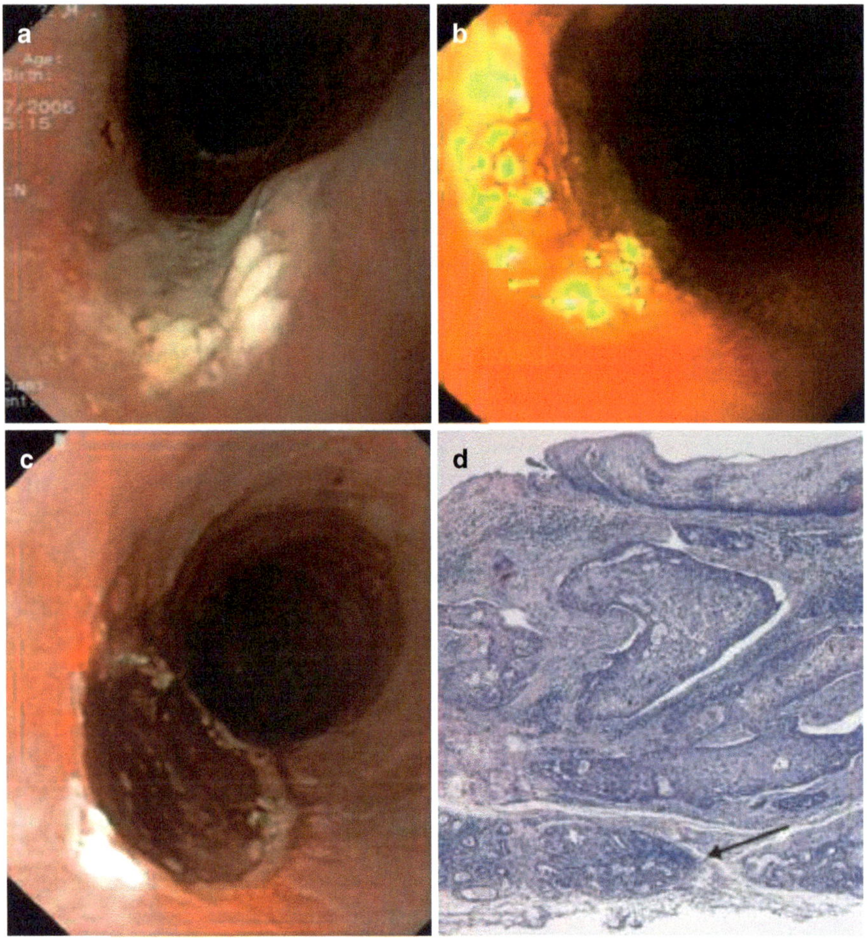

Fig. 7.5 (**a**) Whitish neoplasia 0-IIa in mid-esophagus in a 67-year-old man. Biopsy: keratinizing SCC G2, WLI. (**b**) Lugol-unstained neoplasia 0-IIa, WLI. (**c**) Resection bed after aspiration–endoscopic mucosal resection (EMR) of SCC 0-IIa., (**d**) Keratinizing SCC G2, sm invasive (sm1-2). Basal resection margin positive (R1, *arrow*). Patient was referred for esophagectomy (no residual SCC, pN0)

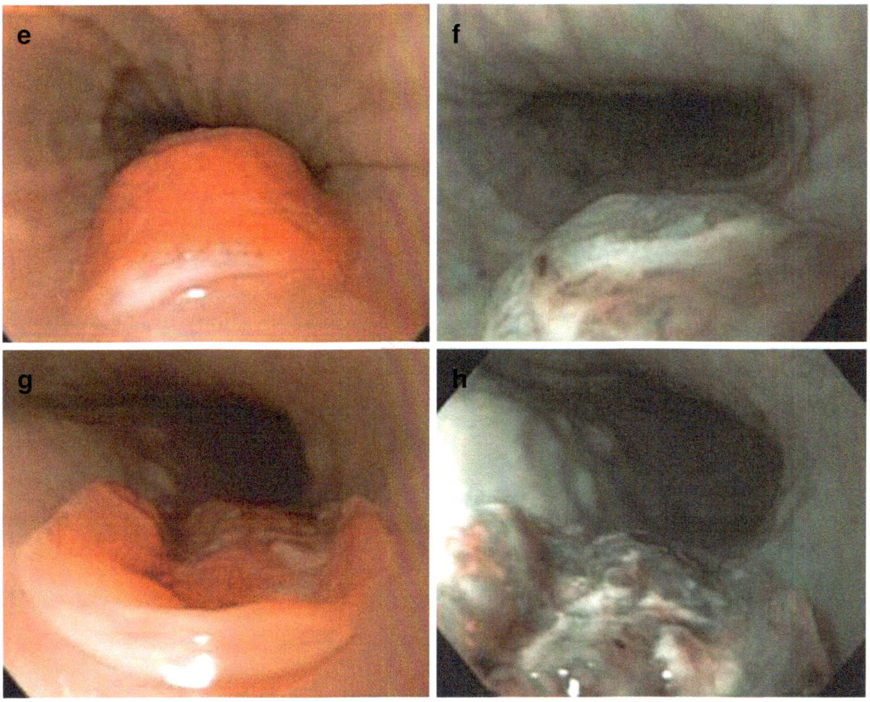

Fig. 7.5 (continued) (**e**) Lesion 0-Is in squamous mucosa, mid-esophagus, WLI. Biopsy: SC-HGIN. (**f**) MV pattern V_N sparse (B_3 JES) appears deeply sm invasive, NBI, 20-fold. (**g**) Same lesion 6 weeks later after one cycle of chemotherapy for myelodysplastic syndrome: Lesion type 0-IIa + III (typical for deep sm invasion), WLI, 20×. (**h**) Ulcerated lesion 0-III with nonstructured surface and VP B3 JES, NBI 20-fold

7.6 Endoscopic Diagnosis of Grade of Invasion of Esophageal SCC

Vertical extension of early squamous cell carcinoma closely correlates with *macroscopic types* of neoplasia and irregularities of *VP* [5, 11, 12]. Early neoplasias in a large series of resected specimens were mostly flat (0-II, 70%), much less protuberant (0-I, 16%), or excavated (0-III, 5%), as detected before the introduction of magnifying NBI (Table 7.1). Squamous cell early cancers type 0-I or 0-III show in ≥80% deep submucosal invasion (sm2-3 or T2 category) and in 50% lymph node metastasis and type 0-IIa and 0-IIa + IIc in about 50% deep submucosal invasion (Fig. 7.6a–h) and irregular IPCL pattern (*see* Figs. 7.2, 7.3, and 7.5g, h). Depressed *type 0-IIc* SCCs had a nearly 30% probability of sm2–3 invasion with high risk of lymph node metastasis [4, 17].

More than 80% of Type 0-IIb completely flat neoplasias show no or minimal vertical invasion and are category T1a (EP or LPM) (Fig. 7.7a–d). Typical cases of superficial neoplasias type 0-IIb exhibiting negative Lugol staining and highly irregular and dense IPCL pattern type B_1 (Fig. 7.7c, d) allow with high certainty the endoscopic diagnosis of HGIN or differentiated squamous cell cancer with low invasion depth (*EP or LPM*) (the so-called *optical biopsy*, specificity >80%).

Experienced endoscopists achieved 84% accuracy for endoscopic prediction of submucosal invasion of SCC in the body of the esophagus, matching the accuracy of high-resolution EUS (20 MHz) [18].

Note Endoscopic signs that indicate *deep submucosal* invasion of SCC:

- Polypoid neoplasms, 0-Ip, 0-Isp, 0-Is (with few exceptions)
- Neoplasms with ulceration (0-III)
- Neoplasias type IIa (~48%), and IIa + IIc (66% sm2 invasion)
- Microvascular pattern type B_3 JES (Inoue V_N)

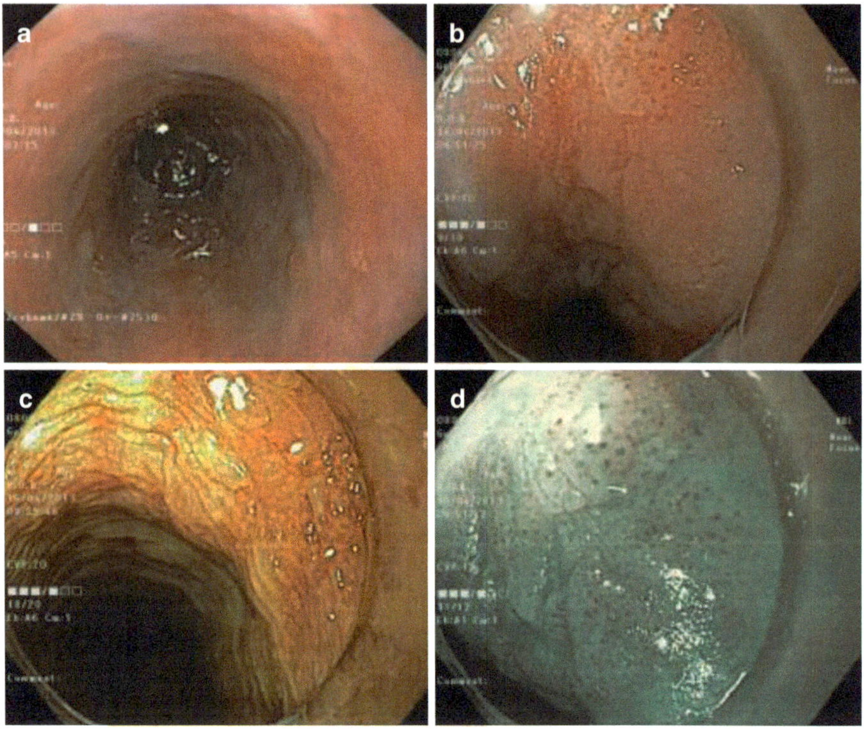

Fig. 7.6 (**a**–**d**) *Squamous epithelial carcinoma* (SCC) type 0-IIb + IIa, proximal esophagus. (**a**) Lesion 0-IIa (from 12 to 4 o'clock), reddish velvety surface (loss of reflex and sm-VP), WLI. (**b**) Reddish lesion (11–5 o'clock) 0-IIa, loss of dendritic sm vascular pattern (magnified WLI, 40×). (**c**) Lugol-unstained SC lesion 0-IIa with "Tatami-no-me Sign" (like "bamboo flooring"). (**d**) Lesion 0-IIa, abnormal loop VP B-1, JES (Inoue V1–V2), M-NBI (40×). ESD (R0): SCC G2, T1a (M2) (Ca in situ)

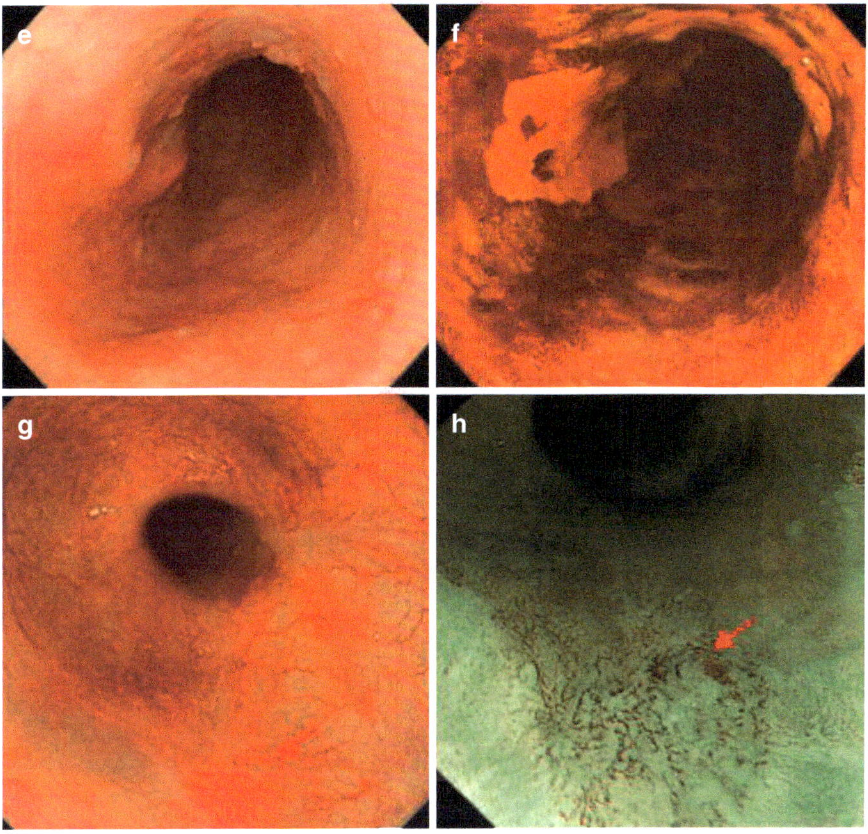

Fig. 7.6 (continued) (**e**, **f**) Bifocal squamous epithelial neoplasia type 0-IIb, 0-IIa [SCC m3 and sm1-2]. (**e**) Reddish lesion with some protrusion, type 0-IIb + IIa, more than semicircumferential (from 8 to 3 o'clock), mid esophagus. WLI. (**f**) Lugol staining reveals two Lugol-voiding mucosal areas next to each other (0-IIb and 0-IIa) and multifocal diminished staining (most likely dysplastic areas). (**g**) Reddish lesion 0-IIb, mid-esophagus, WLI; ICPL pattern. (**h**) *Non-loop B2*, JES (*type V-3*, Inoue) (*red arrow*), M-NBI (40×), Histology: SCC m3 and sm1 (T1b sm1)

7.7 Endoscopic Resection of Early Squamous Cell Cancer

Basically, en bloc resection should be performed. The size of lesions that can be removed by snare endoscopic mucosal resection (EMR) is limited: The *indication for snare-EMR* is:

- Squamous cell cancer T0 m1 (HGIN) or T1 m2, *size* $\leq$ *2 cm*

Larger lesions are technically resectable with rubber-band EMR or snare-EMR in piecemeal technique (e.g., cap-EMR) [19, 20, 21]. The outcome after EMR of T1m SCC of the esophagus is comparable to the outcome after surgical esophagectomy

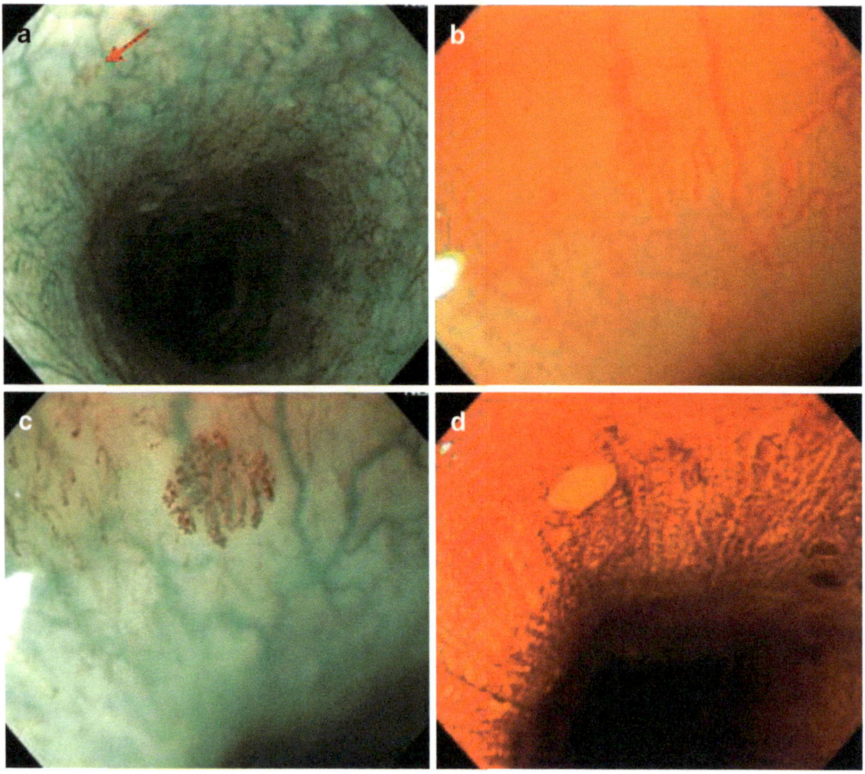

Fig. 7.7 Intramucosal neoplastic lesion 0-IIb. Histology: HGIN. (**a**) Tiny brown spot 0-IIb (*red arrow*), standard NBI mapping of esophagus. (**b**) Minute lesion 0-IIb (abnormal loops, disappearance of sm vessels) on M-WLI (80-fold). (**c**) Abnormal loop pattern B_1, M-NBI (80-fold). (**d**) Lugol stain: Lugol-voiding lesion 0-IIb. *Note*: All features (**a–d**) are consistent with intramucosal cancer or HGIN (diameter 1 mm)

(95% vs. 93.5% disease-specific 5-year survival rate) [21]. However, piecemeal EMR resulted in a high rate of recurrence (over 25%) [20] and therefore is no longer an established indication; comparable esophageal SCCs were resected en bloc with hook-knife endoscopic submucosal dissection (ESD) without recurrence (102 cases, median follow-up 21 (range 3–54) months) [7]. In addition, a retrospective comparison of EMR versus ESD resulted in superior en bloc resection rates for ESD (100%, 97% curative) versus cap-aspiration-EMR (87%, 71% curative) versus two-channel EMR (71%, 46% curative [19]. Cap-aspiration EMR of cancers <15 mm in size yielded an identical en bloc resection rate (100%) but a trend to a lower cure rate (86%) than ESD (97%; difference ns) [19]. Hence, ESD is the treatment of choice even for smaller mucosal SCC.

Table 7.4 Guideline indication (*upper row*) and expanded indications (*both lower rows*) for endoscopic en bloc resection of esophageal early squamous cancer [5, 7, 22]

Histology	Depth (all L0 and V0)	Type	Size
HGIN/SCC G1 or G2	≤M2	0-IIb	Any size
	M3[a]	0-IIa-c, c N0	<50 mm
	sm1 < 200 μm[b]	no ulcer, c N0	

[a, b]Overall risk of LN+ is 9% (M3) and 20% (sm1). However, for low-risk criteria (when ≤G2, L0, V0), risk of LN+ metastasis is only 4.2% for sm1 [6]

ESD en bloc is indicated for larger (≥20-mm) HGIN or early SCC with VP type B1 JES (Inoue type V-1 and V-2). VP type B2 JES (Inoue's VP type V-3) may represent an expanded indication for ESD in patients with high operative risk (Table 7.4). HGIN or SCC G1 or G2 should be confirmed by targeted biopsy prior to ESD.

The *classic indication for ESD* in squamous epithelial esophagus is HGIN or SCC G1 or G2, T0 m1 or T1 m2 involving less than two thirds of the circumference [5, 7]. There are two *relative indications for ESD:* (1) HGIN or SCC G1 or G2, T0 m1 or T1a m2 of the entire circumference; (2) SCC G1 or G2, T1b, sm1 (<200 μm sm invasion, L0 V0), without ulcer and without evidence of lymph node metastasis upon clinical staging.

SCCs deeply invading the sm layer (sm2-3) carry an increased risk of lymph node metastasis (28–49%) [3, 4, 17]. However, differentiated SCCs (G1 or G2, and L0, V0) superficially sm invasive (<200 μm below the muscularis mucosae) had shown lymph node metastases in only 4.2% of cases [6] and are taken as a relative indication for ESD in surgical high-risk patients. Lymph vessel permeation of SCC is a strong predictor of lymph node metastasis and demands additional therapy (esophagectomy or radiochemotherapy) [5, 6].

Contraindications for esophageal ESD:

- Evidence of deep sm invasion (risk of R2 resection)
- Frank bleeding diathesis (e.g., combined antiplatelet-anticoagulant therapy)
- Very poor or impossible technical resectability

ESD indication for squamous epithelial neoplasm in hypo-/pharynx [22, 23]:

- HGIN or SCC G1 or G2, T1a (T0 m1 or T1 m2), technically resectable (under general anesthesia with intratracheal intubation)

Early pharyngeal cancer. There are no large patient series on surgical outcome with respect to metastatic nodal status versus depth of submucosal invasion of early pharyngeal cancer. A recent case series (n = 115, median follow-up 34 months) suggested tumor thickness > 1000 μm as a risk factor for LN metastatic recurrence [24]. Structural differences prohibit extending the criteria for ESD in the esophagus to hypopharyngeal squamous cell cancer. Therefore, the indication for ESD of

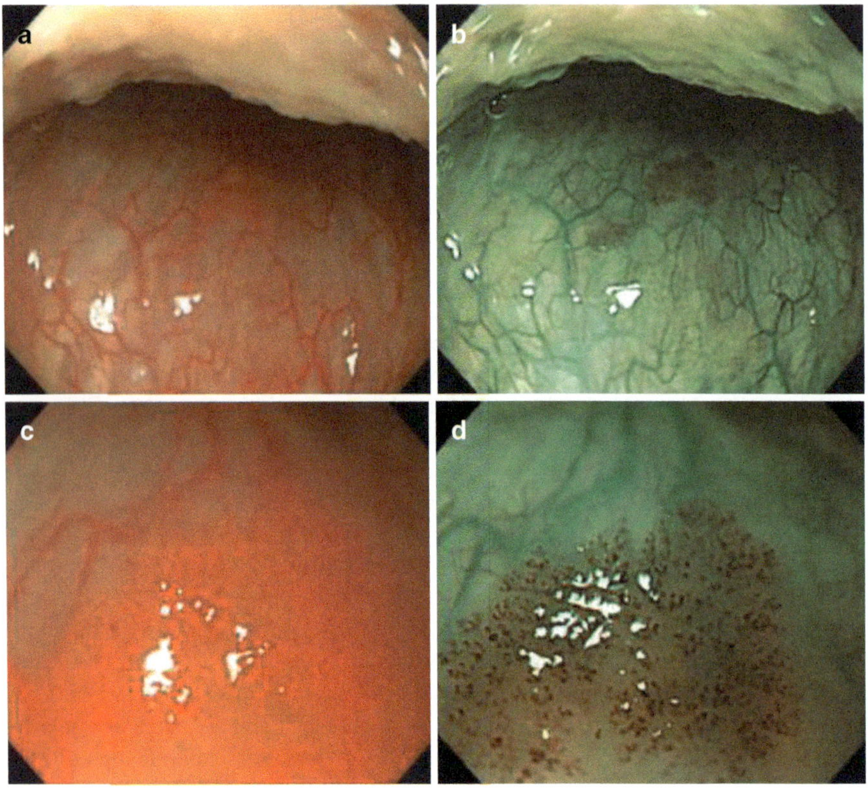

Fig. 7.8 Early pharyngeal SCC, epithelial SCC. (**a**) Small (6.5 × 3 mm) faint reddish spot (lesion 0-IIb) in posterior wall of hypopharynx, WLI. (**b**) A brownish area, NBI (20×). (**c**) Observation of vascular pattern was difficult by WLI (OLYMPUS Lucera). (**d**) *Abnormal loop* B_1, m-NBI (80×). ESD (R0) confirmed SCC pT1a (EP), Ly0, V0

invasive carcinoma is controversial [22]. Small, suitable premalignant neoplasias or epithelial cancers T1a (diameter < 1 cm) may be resectable en bloc with EMR, with larger ones using piecemeal EMR [25]. ESD is technically feasible (Fig. 7.8) and preferable for en bloc resection of lesions larger than 10 mm. The organ-sparing approach is beneficial for pharyngeal function [23, 24].

7.8 Cases: Dysplasia [HGIN] and Early Cancer in Squamous Esophagus and Hypopharynx

Case 1: Minute Esophageal Red Spot

A 72-year-old man underwent screening gastroscopy. On scope insertion, a tiny reddish spot was seen, with brownish appearance on NBI (Fig. 7.9).

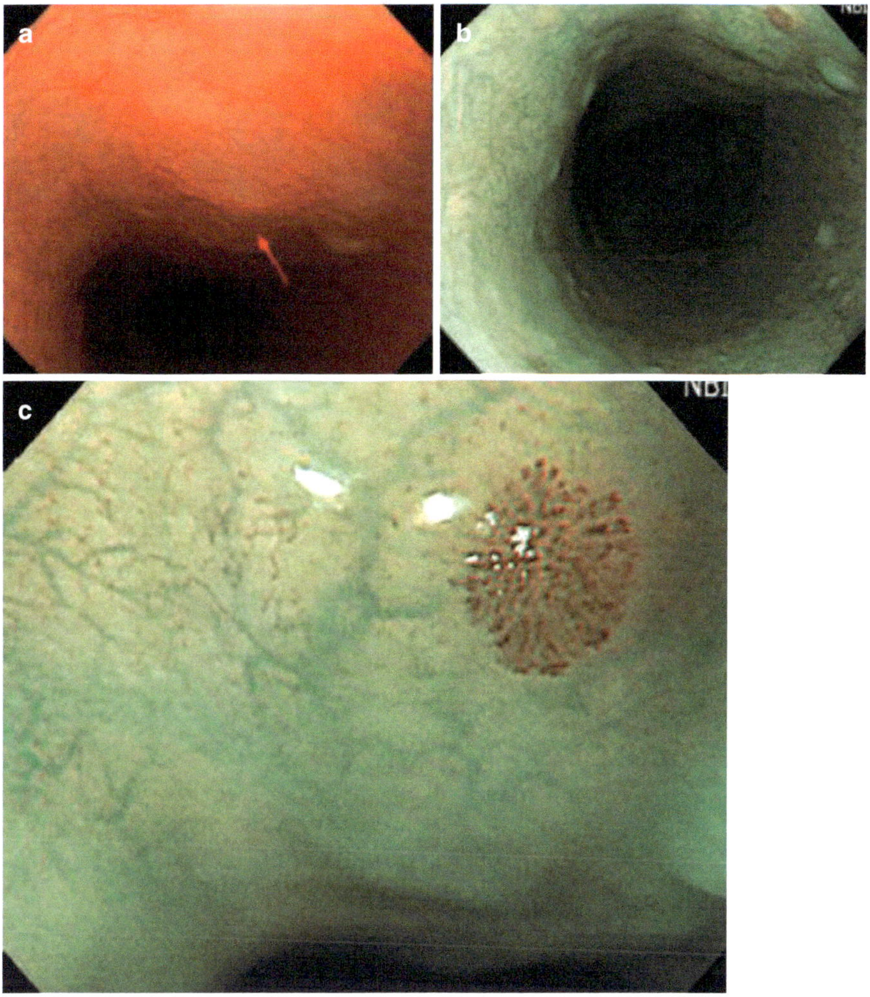

Fig. 7.9 Intramucosal squamous neoplasia (HGIN or SCC T1 m0). (**a**) Small reddish spot on standard WLI (*arrow*), (**b**) Brownish spot on NBI, (**c**) Pattern abnormal loop B1 on m-NBI (80×)

Note Watch for brownish areas during NBI mapping of the esophagus.

Case 2: Flat Reddish Area Oral to the Gastroesophageal Junction
A 65-year-old male smoker presented a reddish depressed lesion at the anterior wall oral to the gastroesophageal (GE) junction. Sophisticated endoscopic analysis favored ESD (Fig. 7.10).

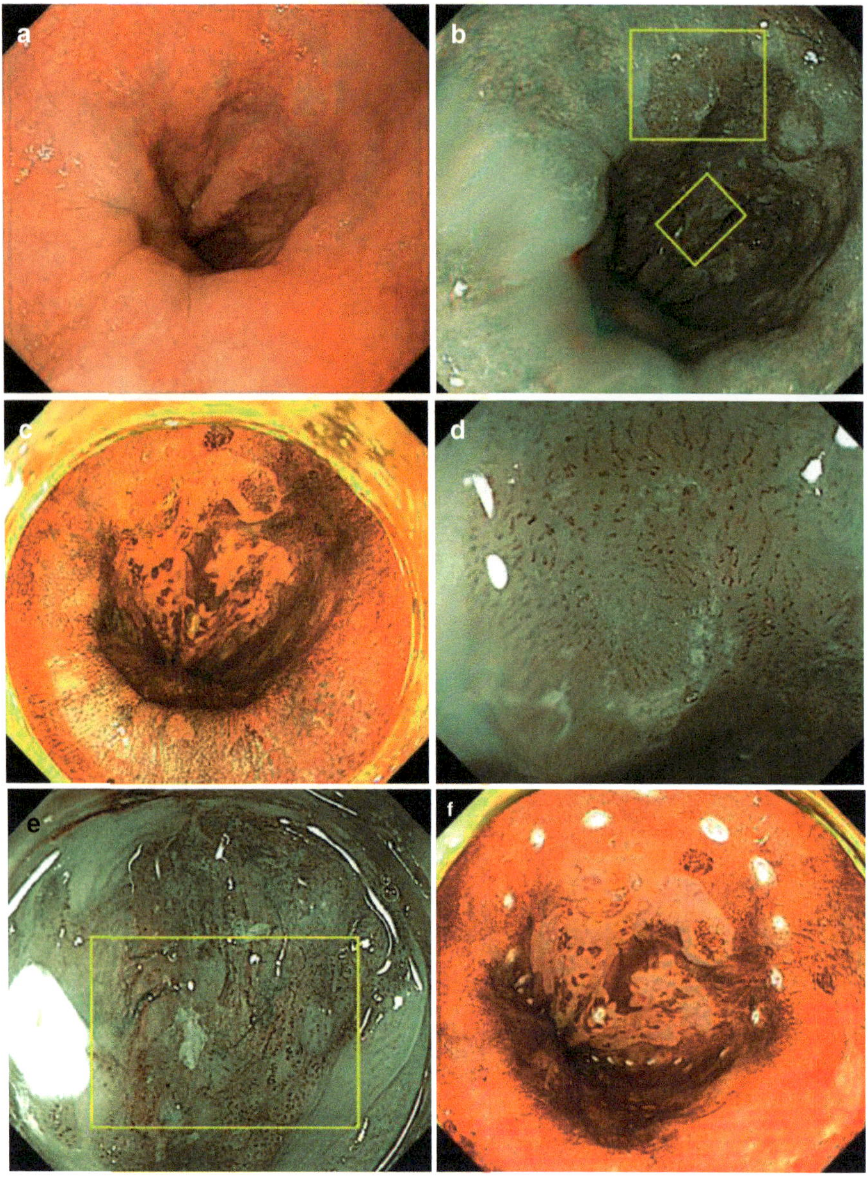

Fig. 7.10 (**a**) Shallow depressed, irregular reddish area, anterior wall of esophagus. (**b**) Irregularly shaped brownish area on NBI (*large* and *small yellow squares* indicate regions shown in (**d**) and (**e**), respectively). (**c**) Lugol-voiding lesion with staining squamous cell (SC) islets. (**d**) Magnifying (80×) NBI analysis of the oral part of the Lugol-voiding lesion showed disappearance of dendritic sm vessel pattern and elongated IPC loops with some dilatation and curling. (**e**) The distal end of the lesion showed disappearance of dendritic sm vessels and some non-loop IPCL pattern (right lower part of square) and thick vessels (middle-left side) without disappearance of sm vessels. *Clinical diagnosis*: cT1 (MM or sm1). *Explanation of M-NBI analysis*: (**d**) The rostral part of the lesion presents pattern type *abnormal loop B1* (JES). (**f**) Lesion (Lugol voiding) and 5 mm safety margin marked for ESD

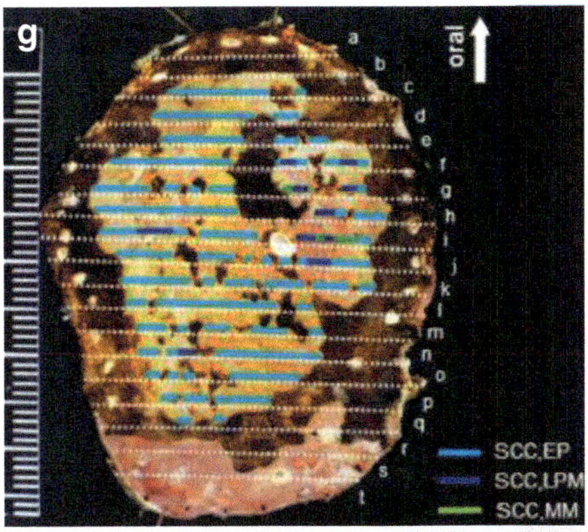

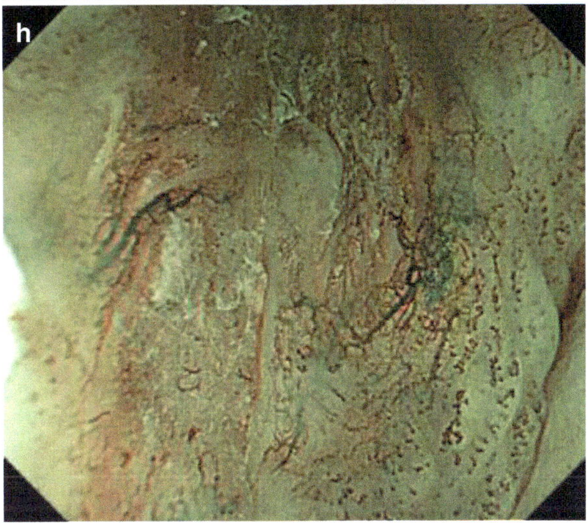

Fig. 7.10 (continued) (**g**) The specimen (Lugol stain), showing invasion depth of cancer on serial section (*color code*). Orientation as on endoscopic image (**f**). *Pathological diagnosis*: SCC type 0-IIc, 38 × 28 mm (in 52 × 40 mm), pT1a(MM, d 1.5 mm), ly(−), v(−), pHM0, pVM0. Resection with free margins R0, curative. (**h**) Magnified view of (**e**), yellow square, shows areas of SCC on right side: disappearance of dendritic sm pattern and pattern non-loop B2 (JES); but on center and left side, "thick" dendritic *sm vessel pattern* (no JES B3!) is visible at GE junction without IPCL pattern, i.e. outside of the neoplasia. (Compare distal margin of GE junction in (**g**) showing Lugol-voiding cylinder cell epithelium at cardia)

Note Do not mistake dendritic sm vessels for thick tumor vessels!

Key Points for SCC:

- *Disappearance* of sm vessel pattern, *and*
- Neoplastic *IPCL patterns B1–B3* are required for endoscopic diagnosis of SCC.

Case 3: Reddish Lesion 0-IIb in Hypopharynx

On gastroscopy, a flat reddish lesion was pointed out at the right recessus piriformis in a 58-year-old man, a chronic cigarette smoker. Endoscopic criteria indicated mucosal SCC resectable by ESD (Fig. 7.11).

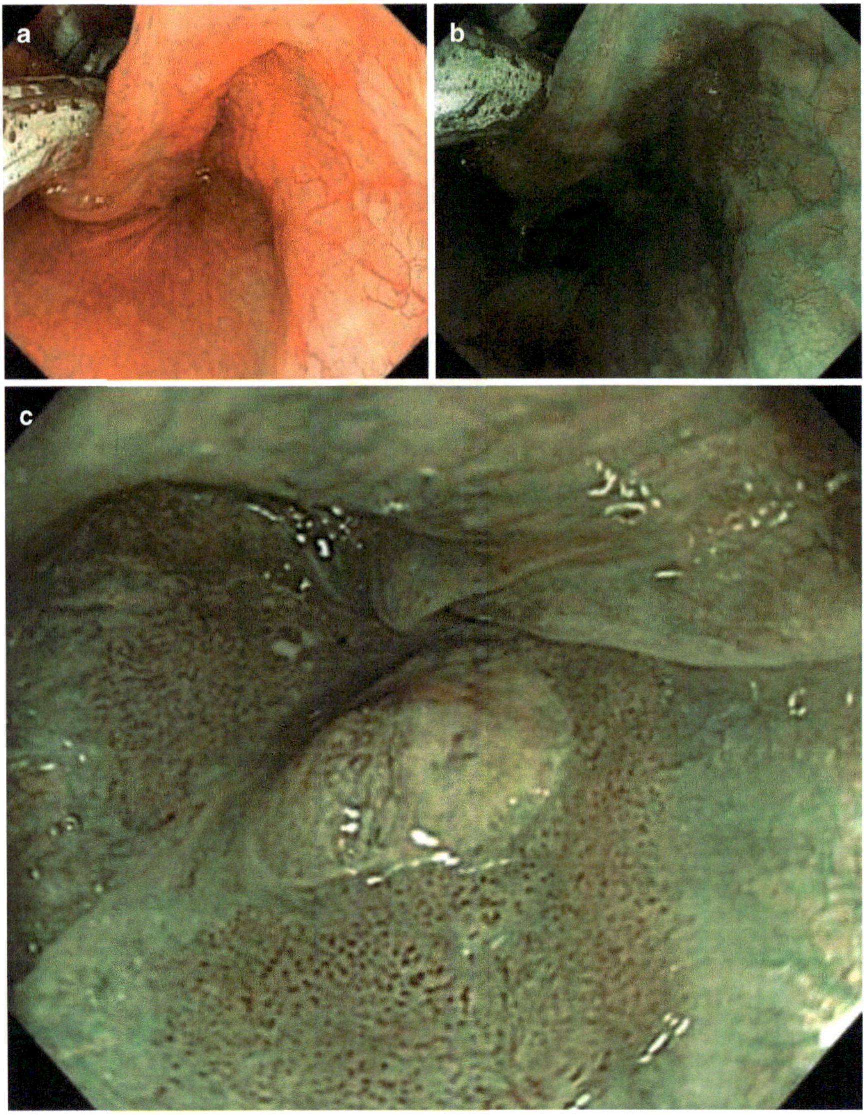

Fig. 7.11 Early SCC in right recessus piriformis of hypopharynx, ESD endoscopic view (**a**) with standard WLI; (**b**) with NBI (tracheal intubation); (**c**) neoplasia 0-IIa + IIb abnormal loop B1, NBI (40×)

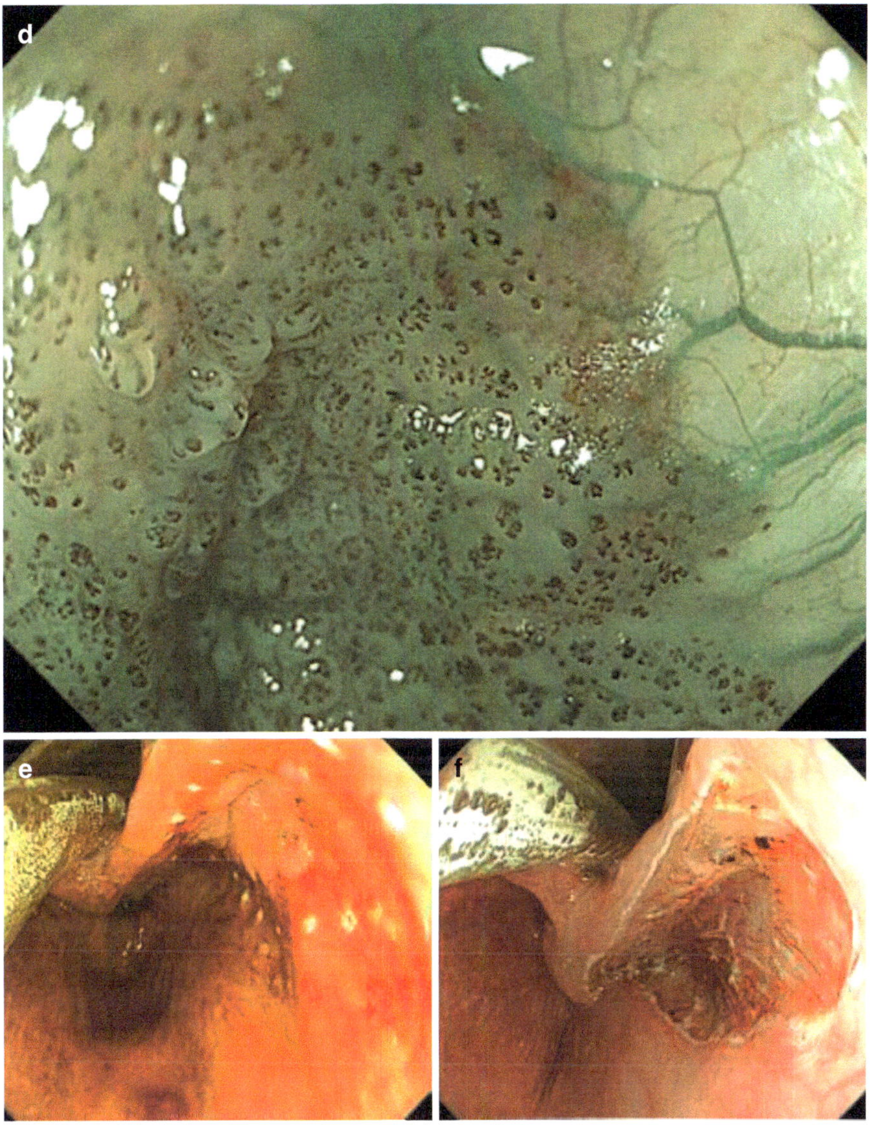

Fig. 7.11 (continued) (**d**) IPCL abnormal loop B1, non-loop B2, M-NBI (80×). (**e**) Lugol-voiding SCC and markings of safety margin (WLI). (**f**) Resection bed after hook-knife ESD (WLI)

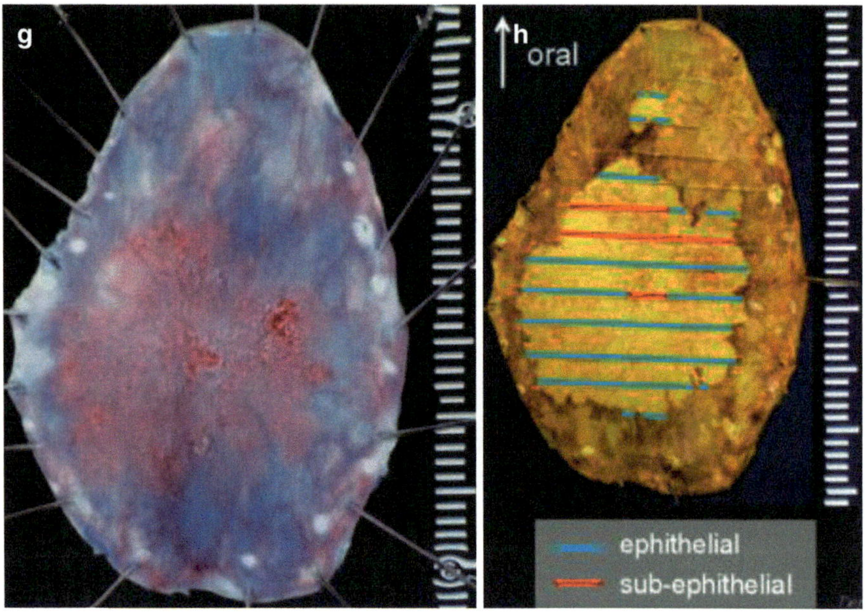

Fig. 7.11 (continued) (**g**) Specimen (50 × 39 mm, for histological workup). (**h**) Two SCC: *no. 1 (top)*, hypopharyngeal SCC, subepithelial invasion (depth 1000 μm, width 2.5 mm), and *no. II* (larger) hypopharyngeal epithelial SCC, ly 0, v0, HM0, VM0, 0-IIa + IIb, 22 × 19 mm. *SCC no. 2*, hypopharyngeal SCC, epithelial, ly0, v0, HM0, VM0, 0-IIb, 4 × 3 mm

Note Provided special expertise and equipment is available, ESD of early SCC in hypopharynx/glottis is organ-sparing and may be curative (although criteria need prospective evaluation).

Acknowledgments We acknowledge the contribution of cases by Dr. Hans-Peter Allgaier, Freiburg, Germany; Dr. Gerhard Kleber, Aalen, Germany; and Dr. Daniel Neureiter and Dr. Frieder Berr, Salzburg, Austria.

References

1. Muto M, et al. Early detection of superficial squamous cell carcinoma in the head and neck region and esophagus by narrow band imaging: a multicenter randomized controlled trial. J Clin Oncol. 2010;28:1566–72.
2. Yokoyama A, et al. Risk appraisal and endoscopic screening for esophageal squamous cell carcinoma in Japanese populations. Esophagus. 2007;4:135–43.
3. Takubo K, et al. Early squamous cell carcinoma of the oesophagus: the Japanese viewpoint. Histopathology. 2007;51:733–42.
4. Kodama M, et al. Treatment of superficial cancer of the esophagus: a summary of responses to a questionnaire on superficial cancer of the esophagus in Japan. Surgery. 1998;123:432–9.

5. Kuwano H, et al. Guidelines for diagnosis and treatment of carcinoma of the esophagus April 2012 edited by the Japan Esophageal Society. Esophagus, 2015;12:1–30.
6. Oyama T, et al. Diagnosis and long-term results and prognosis of m3 and sm1 Esophageal Cancer. Lymph nodal metastasis of m3, sm1 esophageal cancer. Stomach Intestine. 2002;37:71–4.
7. Oyama T, et al. Endoscopic submucosal dissection of early esophageal cancer. Clin Gastroenterol Hepatol. 2005;3:S67–70.
8. Ishihara R, et al. Significance of each narrow-band imaging finding in diagnosing squamous mucosal high-grade neoplasia of the esophagus. J Gastroenterol Hepatol. 2010;25:1410–5.
9. Inoue H, et al. Lugol chromoendoscopy for esophageal squamous cell cancer. Endoscopy. 2001;33:75–9.
10. Ishihara R, et al. Quantitative analysis of the color change after iodine staining for diagnosing esophageal high-grade intraepithelial neoplasia and invasive cancer. Gastrointest Endosc. 2009;69:213–8.
11. Oyama T, et al. Prediction of the invasion depth of superficial squamous cell carcinoma based on microvessel morphology: magnifying endoscopic classification of the Japan Esophageal Society. Esophagus. 2017;14:105–12.
12. Inoue H, et al. Magnification endoscopy in esophagela squamous cell carcinoma: a review of the intrapapillary capillary loop classification. Ann Gastroenterol. 2015;28:41–8.
13. Arima M, et al. Evaluation of microvascular patterns of superficial esophageal cancers by magnifying endoscopy. Esophagus. 2005;2:191–7.
14. Yoshida T, et al. Narrow-band imaging system with magnifying endoscopy for superficial esophageal lesions. Gastrointest Endosc. 2004;59:288–95.
15. Yokoyama A, et al. Esophageal melanosis, an endoscopic finding associated with squamous cell neoplasms of the upper aerodigestive tract, and inactive aldehyde dehydrogenase-2 in alcoholic Japanese men. J Gastroenterol. 2005;40:676–84.
16. Pham AM, et al. Endoscopic removal of a giant fibrovascular polyp of the esophagus. Ann Otol Rhinol Laryngol. 2008;117:587–90.
17. The Paris endoscopic classification of superficial neoplastic lesions: esophagus, stomach, and colon: November 30 to December 1, 2002. Gastrointest Endosc. 2003;58:S3–43.
18. May A, et al. Accuracy of staging in early oesophageal cancer using high resolution endoscopy and high resolution endosonography: a comparative, prospective, and blinded trial. Gut. 2004;53:634–40.
19. Ishihara R, et al. Comparison of EMR and endoscopic submucosal dissection for en bloc resection of early esophageal cancers in Japan. Gastrointest Endosc. 2008;68:1066–72.
20. Pech O, et al. Curative endoscopic therapy in patients with early esophageal squamous-cell carcinoma or high-grade intraepithelial neoplasia. Endoscopy. 2007;39:30–5.
21. Shimizu Y, et al. Long-term outcome after endoscopic mucosal resection in patients with esophageal squamous cell carcinoma invading the muscularis mucosae or deeper. Gastrointest Endosc. 2002;56:387–90.
22. Fujishiro M. Perspective on the practical indications of endoscopic submucosal dissection of gastrointestinal neoplasms. World J Gastroenterol. 2008;14:4289–95.
23. Shimizu Y, et al. Endoscopic submucosal dissection for treatment of early stage hypopharyngeal carcinoma. Gastrointest Endosc. 2006;64:255–9; discussion 260-252.
24. Kinjo Y, et al. The short-term and long-term outcomes of the endoscopic resection for the superficial pharyngeal squamous cell carcinoma. Endosc Int Open. 2015;3:E266–73.
25. Fujishiro M, et al. Application of endoscopic mucosal resection for hypopharyngeal cancer. Dig Endosc. 2001;13:220–4.

Chapter 8
Columnar Epithelium-Lined (Barrett's) Esophagus: Mucosal Neoplasias

Pierre H. Deprez and Takashi Toyonaga

The incidence of adenocarcinoma of the esophagogastric junction (EGJ) and lower esophagus has steadily increased during the past five decades in Western industrialized countries, probably due to the increasing prevalence of chronic gastroesophageal reflux disease (GERD) [1]. An adaptive reaction to chronic inflammatory stimuli in the squamous epithelium at the EGJ is the formation of columnar epithelium that can lead to field cancerization [2]. Barrett's esophagus (BE) carries an annual risk (0.12–0.5%) of transformation to adenocarcinoma (BE-AC) [3]. The incidence of AC at the EGJ is five-fold to ten-fold lower in Japan and East Asia but is also rising, and BE is becoming a target for surveillance [4]. Patients with chronic GERD should be on proton pump inhibitor therapy for 4 weeks prior to surveillance endoscopy, to improve detection of neoplastic lesions in the absence of flat inflammatory lesions. On BE surveillance, BE-AC has often been diagnosed as early BE-AC in stage 0 (66%) or stage 1 (26%), and overall survival of the patients was normal [5]. Recommendations for screening and surveillance are detailed in Chap. 6.

Note Barrett's neoplasia can be treated by resection and ablation, depending on the presence of visible lesions. Endoscopic imaging is therefore crucial to detect subtle mucosal abnormalities that will need endoscopic mucosal resection (EMR) or endoscopic submucosal dissection (ESD) before ablation of the remaining Barrett's extent.

P. H. Deprez (✉)
Department of Hepato-Gastroenterologie, Cliniques Universitaires Saint-Luc, Université Catholique de Louvain, Brussels, Belgium
e-mail: pdeprez@uclouvain.be

T. Toyonaga
Department of Endoscopy, Kobe University Hospital, Kobe, Japan

F. Berr et al. (eds.), *Atlas of Early Neoplasias of the Gastrointestinal Tract*,
https://doi.org/10.1007/978-3-030-01114-7_8

8.1 Diagnosis and Examination of Barrett's Esophagus

Endoscopic examination requires a standardized approach to define the extent of Barrett's esophagus with Prague chromoendoscopy (CE) criteria [6–8]. The diagnosis of BE is made if the distal esophagus is lined with *columnar epithelium* with a minimum length of 1 cm (tongues or circular) and containing *specialized intestinal metaplasia* (histopathological examination; *see* Chap. 2) (Fig. 8.1) [8]:

- On white light endoscopy (WLI), columnar-appearing mucosa, slightly reddish, contrasts with cardiac columnar and esophageal squamous mucosa.
- Identify the EGJ as at the tops of the gastric mucosal folds (Western definition) or the distal end of esophageal palisade vessels (East Asian definition) [2].
- If hiatus hernia is present, do not mistake the diaphragmatic hiatal impression for the EGJ.
- For circumferential columnar-appearing mucosa, define its extent in centimeters above the EGJ: report as the C value.

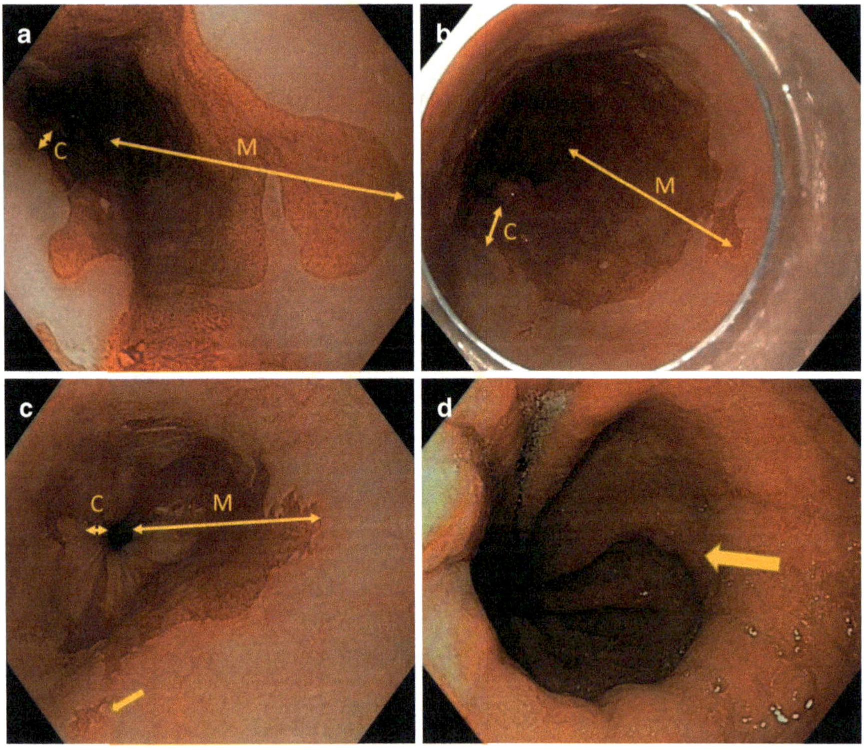

Fig. 8.1 Barrett's cases examined in white light endoscopy (WLI), using Prague classification. (**a**) C1M5. (**b**) C1M4. (**c**) C0M3. The *small arrow* shows a small islet above the maximum extent of BE. (**d**) *Large arrow* shows top of gastric folds at site of esophagogastric sphincter

- For any tongue-like areas of columnar-appearing mucosa, measure the maximum extent in centimeters above the EGJ: report as the M value.
- Islets of BE above the maximum extent should be reported separately.

Mucosal surface and vascular patterns may widely differ in BE. They will be better defined using magnification and optical chromoendoscopy techniques. Mucosal surface will even be better analyzed with acetic acid combined with optical chromoendoscopy and magnification. The examination technique involves cleaning the mucosa with water or saline, using a cap if needed, and describing the vascular pattern (VP) and surface pattern (SP). To this end, use magnification before acetic acid staining (for VP and SP) and after the staining (SP, and loss of VP). Examples are shown in Fig. 8.2. Various classifications have been proposed by Japanese authors, such as M-NBI with five different SPs, and the corresponding VPs. To simplify, the mucosal pattern can either be flat and atrophic or it can be "rich" with tubuli, villi, and ridges. Intestinal metaplasia can show the same pattern as in the stomach, with the light blue crests (LBC). Vessels are better seen in the atrophic type (arborized brown capillaries and larger greenish submucosal veins), but regular capillaries can also be observed in the villi-type mucosa. Figure 8.2 shows some

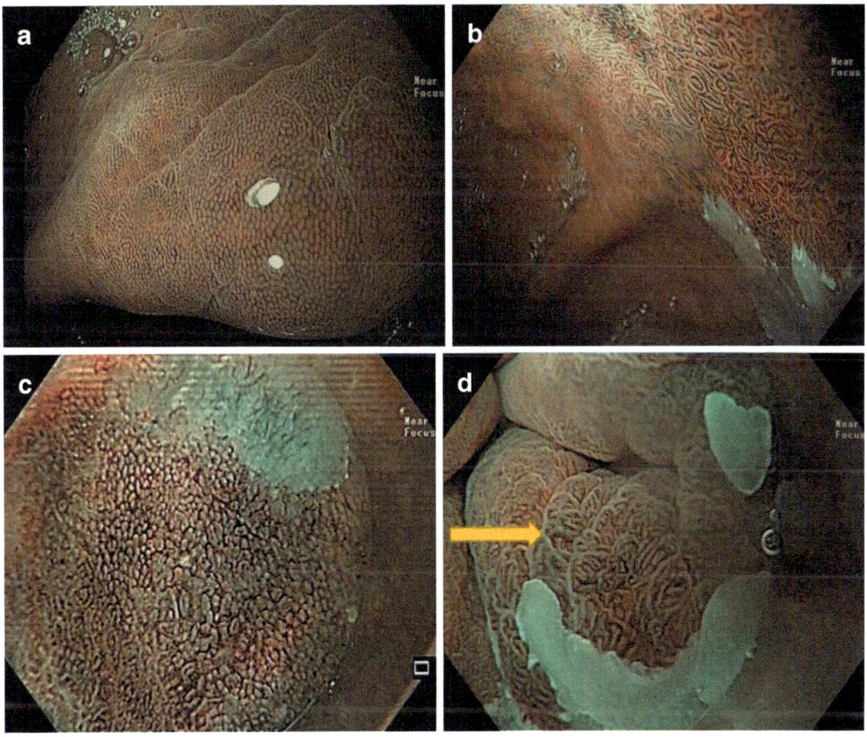

Fig. 8.2 NBI imaging of *Barrett's cases* showing (**a**) junction between normal gastric (pits) and regular ridges from Barrett's esophagus; (**b**) regular mucosal surface (ridges), and vascular pattern; (**c**) regular mucosal surface (villous, some pits) and vascular pattern; (**d**) more abundant villi mucosal surface with LBC (light blue crest) typical of intestinal metaplasia (*arrow*)

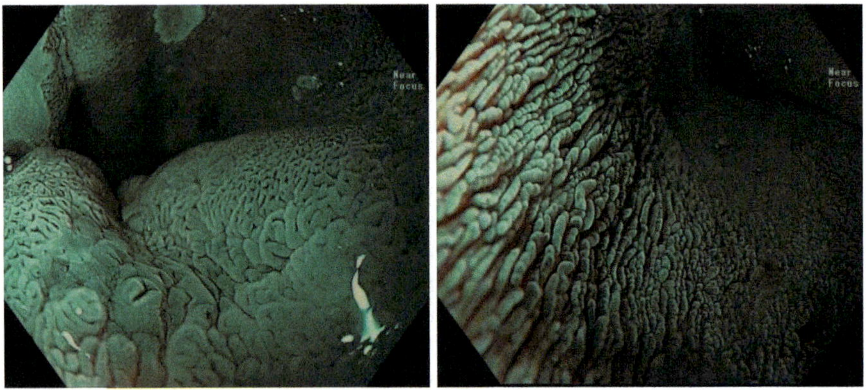

Fig. 8.3 Acetic acid chromoendoscopy (CE) with NBI and magnification showing a surface pattern of villi and ridges (*left panel*) and tubuli pattern (*right panel*)

examples. For imaging examples, the Nottingham classification (not validated) is given in the Appendix of this chapter.

Note *Acetic acid* amplifies the surface structure but loses the vascular pattern, as shown in Fig. 8.3.

8.2 Procedure for Detection and Analysis of Barrett's Neoplasia

A diagnosis of esophageal adenocarcinoma is virtually always associated with an endoscopically *visible lesion*, which requires endoscopic resection for staging and treatment. To detect these lesions, examination should start in WLI, then optical chromoendoscopy without and with magnification, and finally acetic acid chromoendoscopy (CE). Maximum magnification and sharpness of still images is achieved using a distal hood combined with water immersion (Compare Sects. 1.5.1, 1.5.2, 1.7.3, 2.5.1). Neoplastic lesions have a predilection to be found in the right upper and lower quadrant in the left lateral position. The aim is to detect subtle changes in color (*reddish with WLI*) or surface relief, and to characterize any visible lesion for location, color, size, and type, according to the Paris classification (*see* Fig. 1.2) [9–11]. Visible lesions show up as color changes (mostly reddish or glossy-pale; brownish on NBI), elevation or depression (0-IIa or 0-IIc; rarely [15%] 0-Is/p or 0-III), and surface irregularity with type 0-IIb (Fig. 8.4).

Most (85%) early malignant Barrett's neoplasias are diminutive and flat lesions (0-IIa,b,c) and are difficult to detect [12, 13]. When there are no visible lesions on WLI or magnifying NBI endoscopy (M-NBI), chromoendoscopy with 2.5% acetic acid may reveal covert lesions as *focal loss of acetowhitening* on standard WLI, i.e.

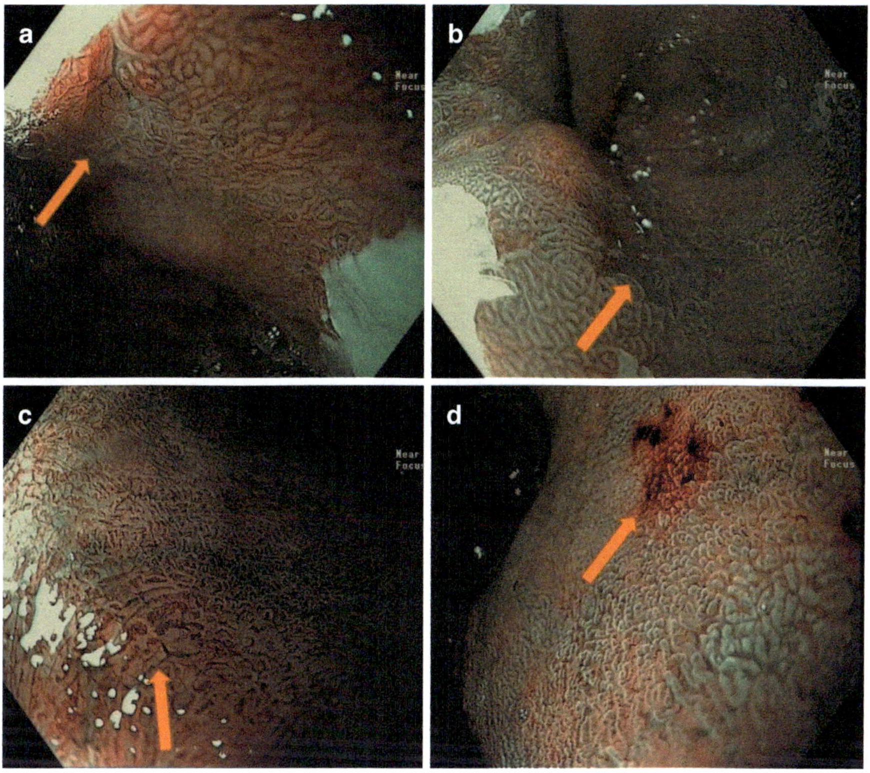

Fig. 8.4 M-NBI (near focus, Olympus HQ190) showing focal visible lesions (*arrows*). (**a**, **b**) Paris 0-II b or c with mucosal irregularity; (**c**) irregular capillaries; or (**d**) small bleeding site with acetic acid CE

as slightly reddish spots in whitish-staining regular Barrett mucosa. Portsmouth Acetic Acid Classification (PREDICT) detected neoplastic Barrett's lesions as *focal loss of acetowhitening* with 98% sensitivity and 97% negative predictive value [14] (*see* Fig. 8.11b).

Note Any suspect Barrett's lesion must be analyzed for VP in M-NBI, followed by 2.5% acetic acid stain to diagnose SP. This procedure is essential to characterize *irregular VP* and *irregular SP* and *demarcation line* around any Barrett's neoplasia (analogous to early gastric cancer [15]) (Fig. 8.5).

Figure 8.6 illustrates the difference between regular and irregular vascular and mucosal patterns, following a simplified classification (BING) more often used in the Western world [16–18]. Experts and nonexperts distinguished these two categories with very high sensitivity (90–95%) and accuracy (93–97%) [19]. Basically, this differential diagnosis is feasible, but prospective evaluation of V/S pattern classification in clinical studies is still pending for accurate diagnosis of Barrett's lesions.

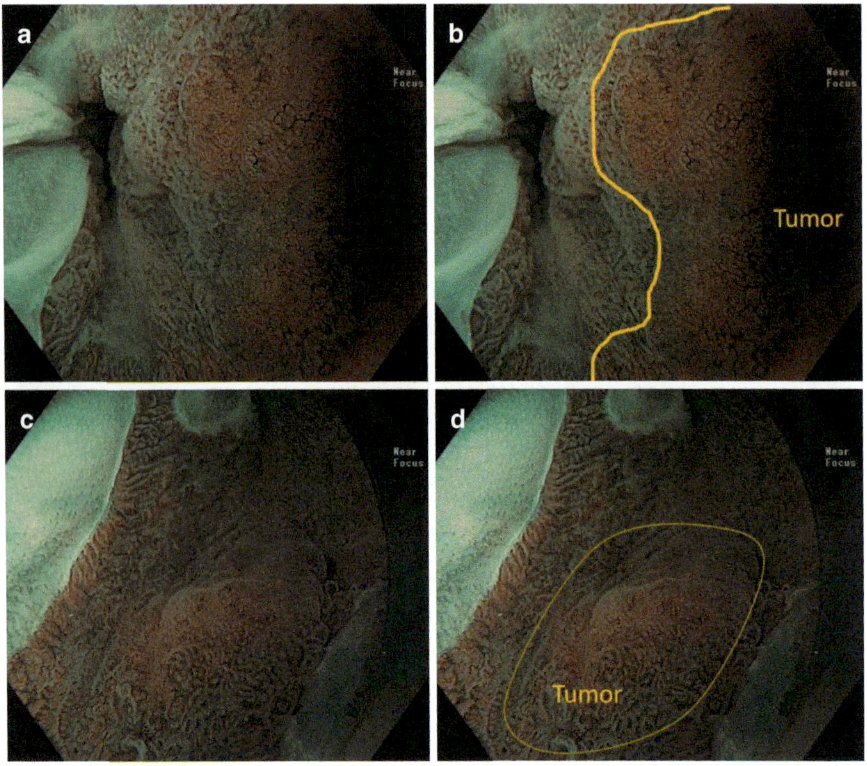

Fig. 8.5 Illustration of the role of M-NBI with water immersion (in an intubated anesthetized patient) to demarcate visible lesions. (**a**, **b**) Paris 0-IIb high-grade neoplasia. (**c**, **d**) Paris 0-IIa, pT1m2 adenocarcinoma

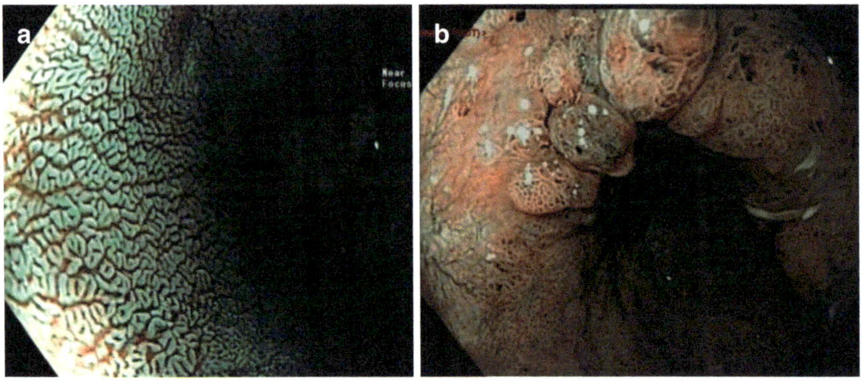

Fig. 8.6 (**a**) A regular mucosal pattern. (**b**) Irregularities and nodularity (pT1m3 adenocarcinoma)

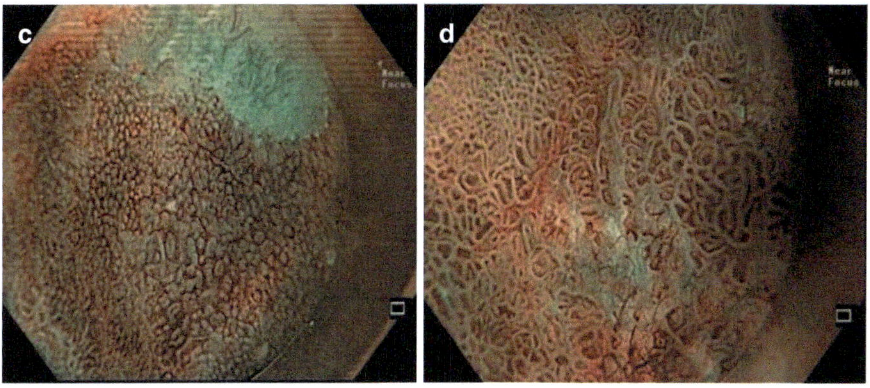

Fig. 8.6 (continued) (**c**) A regular vascular network. (**d**) A small area with an irregular vascular pattern corresponding to focal high-grade neoplasia

Table 8.1 Distribution of Macroscopic Types in Early Barrett Neoplasias, and sm Invasiveness and Poorly Differentiated Grading per Type[a]

	Lesions, *n*	**Macroscopic type**					
		I	**IIa**	**IIb**	**IIc**	**IIa + c**	**III**
Early Barrett neoplasia	380	13%	37%	28%	5%	16%	2%[b]
sm invasive (*n* = 42)	Per type	10%	14%	3%	24%	18%	(0)[b]
G3 (*n* = 21)	Per type	10%	6%	2%	(0)[b]	8%	(0)[b]
Neoplasia category according to macroscopic type							
HGIN	30	7%	17%	70%	3%	0	3%
T 1a	308	14%	37%	27%	4%	17%	2%
T 1b	42	12%	45%	7%	10%	26%	(0)[b]

HGIN high-grade intraepithelial neoplasia, *sm* submucosa
[a]According to Pech et al. [12]
[b]Type 0-III lesions and G3 are prone to referral bias (underestimation)

8.3 Endoscopic Diagnosis of sm-Invasive Cancer in Barrett's Esophagus

Most samples of BE mucosa show duplication or multilayering of the MM layer because myofibroblasts formed a superficial layer (SMM) in the LPM above the original MM (deeper MM, DMM). Depth of sm invasion is measured from the lower end of the DMM. Barrett cancers pT1a show mainly low-risk criteria (95%). However among BE-AC pT1b, high-risk criteria—budding Bd $\geq$ 2; grading G3; L(+), V(+)—are frequent, up to about 30%, and risk of LN metastasis rises to 30–50% with T1b-SM2-3 [20].

Macroscopic types have close association with the risk of submucosal invasion of that neoplastic lesion [12] (Table 8.1). In a large prospective series of 380 early Barrett's neoplasias, most of the high-grade intraepithelial neoplasia (HGIN) lesions were type 0-IIb (70%) and 0-IIa (17%). The likelihood of submucosal invasive early cancer was lowest for lesions type 0-IIb (3%); it progressively increased for lesions type 0-I (10%), 0-IIa (14%), IIa + c (18%), and 0-IIc (24%) [12]. In spite of high risk of deep sm invasion for protruded type 0-Is early cancer, softness on palpation and flattening on distension by air insufflation (AID +) suggest mucosal neoplasia without or with only superficial sm invasion, suitable for diagnostic ESD. Because of difficult recording at the EGJ, high-frequency EUS (20–30 MHz) was not reliable enough to detect submucosal invasion in neoplastic Barrett's lesions at that location (sensitivity only 27%) [21].

The simplified M-NBI classification (*BING classification*) for changes of SP and VP gives no information as to any characteristics for sm-invasion of adenocarcinoma [16]. In contrast to the BING classification, the previous *Nottingham classification* uses similar simplified descriptors for non-neoplastic lesions; descriptors for neoplastic lesions include "irregular SP & irregular VP" or "absent SP & irregular VP," and for sm-invasive adenocarcinoma, "severely irregular SP & VP," with specifically detailed description and excellent magnifying NBI endoscopic images [22] (*see* Fig. 8.18). Corresponding to these SP types, the VP types have been detailed by Goda et al. [23]. Therefore, the Nottingham classification supplemented with Goda's VP types (*See* Sect. 8.6, Table 8.2) better tries to define whether superficial Barrett cancer is indicated for endoscopic resection or already contraindicated when showing signs of deep sm invasion [22–24]. Evaluation in prospective clinical studies would be essential to create a diagnostic algorithm like that established for differentiated gastric cancer [15]. (Compare Fig. 9.9a.)

Signs suspect for sm-invasion are summarized below and shown in Figs. 8.7, 8.8 and 8.9 and in the Sect. 8.5 Cases. All provide examples of endoscopic signs corresponding to proven histology. These signs are taken in analogy to endoscopic diagnostics for early gastric adenocarcinoma [15, 25], but they have not been prospectively evaluated for Barrett's neoplasias.

Note *Superficial sm invasion* may show:

- Macroscopic types 0-Is (soft consistency), 0-IIa, IIc, IIa + c
- *and*
- Highly irregular villous surface pattern (high density, variable sizes, fused villi)
- Irregular dense vascular pattern

Deep sm-invasion may show:

- Types 0-Is (firm consistency), 0-IIa, IIc, IIa + c −/+ nodule, or 0-III
- *and*
- Highly irregular vascular pattern (variable, loose density, long runs, and thick vessel)
- Amorphous or irregular absent surface pattern

BE-AC lesions bordering at squamous epithelium (SCE) very often (50–80%) extend underneath SCE for up to 5 mm distance; they are sometimes even detectable on M-NBI by *minimal elevation* and faintly *brownish, translucent VP* beneath SCE [26]. Therefore, an extended safety distance of 10 mm around BE neoplasia is good practice for resection, especially ESD [11].

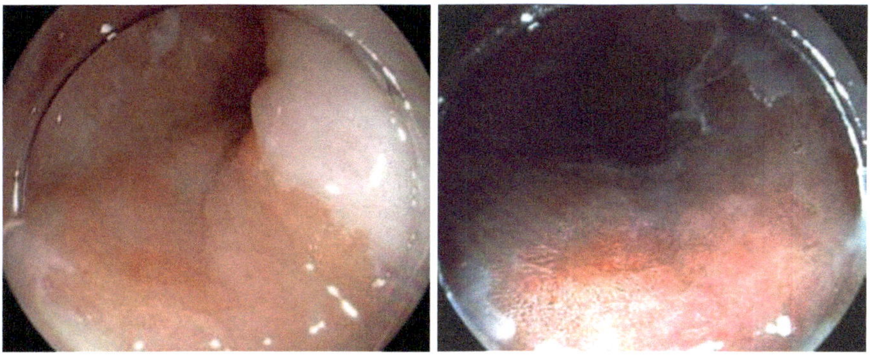

Fig. 8.7 Barrett's esophagus, depressed lesion type 0-IIc with microinvasion of the submucosa, irregular pit pattern. [Pentax WLI (*left*) and i-scan (*right*), ˜20-fold.]. (Courtesy of Dr. Ralf Kiesslich, Germany.)

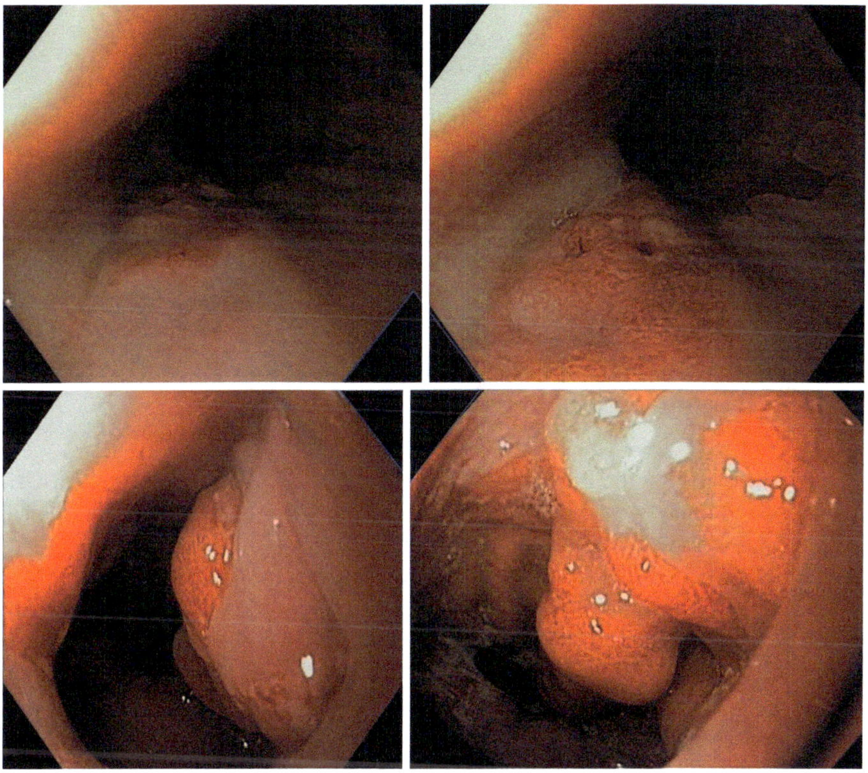

Fig. 8.8 Barrett's esophagus. (**Top panel**) pT1sm1, G3, LV- adenocarcinoma (Paris 0-IIa, soft consistency, irregular vessels. **(Bottom panel)** pT1sm2, G2, L+ adenocarcinoma (Paris 0–1 s, firm consistency, irregular vessels)

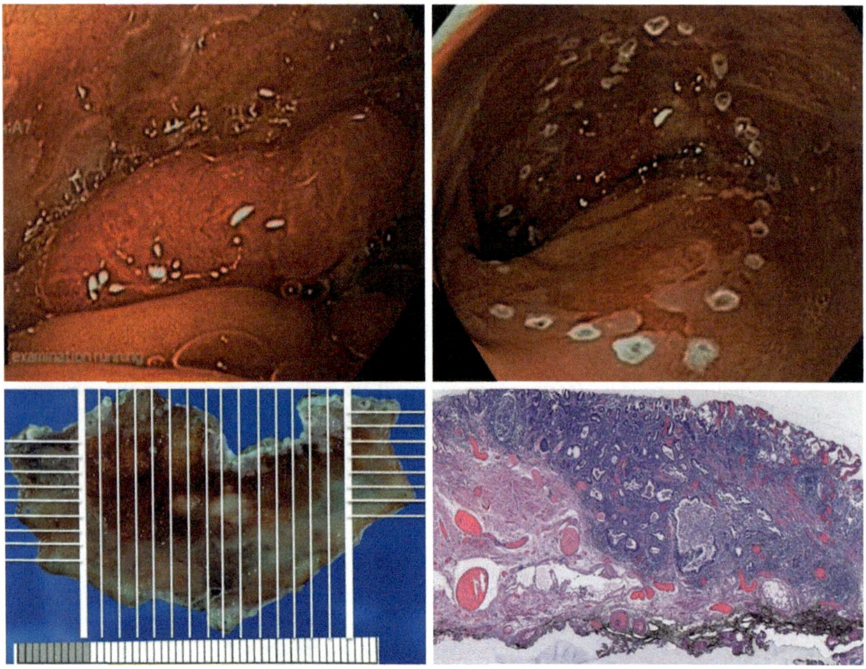

Fig. 8.9 C2M3 Barrett's esophagus, 2-cm elevated lesions Paris 0-IIs, with en bloc and curative ESD in a 60-year-old patient. Macroscopic view of en bloc specimen measuring 5.6 × 3.6 cm shows two central brownish lesions; white lines indicate axis of cut. Histologic appearance shows an esophageal adenocarcinoma with limited invasion of the submucosa, and with free vertical and horizontal margins. Final diagnosis and staging: pT1sm1, G1, L–, V–

8.4 Endoscopic Resection of Early Neoplasias in Barrett's Esophagus

Guidelines issued by the European Society of Gastrointestinal Endoscopy (ESGE) (supported in many Western countries) still give credit to EMR, even in piecemeal fashion, for complete endoscopic resection of *mucosal* BE-AC [27]. This is evidence-based, because outcome of EMR in a large cohort with *mucosal* BE-AC (n = 1000) was favorable, with a 96% rate of complete resection, 14% local or metachronous recurrence, 86% disease-free survival (DFS), and 94% complete remission at 5 years [28]. Thus, complete remission 5 years after EMR was similar to the rate of DFS after ESD, at lower procedure costs, less effort, and lower risk of complications (*see* Table 3.2), assuming accurate diagnosis of mucosal BE-AC. The ESGE has given preference to ESD only for Barrett lesions larger than 15 mm with signs of superficial sm invasion or when lifting of the lesion is inadequate for EMR (e.g. due to sm fibrosis or scarring after previous resection) [27].

In fact, Manner et al. had proposed to expand EMR criteria for low-risk BE-AC (G1, G2, L0, V0) to T1b-SM1 (<500 μm), because only 1.4% of this subgroup had

LN metastasis [29]. In the meantime, eight prospective series (431 patients, mainly from Western centers) were reported on ESD for superficial BE-AC, with median rates of 91% en bloc resection, 99% DFS at 3 years, and zero perforation, mortality, or recurrence (*see* Table 3.2). Hence, ESD achieves curative resection and close to zero recurrence for BE-AC, and could avoid frequent follow-up endoscopies (four times in the first year and annually thereafter) as recommended for PM-EMR. Besides endoscopic follow-up, complete thermal ablation, such as with radiofrequency ablation, is generally recommended for any residual Barrett epithelium after endoscopic resection of HGIN or cancer [6, 8, 27, 30]. For outcome of ESD and complications, in particular esophageal stenosis, compare Chap. 3.

Barrett's adenocarcinoma is rare in Japan, and *guideline criteria* of the Japan Esophageal Society (JES) for endoscopic en-bloc resection [4] are based on risk of LN metastasis reported in the literature:

ESD – classic indication[a, c]

- Barrett AC type 0-II (HGIN, G1, G2), intramucosal (m1, *LPM*), no ulcer.

ESD – expanded indication[b, c]

- Barrett AC type 0-II (HGIN, G1, G2), mucosal (*MM*), clinical N 0.

[a]Indications with risk of LNM < 1%

[b]Indications with risk of LNM or systemic M < 4%

[c]Increased risk for stricture formation, when ESD extends for ≥70% of circumference

Two series of esophagectomy for early BE-AC observed LN metastasis in category pT1a in 1.9% (26/1350 patients) [31], and 1.3% (1/75) with one case of undifferentiated AC G3 pT1a-MM, whereas 22% of category T1b had LN metastasis [32]. The risk factors for LN metastasis (tumor histology, size, ulceration) have not been clarified in detail, so the JES established these ESD criteria (LPM/MM) [4]. By contrast, the Paris Workshop consensus adopted T1b sm1 ≤ 500 μm below the deeper muscularis mucosae (DMM) for low-risk BEAC (G1 or G2, L0, V0, Bd ≤ 1), similar to gastric cancer [10]. Nevertheless, the data basis for sm-invasive Barrett carcinoma resected with lymphadenectomy is too scarce to *prove* any depth limit of sm-invasion permissible for curative endoscopic R0 resection [11].

Lately for superficial sm-invasive early cancer in the esophagus and EGJ, ESD has been recommended as the *diagnostic procedure,* before major curative surgery is considered, especially in very elderly or comorbid patients. ESD is a low-risk, minimally invasive resection technique, even in poor surgical-risk patients, and is increasingly becoming part of adjuvant and even palliative anticancer therapy protocols [33, 34]. Nevertheless, the data basis of ESD for adenocarcinoma at the EGJ and in BE is underpowered to issue strong guideline recommendations; prospective clinical studies are still required, both for accuracy of endoscopic diagnosis and indication and for the outcome of ESD with curative or diagnostic intent.

Contraindications for endoscopic resection:

- Undifferentiated carcinoma G3 > 1 cm in size
- Evidence of deep SM invasion (>SM1)

Relative contraindications (depending on experience of the operator):

- Very poor technical resectability (e.g. difficult-to-manage esophageal varices)
- Frank bleeding diathesis (e.g. combined antiplatelet and anticoagulant therapy)

Indications for esophagectomy and LN dissection after diagnostic ESD:

- Differentiated AC G1 or G2 with deep sm-invasion (≥500 μm)
- Lymphatic or vascular invasion (L1 or V1)
- Poorly differentiated AC G3 with tumor size >10 mm
- Resection R1 at vertical margin (but follow-up for R1 lateral margin)

8.5 Cases: Dysplasia and Early Cancer in Barrett's Esophagus

Case 1: Early Barrett neoplasia type 0-Is
A 72-year-old, healthy man (ASA II°) with short-segment Barrett's esophagus presented a sessile neoplastic lesion type 0-Is within a hiatal hernia (Fig. 8.10). The sessile lesion showed irregular S and V patterns (+ few loose, thick vessels → sm invasion) but was soft and well-lifting on injection. Diagnostic ESD en-bloc revealed BE-AC pT1b-sm2 (723 μm). He was referred for esophagectomy.

Note With borderline signs of sm-invasion, avoid R2 resection! Diagnostic ESD en bloc was justifiable and yielded adequate histopathology for a management decision.

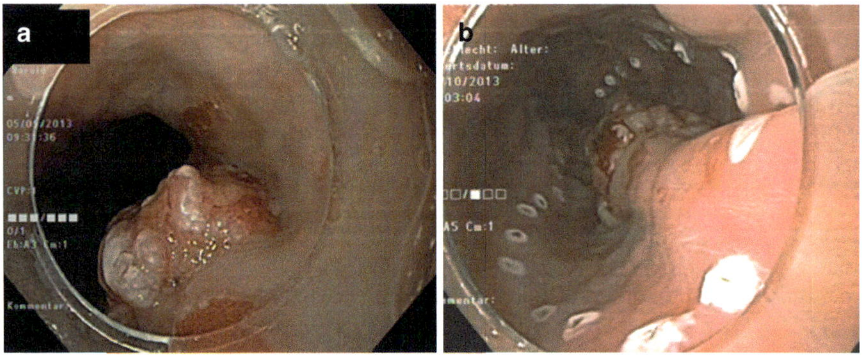

Fig. 8.10 (**a**) Neoplasia 0-Is in short-segment BE C0M4, WLI, and (**b**) with electromarkings of wide safety margin for ESD. (**c**, **d**) Irregular SP and VP typical for carcinoma, VP with few loose thick vessels. (*Diagnosis*: cT1b-sm1/sm2: borderline sm1 invasion?); M-WLI and M-NBI, on (d) margin to BE. (**e**) Diagnostic ESD without visible deep sm-invasion: resection bed. (**f**) Specimen (6.3 × 4.3 cm), WLI. (**g**) Adenocarcinoma G2, pT1b (sm 729 μm), L0 v0, resected R0. Deep sm2-invasion was indication for distal esophagectomy

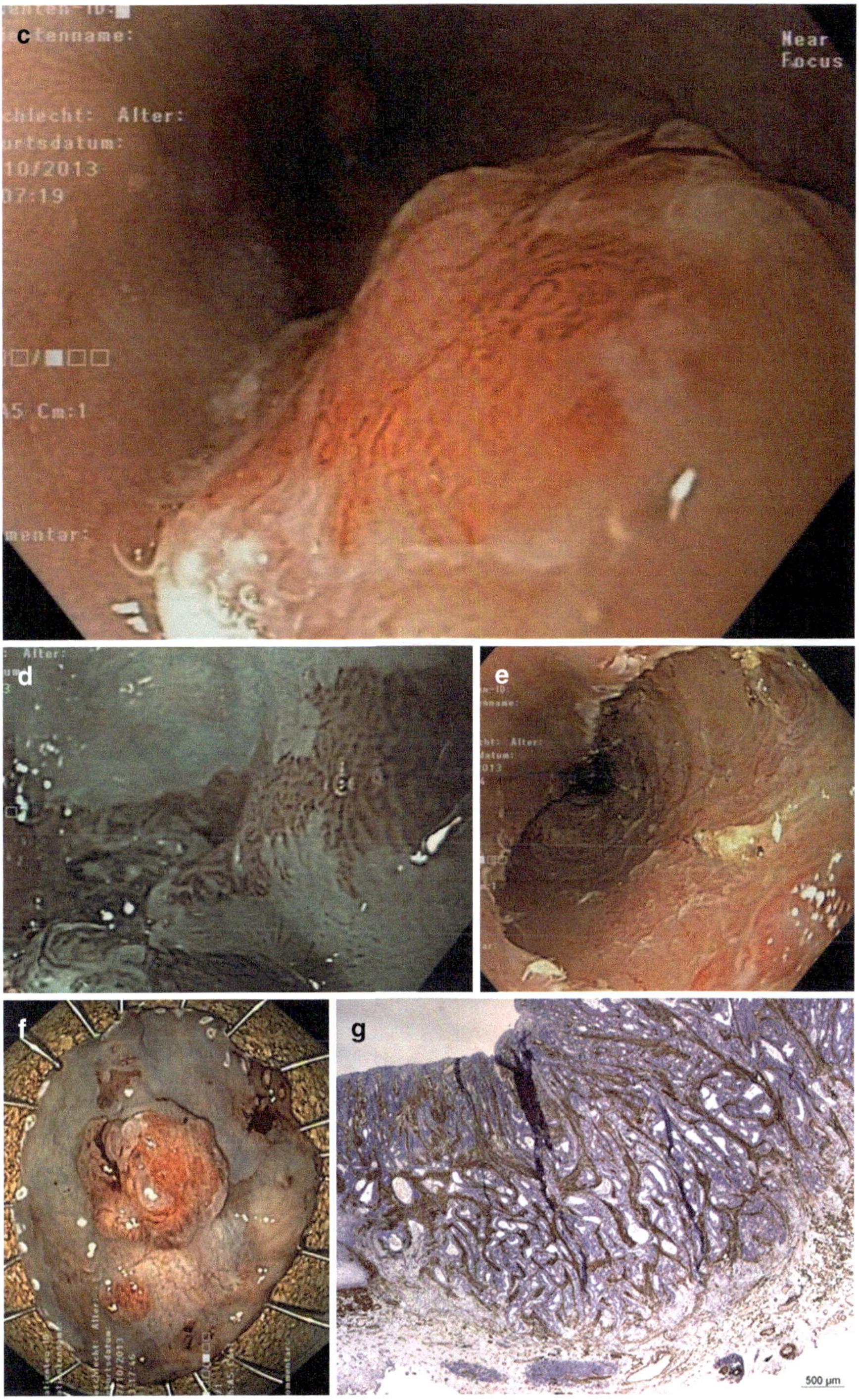

Fig. 8.10 (continued)

Case 2: Barrett's lesion type 0-IIa

In a 69-year-old, healthy man, a lesion 0-IIa, 14 × 10 mm, was seen in short-segment BE (C0M4 at 5 o'clock) (Fig. 8.11). EUS did not show enlarged regional lymph nodes, nor a break of the sm echo band in the organ wall.

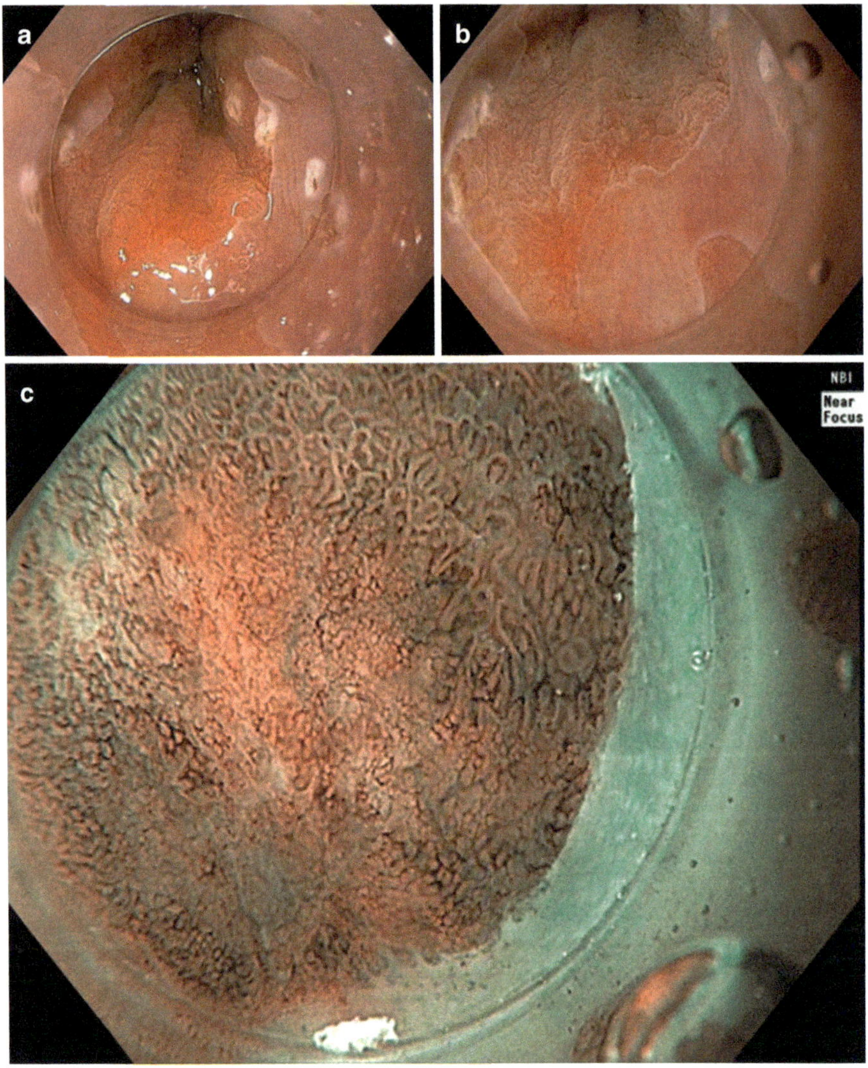

Fig. 8.11 (**a**) Lesion 0-IIa at 5 o'clock (posterior wall) close to the oral end of the short-segment BE tongue. (**b**) Lack of accetowhitening (reddish discoloration) on acetic acid CE, standard WLI. (**c**) M-NBI (60-fold), irregular network VP. (**d**) M-NBI and acetic acid show villi that are irregular to sparse, some larger-sized (fused?, center-right); and faint network VP. *Diagnosis*: superficial cancer, non-invasive. → ESD en-bloc for curative intention: Specimen size was 63 × 43 mm; safety rim markings were intact. Histology: Moderately differentiated AC G2, pT1a-LPM, L0 V0; R0 curative. (Courtesy of Dr. Hans Allgaier and Dr. Tsuneo Oyama)

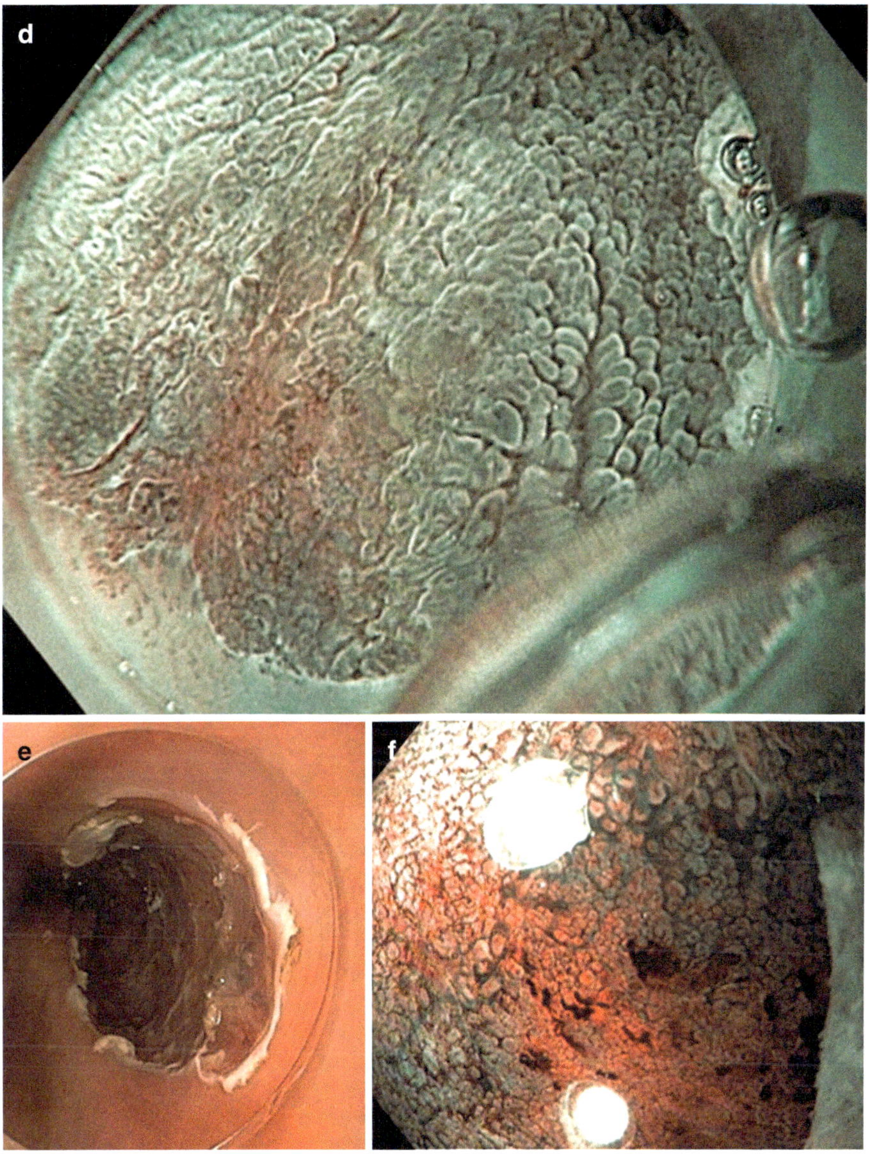

Fig. 8.11 (continued) (**d**) m-NBI with acetic acid; (**e**) Resection bed after ESD en bloc. (**f**) Specimen, M-NBI, lesion center showing caliber changes and fine, irregular network VP (non-invasive)

Note Small inapparent lesion 0-IIb, yet moderately differentiated AC (pT1a, G2).

Case 3: Circular Barrett's carcinoma 0-Ip/s + IIa in EG junction
This 82-year-old woman (ASA III) had intermittent dysphagia of solids for 1 month. UGI endoscopy revealed a circular lesion that extended from the squamo-columnar junction for 4.5 cm to the end of the EGJ (Fig. 8.12).

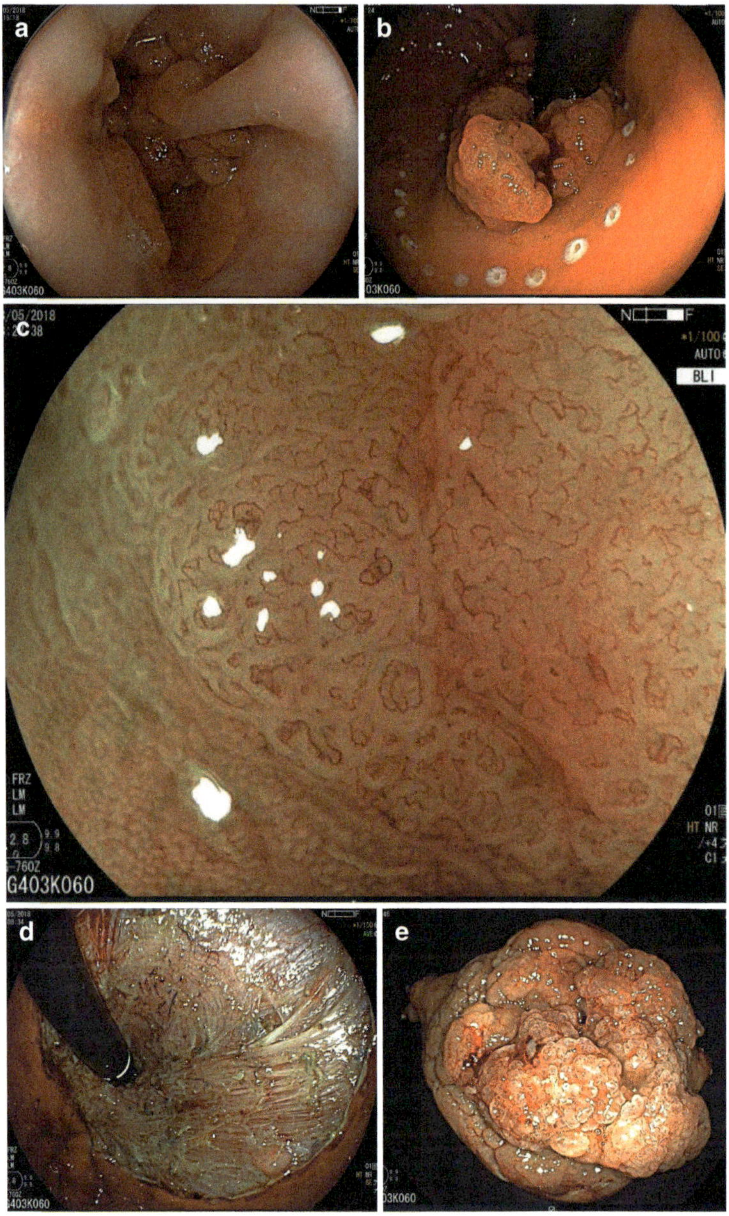

Fig. 8.12 (**a**, **b**) Soft lesion type 0-IIa + Is/p with a polypoid part on the fornix fold. (**c**) Magnified BLI (120-fold) shows irregular villi (irregular SP [ISP], in density and size; white zone [WZ] about even) with tortuous, crowded vessels (IVP with V/S concordance) and clear demarcation line (DL, in pattern and relief). EUS did not show enlarged LN, and the sm echo band seemed preserved. Biopsy revealed well-differentiated adenocarcinoma (WDAC). *Clinical diagnosis:* Early WDAC, no proof of sm invasiveness. (**d**) Diagnostic ESD, circular and en-bloc (Flush Knife BT, with 3 clip lines). (**e**) Intact specimen (after longitudinal cut 11.6 × 6.0 cm) with lesion (7.7 × 2.4 × 0.8 cm). *Histology:* WDAC G1, pT1a-DMM, Bd 1, L0 V0 Pn0; resection R0 → curative ESD

Note Large BE-AC with relatively favorable endoscopic signs → diagnostic ESD.

Case 4: Multifocal Paris 0-Is lesions

The patient was a 65-year-old man with a long Barrett classified C4M5 and several soft Paris 0-Is/IIa lesions 5–12 mm. Resection was performed by ESD all en-bloc, removing 80% of the esophageal circumference. Pathological staging: adenocarcinoma pT1a-m2 multifocal, G1, LV(−), R0. Resection was considered curative and the remaining Barrett was ablated by Halo 90 radiofrequency ablation (RFA) (Fig. 8.13).

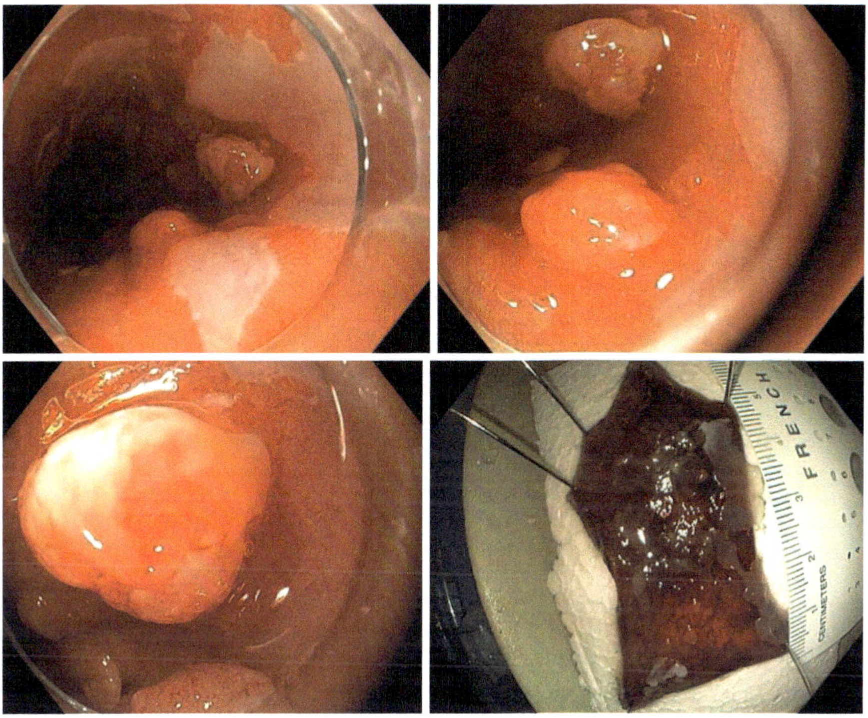

Fig. 8.13 Multiple lesions Paris 0-Is/p with multifocal pT1m2 adenocarcinoma

Case 5: Barrett's esophagus and submucosal lesion
A 60-year-old male patient was followed for a long BE classified as C4M6 with a Paris 0-IIa lesion, resected en bloc by ESD. Final pathology result was pT1sm1 adenocarcinoma, R_0 resection, G2 differentiation, but D2–40+ so L(+). Resection was considered as non curative, so the patient was sent for surgery (Fig. 8.14).

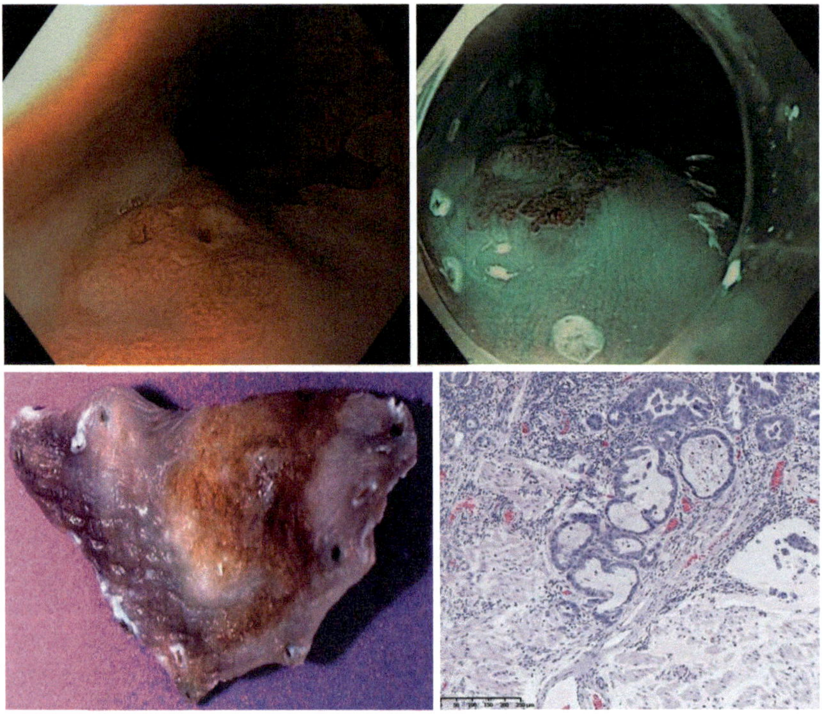

Fig. 8.14 Paris 0-IIa lesion, with irregular mucosal and vascular patterns, and surrounding elevation suggestive of submucosal invasion. Pathology confirms sm1 extent

Case 6: Underwater and acetic acid delineation of mucosal adenocarcinoma
An 82-year-old man had a Prague C1M5 long Barrett's esophagus and a Paris 0-IIa that was removed en bloc by ESD, with a final pathology stage pT1m3 adenocarcinoma, well-differentiated G1, and no lymphovascular invasion; it was considered a curative R0 resection (Fig. 8.15).

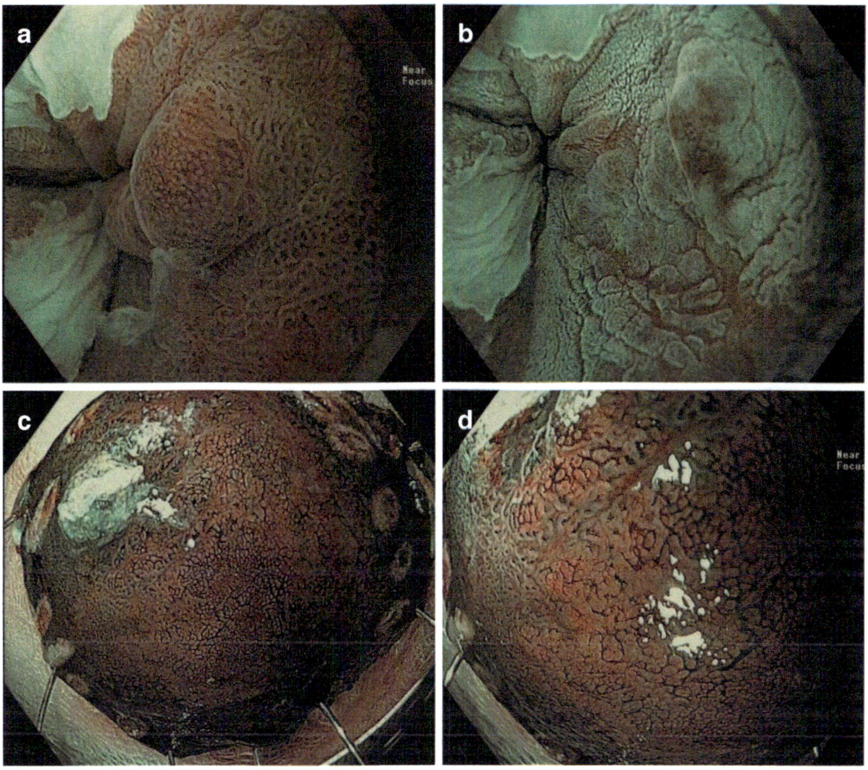

Fig. 8.15 Paris 0-IIa lesion examined underwater (**a** and **b**), with acetic acid CE. The post-ESD specimen (**c** and **d**) confirms free lateral margins and the irregular vascular network pattern typical of mucosal cancer (pT1m3)

Case 7: Barrett's esophagus with a Paris 0-Is submucosal lesion
The patient presented with a newly discovered Barrett's esophagus C5M6 and a Paris 0-Is/p of 2 cm, suspicious for sm invasion (large bulging tumor and vascular pattern showing large irregular vessels) (Fig. 8.16).

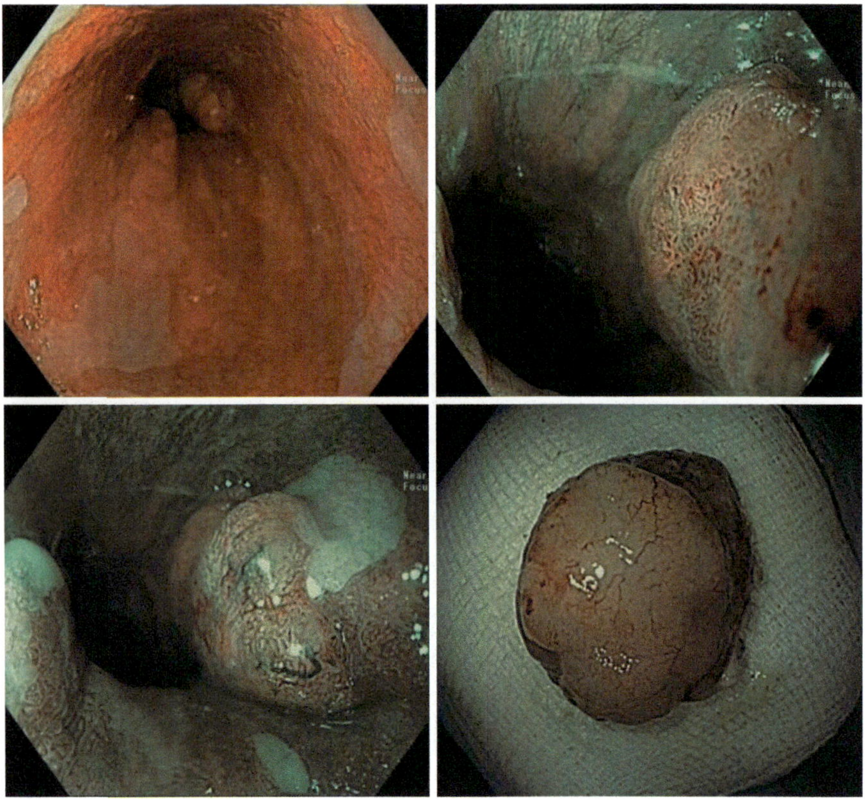

Fig. 8.16 Resection by en bloc ESD (with diagnostic intention). The pathology specimen confirms a pT1sm1 adenocarcinoma, G1–2, LV(−), R0, considered a curative resection

Note ESD with diagnostic intention is important in borderline sm invasive Barrett AC for histologic diagnosis to plan additional treatment; it can prevent overtreatment in some cases.

Case 8: Long BE with mucosal cancer (whitish elevation and thick irregular vessels) with lymphatic mucosal invasion

The patient is an 82-year-old man, with long BE C11M12, Paris 0-IIa lesion in two nodules. Resection was performed by ESD, with en-bloc specimen of 3.4 × 2.7 cm, pT1m2, Vienna classification 5.1, G2, and positive lymphatic invasion, confirmed by D2–40 positive immunohistochemistry. The resection was considered to be non-curative, but the patient refused "adjuvant" surgery (Fig. 8.17).

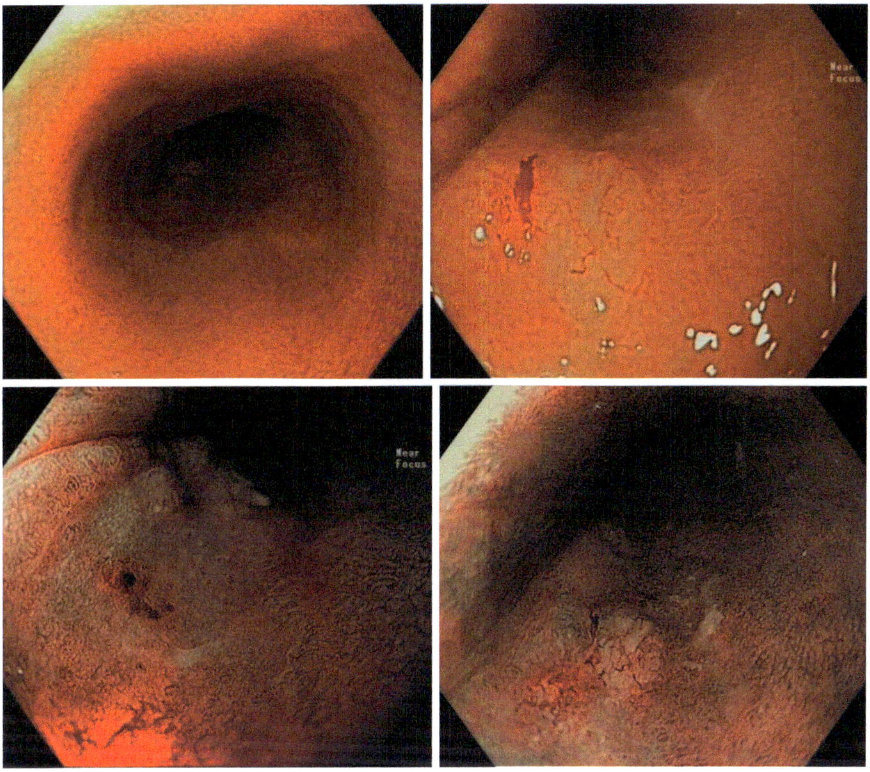

Fig. 8.17 Subtle elevation, whitish aspect corresponding to a Paris 0-IIa lesion, with irregular mucosal and vascular patterns, some thicker vessels

Acknowledgments We gratefully acknowledge the contribution of ESD cases by Dr. Tsuneo Oyama, Nagano, Japan; Dr. Hans P. Allgaier, Freiburg and Dr. Micheal Anzinger, Munich, Germany; and Dr. Frieder Berr and Dr. Daniel Neureiter, Salzburg, Austria.

8.6 Appendix

The morphology of surface and vascular patterns of Barrett's epithelium and BE neoplasias have been analyzed by Kara [35], Goda [23, 24], Anagnostopoulos [22], Sharma [16, 17], and others. The Nottingham classification supplemented with Goda's VP types (Table 8.2) tries to define whether Barrett cancer is superficial and an appropriate indication for endoscopic resection, or if it shows signs of deep sm invasion, an indication for esophagectomy [22–24]. (*See* Table 8.2 and Fig. 8.18.) Capillary (VP) and surface relief architecture (SP) of BE-AC bear analogies to early gastric cancer, but have not been prospectively validated for BE-AC.

Table 8.2 Surface pattern of esophageal columnar epithelium (M-NBI)

SP type[a]	Surface pattern	Likely histopathology	Vessel VP type[a]	Fig. no.
Regular	Uniform pits	Columnar-lined mucosa:		8.18a
	Small pits, round	"Fundus" type	I mesh-like	
	~, slit-like oval	"Corpus" type		
Regular	Uniform tubuli	Normal columnar epithelium, LBC = intestinalized (IM)[b]	II coiled, curly haired	8.18b
	Tubular			
Regular	Uniform folds, villi	Normal columnar epithelium		8.18c 8.18d
	Linear/ridges (top)	"Cardia" type	III vine-like	
	Villous (bottom)	"Antrum" type	IV DNA-spiral-like	
	−/+ *LBC* on NBI	LBC ≈ apical brush border (intestinalized cells) (IM)[b]		
Atrophic-regular	Absent SP (atrophic CL mucosa) with arborized VP & SMVs[c], *unclear* demarcation	"Flat intestinal metaplasia" (SIM)[c]	0 branched VP & cyan sm-veins	8.18e, f
Irregular (& irregular. V)	Irregular SP micrified villous/ gyrous, smooth WZ, clear demarcation line[a]	HGIN/carcinoma T1a	V irregular (caliber, tortuous, crowded, *V/S concordance*)	8.18g
Severely irregular	Severely irregular SP with destroyed pits/ fused villi and clear demarcation line (DL)	Carcinoma, likely deep sm invasive	Severely irregular (corkscrew, non-network, sparse, thick vessel, and *V/S discordance*)	8.18h
Absent (& irregular V)	Absent SP, sharp DL[a]	Carcinoma, sm-invasive or poorly differentiated AC (grading G3)	Severely irregular (as above), sm-veins invisible, clear DL	8.18h

Modified from [10, 16, 19, 22, 23, 35]; Permission by Blackwell Publishing. Ltd. [22]
[a]VP types I–V according to Goda [23], and absent SP according to Kara [35]
[b]"Light blue crest" aspect (=apical brush border) of IM on M-NBI of SP [23]
[c]Flat smooth surface without pits, villi, or folds, but with visible arborized submucosal vascular pattern (VP) in up to 20% of columnar mucosa with intestinal metaplasia (flat-type IM) [35]

Fig. 8.18 Surface patterns of esophageal columnar epithelium (M-NBI). (**a**) Normal fundus-type columnar-lined mucosa (uniform round pits). (**b**) Uniform tubular-type Barrett epithelium with light blue crests (LBC), indicating flat intestinal metaplasia (SIM). (**c**) Uniform cardia-type columnar epithelium with LBC (Barrett's mucosa). (**d**) Uniform villous-type columnar epithelium with LBC (Barrett's mucosa). (**e**) Columnar epithelium with absent microsurface pattern (MSP), arborized submucosal veins (SMV). (**f**) Absent surface pattern (ASP) (center-left) with acetic acid surface enhancement (lower right margin: pit and villous) (M-NBI, 60×, OLYMPUS Excera III). (**g**) Irregular micrified villous MSP with irregular white opaque substance (WOS), typical of HGIN/M2 carcinoma. (**h**) Severely irregular SP (ISP) and IVP (or absent SP on M-CE), fused villi indicative of sm-invasive AC; *arrows* mark demarcation line. OLYMPUS Lucera, M-NBI (100-fold). Permission of Blackwell Publishing Ltd. [22]. (Part **f** courtesy of Dr. Tsuneo Oyama.)

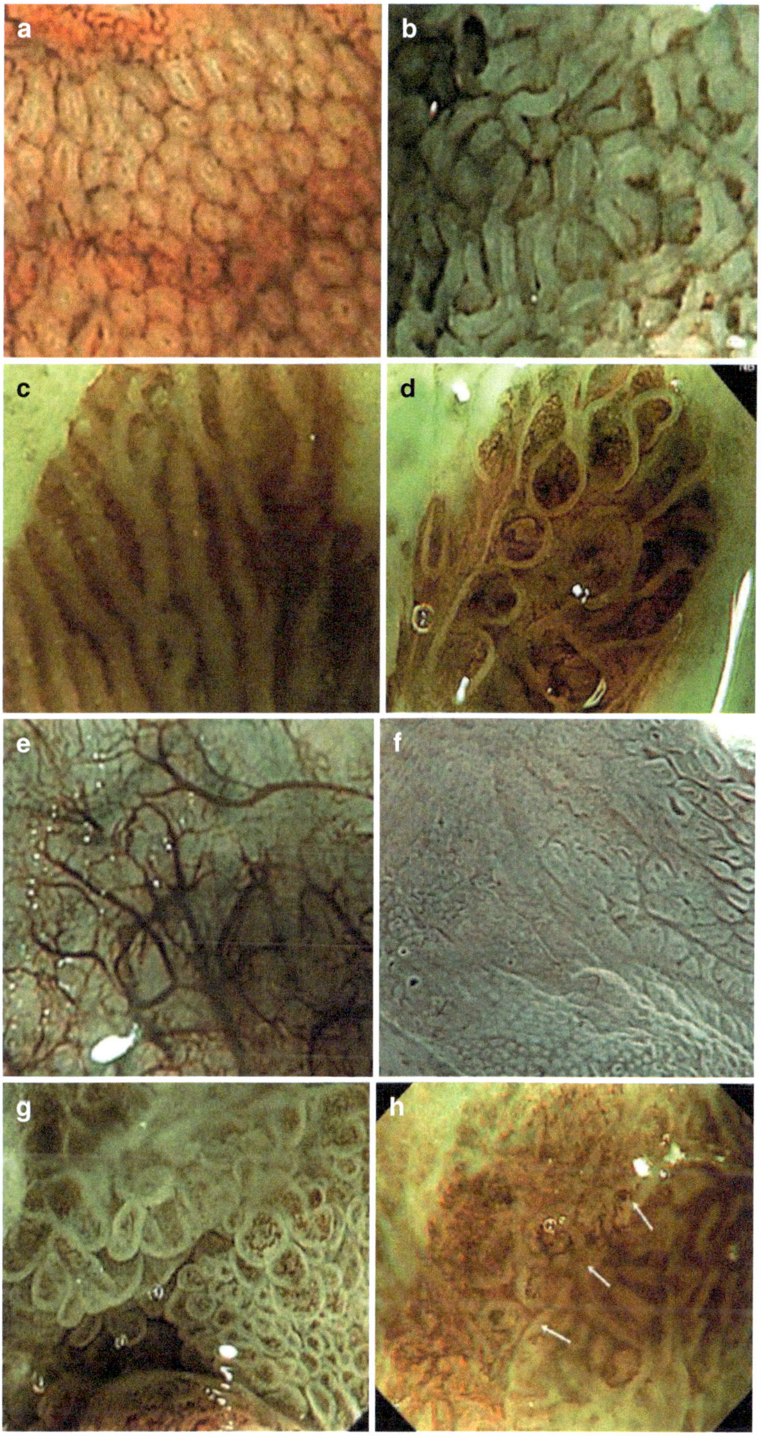
a
b
c
d
e
f
g
h

References

1. van Blankenstein M, et al. The incidence of adenocarcinoma and squamous cell carcinoma of the esophagus: Barrett's esophagus makes a difference. Am J Gastroenterol. 2005;100:766–74.
2. Spechler SJ, et al. American Gastroenterological Association medical position statement on the management of Barrett's esophagus. Gastroenterology. 2011;140:1084–91.
3. Kelty CJ, et al. Barrett's oesophagus: intestinal metaplasia is not essential for cancer risk. Scand J Gastroenterol. 2007;42:1271–4.
4. Kuwano H, et al. Guidelines for diagnosis and treatment of carcinoma of the esophagus April 2012 edited by the Japan Esophageal Society. Esophagus. 2015;12:1–30.
5. Kastelein F, et al. Impact of surveillance for Barrett's oesophagus on tumor stage and survival of patients with neoplastic progression. Gut. 2016;65:548–54.
6. Shaheen NJ, et al. ACG clinical guideline: diagnosis and management of Barrett's esophagus. Am J Gastroenterol. 2016;111:30–50.
7. Sharma P, et al. The development and validation of an endoscopic grading system for Barrett's esophagus: the Prague C & M criteria. Gastroenterology. 2006;131:1392–9.
8. Weusten B, et al. Endoscopic management of Barrett's esophagus: European Society of Gastrointestinal Endoscopy (ESGE) position statement. Endoscopy. 2017;49:191–8.
9. Lambert R. The Paris endoscopic classification of superficial neoplastic lesions: esophagus, stomach, and colon: November 30 to December 1, 2002. Gastrointest Endosc. 2003;58:S3–43.
10. Paris Workshop on columnar metaplasia in the esophagus and the esophagogastric junction, Paris, France, December 11–12 2004. Endoscopy. 2005;37:879–920.
11. Oyama T. Diagnostic strategies of superficial Barrett's esophageal cancer for endoscopic submucosal dissection. Dig Endosc. 2013;25(Suppl 1):7–12.
12. Pech O, et al. Prospective evaluation of the macroscopic types and location of early Barrett's neoplasia in 380 lesions. Endoscopy. 2007;39:588–93.
13. Theisen J, et al. Preferred location for the development of esophageal adenocarcinoma within a segment of intestinal metaplasia. Surg Endosc. 2006;20:235–8.
14. Kandiah K, et al. International development and validation of a classification system for the identification of Barrett's neoplasia using acetic acid chromoendoscopy: the Portsmouth acetic acid classification (PREDICT). Gut 2018;67:2085–91.
15. Muto M, et al. Magnifying endoscopy simple diagnostic algorithm for early gastric cancer (MESDA-G). Dig Endosc. 2016;28:379–93.
16. Sharma P, et al. Development and validation of a classification system to identify high-grade dysplasia and esophageal adenocarcinoma in Barrett's esophagus using narrow-band imaging. Gastroenterology. 2016;150:591–8.
17. Sharma P, et al. Standard endoscopy with random biopsies versus narrow band imaging targeted biopsies in Barrett's oesophagus: a prospective, international, randomised controlled trial. Gut. 2013;62:15–21.
18. Singh M, et al. Observer agreement in the assessment of narrowband imaging system surface patterns in Barrett's esophagus: a multicenter study. Endoscopy. 2011;43:745–51.
19. Kato M, et al. Image assessment of Barrett's esophagus using the simplified narrow band imaging classification. J Gastroenterol. 2017;52:466–75.
20. Zemler B, et al. Early Barrett's carcinoma: the depth of infiltration of the tumour correlates with the degree of differentiation, the incidence of lymphatic vessel and venous invasion. Virchows Arch. 2010;456:609–14.
21. Pech O, et al. The impact of endoscopic ultrasound and computed tomography on the TNM staging of early cancer in Barrett's esophagus. Am J Gastroenterol. 2006;101:2223–9.
22. Anagnostopoulos GK, et al. Novel endoscopic observation in Barrett's oesophagus using high resolution magnification endoscopy and narrow band imaging. Aliment Pharmacol Ther. 2007;26:501–7.

23. Goda K, et al. Usefulness of magnifying endoscopy with narrow band imaging for the detection of specialized intestinal metaplasia in columnar-lined esophagus and Barrett's adenocarcinoma. Gastrointest Endosc. 2007;65:36–46.
24. Goda K, et al. Current status of endoscopic diagnosis and treatment of superficial Barrett's adenocarcinoma in Asia-Pacific region. Dig Endosc. 2013;25(Suppl 2):146–50.
25. Oyama T. Diagnosis of gastric adenocarcinoma with magnified endoscopy. In: Oyama T, editor. Endoscopic diagnosis of superficial gastric cancer for ESD. Tokyo, Japan: Springer; 2016. p. 39–51.
26. Yamagata T, et al. Efficacy of acetic acid-spraying method in diagnosing extension of Barrett's cancer under the squamous epithelium. Dig Endosc. 2012;24:309–14.
27. Pimentel-Nunes P, et al. Endoscopic submucosal dissection: European Society of Gastrointestinal Endoscopy (ESGE) guideline. Endoscopy. 2015;47:829–54.
28. Pech O, et al. Long-term efficacy and safety of endoscopic resection for patients with mucosal adenocarcinoma of the esophagus. Gastroenterology. 2014;146:652–660.e651.
29. Manner H, et al. Early Barrett's carcinoma with "low-risk" submucosal invasion: long-term results of endoscopic resection with a curative intent. Am J Gastroenterol. 2008;103:2589–97.
30. Phoa KN, et al. Multimodality endoscopic eradication for neoplastic Barrett oesophagus: results of an European multicentre study (EURO-II). Gut. 2016;65:555–62.
31. Dunbar KB, et al. The risk of lymph-node metastases in patients with high-grade dysplasia or intramucosal carcinoma in Barrett's esophagus: a systematic review. Am J Gastroenterol. 2012;107:850–62; quiz 863.
32. Leers JM, et al. The prevalence of lymph node metastases in patients with T1 esophageal adenocarcinoma a retrospective review of esophagectomy specimens. Ann Surg. 2011;253:271–8.
33. Kawaguchi G, et al. The effectiveness of endoscopic submucosal dissection followed by chemoradiotherapy for superficial esophageal cancer. Radiat Oncol. 2015;10:31.
34. Takeuchi M, et al. Technical feasibility and oncological safety of diagnostic endoscopic resection for superficial esophageal cancer. Gastrointest Endosc. 2018;88:456–65.
35. Kara MA, et al. Detection and classification of the mucosal and vascular patterns (mucosal morphology) in Barrett's esophagus by using narrow band imaging. Gastrointest Endosc. 2006;64:155–66.

Chapter 9
Stomach: Mucosal Neoplasias

Tsuneo Oyama

9.1 Introduction

High prevalence of high-risk chronic gastritis and gastric cancer justifies screening gastroscopy that has led to the frequent diagnosis of early gastric cancer in Japan [1]. In Western countries, as detailed in Chap. 6, opportunistic screening gastroscopy of high-risk individuals and surveillance of high-risk conditions increasingly reveals HGIN or early cancer of the stomach [2]. The miss rate of minute and small flat gastric neoplasias (0-IIa/b/c) was considerable even in Japan [3]. Therefore, endoscopic detection and diagnosis of small and minute gastric neoplasias (HGIN and cancer T1 m) is the goal – see also recent atlas for more detailed explanation and analyzed cases [4].

9.1.1 Individuals with Increased Risk for Gastric Cancer

Surveillance gastroscopy (Chap. 6) is justified for risk groups [2, 5] with:

- chronic atrophic gastritis with Helicobacter pylori infection,
- chronic atrophic autoimmune gastritis,
- chronic gastric remnant gastritis after Billroth-II gastrectomy,
- protruded or flat type neoplasia in FAP or HNPCC, respectively.

T. Oyama (✉)
Department of Endoscopy, Saku Central Hospital Advanced Care Center, Saku, Nagano, Japan
e-mail: oyama@coral.ocn.ne.jp

F. Berr et al. (eds.), *Atlas of Early Neoplasias of the Gastrointestinal Tract*,
https://doi.org/10.1007/978-3-030-01114-7_9

9.2 Gastroscopy for Detection of Early Gastric Cancer (EGC)

Preparation is essential (Sect. 6.4.2). The patient receives intravenous sedation and anticholinergics. When the scope has passed the cardia, you have to assess the general condition of the stomach – normal mucosa or chronic gastritis –/+ atrophy which signifies increased risk of gastric cancer. You must rinse the mucosa clean. While changing the amount of air insufflation/desufflation search for subtle alterations of surface structure or color. Proceed as follows with

- standard WL imaging and mapping of all anatomic areas of stomach (Fig. 6.3) when you diagnose high risk chronic gastritis,
- search for surface change (flat, ulcerated or protruded lesion) and color change (reddish or whitish) [6]
- magnifying NBI (M-NBI) of surface (SP) and microvascular pattern (VP) of any lesion, acetic acid-indigo carmine magnifying CE, when the lesion remains indiscriminate [7–9]
- biopsy of suspicious lesions, but only very few and targeted biopsies, because scars will later interfere with ESD.

Most early gastric cancers develop on a background of chronic gastritis rendering detection of minute cancers even more difficult. Therefore, you must know the endoscopic structure of gastric mucosa and its alterations on standard WLI- and M-NBI endoscopy. Furthermore, experience with the features of EGC on conventional WLI endoscopy increases detection rate [6].

9.2.1 Basic Structure of Gastric Mucosa

Gastric mucosa is lined with columnar cell epithelium, and there are three types of glands including cardiac, fundic and pyloric gland. And, the length of cardiac gland mucosa is only about 5 mm at the cardia. Therefore, the majority of gastric mucosa is composed by fundic or pyloric glands (Fig. 9.1c, d). Usually, gastric folds can be observed only within fundic gland area. Therefore, you can recognize fundic gland area by the gastric folds (Fig. 9.1a).

Sometimes, H. pylori infection causes atrophic gastritis, and gastric folds will disappear. Usually, the atrophy started from lesser curvature side. Therefore, you must observe the gastric folds of lesser curvature, when you insert a scope into the stomach. And, if you find folds in lesser curvature, the risk of gastric cancer is low (Fig. 9.1a). However, if the folds disappeared, that means atrophic gastritis (Fig. 9.1e–h), and the risk of gastric cancer is high.

The other important risk factor is *H. pylori infection*. Usually, you can observe red dots in the lesser curvature of gastric body (Fig. 9.1b). It is named **r**egular **a**rrangement of **c**ollecting venules (*RAC*) by K. Yagi [10]. If you can observe RAC, the risk of H.pylori infection is low, that means the risk of gastric cancer also is low. But if you can't observe RAC pattern (Fig. 9.1h), that means H.pylori infection yielding higher risk of gastric cancer.

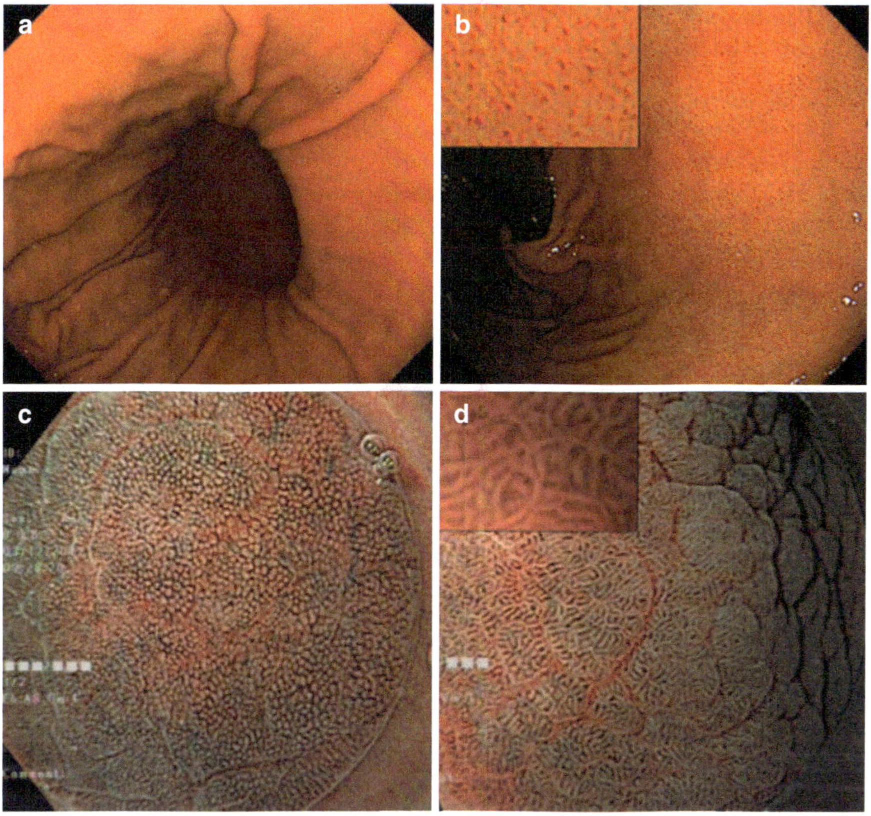

Fig. 9.1 (**a**, **b**) Normal fundic gland mucosa extends in the area of gastric folds and shows fine red dots on WLI (lesser curvature), i.e. starfish-like, regular arrangement of thicker collecting venules (RAC; insert 20x WLI), as characteristic aspect of intact fundus/corpus mucosa devoid of chronic gastritis. (**c**) M-NBI (40x) of fundic type mucosa shows well-defined roundish, pit-like S pattern and regular network-like V pattern, and (**d**) pyloric-type mucosa in antrum shows villous surface pattern with fine helix-like VP surrounded by even, belt-like white marginal crypt epithelium (MCE i.e. white zone, WZ); insert 60x

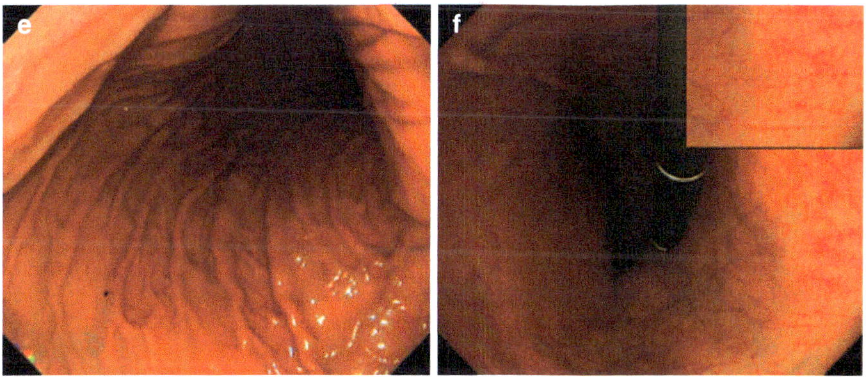

Fig. 9.1 (continued) (**e**, **f**) Chronic atrophic gastritis displays (**e**, **f**) reduction and loss of gastric mucosal folds and (**f**) permeation of regular pattern of larger collecting submucosal venules on standard WLI endoscopy due to atrophy of mucosal glands

Key Points
1. **Folds of gastric body**
2. **RAC**

Chronic atrophic gastritis – of Helicobacter / biliary reflux / autoimmune etiology- with translucent arborizing submucosal vein pattern often presents intestinal metaplasia (IM), i.e. slightly elevated *whitish areas* with *uncertain margins* on WLI, and "*light blue crests*" (LBC, i.e. intraepithelial brush border) in surface pattern on M-NBI (Fig. 9.1 i–l). LBC predict IM (90% accuracy). Annual cancer risk of atrophic gastritis with IM is about 1 % [11].

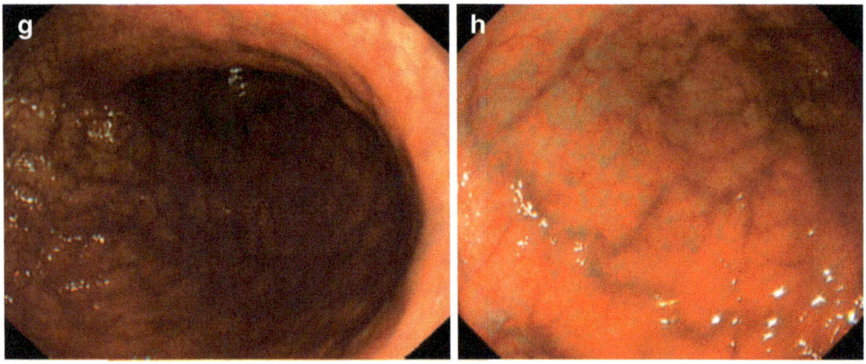

Fig. 9.1 (continued) (**g, h**) Chronic gastritis caused by Helicobacter pylori leads to typical changes with (**g**) loss of gastric folds and (**h**) loss of RAC pattern (most prominent on lesser curvature side)

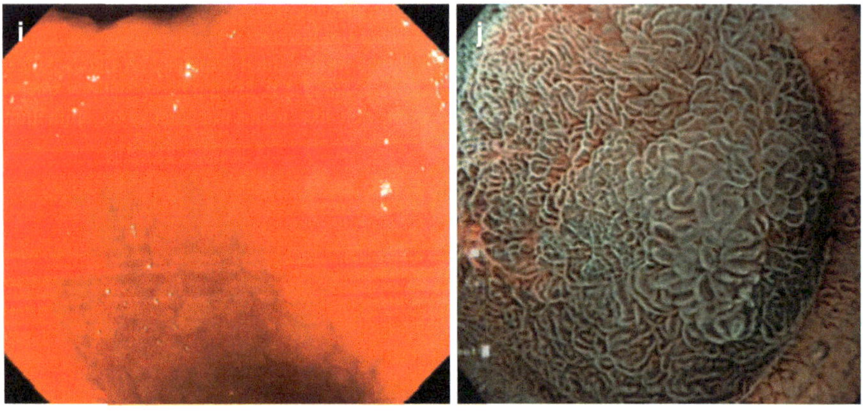

Fig. 9.1 (continued) (**i**) *Intestinal metaplasia* (IM) in chronic gastritis exhibits slightly elevated whitish areas with uncertain margins on standard WLI. (**j**) *Intestinal metaplasia* (IM) in pyloric type mucosa exhibits villous surface pattern with augmented WZ and "*light blue crests*" (LBC) that diminish regular spiral microvascular pattern on magnifying NBI

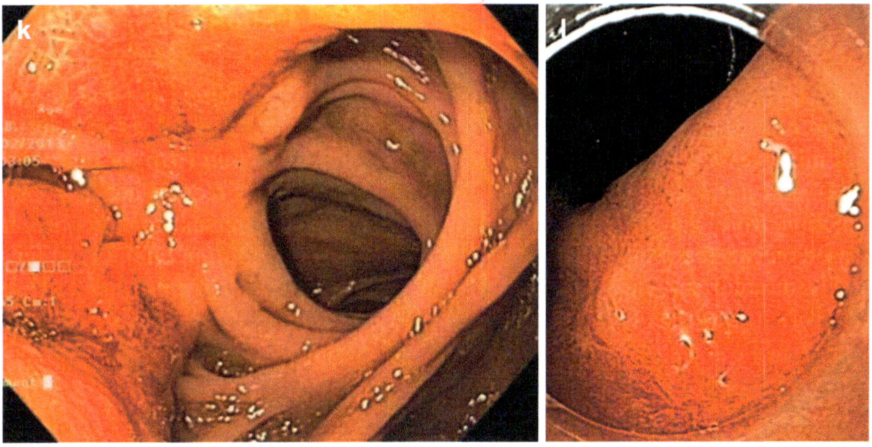

Fig. 9.1 (continued) (**k**) Chronic remnant gastritis 30 yrs after distal gastrectomy with B-II anastomosis. (**l**) chronic gastritis at anastomosis with whitish IM, unclear margins (for M-NBI see Fig. 9.1j)

9.2.2 Basic Endoscopic Structure of Early Gastric Neoplasia (See Sect. 1.6.2)

Non-neoplastic polyps show surface pattern of *adjacent mucosa* (Fig. 9.3a–f).

Gastric adenomas usually present as [9, 12] (Fig. 9.4):

- protruded (0-Is;-Isp) or elevated (0-IIa) lesions,
- more pale aspect on WLI,
- nodular pattern with indigocarmine spreading, and
- regular villous pattern by magnified NBI (M-NBI).

Differentiated adenocarcinomas [4, 8, 13, 14] (Figs. 1.8, 1.9, 9.5d, and 9.6)

- form all type-0 lesions (Is, IIa/b/c, III) with clear margins,
- appear reddish on WLI,
- present demarcated margins (*DL = demarcation line*) on M-NBI, and
- irregular pit or villous surface pattern (SP) &
- fine microvascular network pattern (VP) by M-NBI.

Undifferentiated gastric cancers (*PDAC*, small size) [4, 14, 15] (Figs. 1.11 and 9.8):

- mostly show 0-IIc and 0-IIb lesions,
- pale color on WLI endoscopy,
- well demarcated margin (DL) in fundic gland area – but
- uncertain margin (uncertain or missing DL) in atrophic area.
- Surface pattern is uncertain, vessels are corkscrew-like by M-NBI.

9.3 Observation with Conventional WLI Endoscopy

On *WLI endoscopy*, any lesion is defined by *color*, *macrosopic type*, and *lateral margins*. Reddish color reflects permeation of augmented mucosal and submucosal microvessels. The first distinction is between *protuberant* (Is/p) or ulcerated (III), and *flat lesions* (IIa/IIb/IIc). *Flat cancerous lesions* require accurate distinction from gastritis-like alterations (i.e. neoplastic versus non-neoplastic) based on two features: (a) demarcated border (*DL, demarcation line*), (b) irregularity in color/surface pattern. However, early EGC of *undifferentiated diffuse* type often shows alteration in color (whitish) without DL on WLI or even M-NBI [4, 14, 15].

9.3.1 Differential Diagnosis of Protuberant Lesions on WLI

Protuberant lesion, when reddish with uncertain margin, most likely is an inflammatory lesion (Fig. 9.3a, b). Clear margins of red protuberant lesion strongly support hyperplastic polyp (non-neoplastic) (Fig. 9.3b) or well differentiated adenocarcinoma (algorithm, Fig. 9.2a). Diagnosis is made by biopsy and M-NBI, because hyperplastic polyp shows regular surface and vascular patterns (Fig. 9.3b).

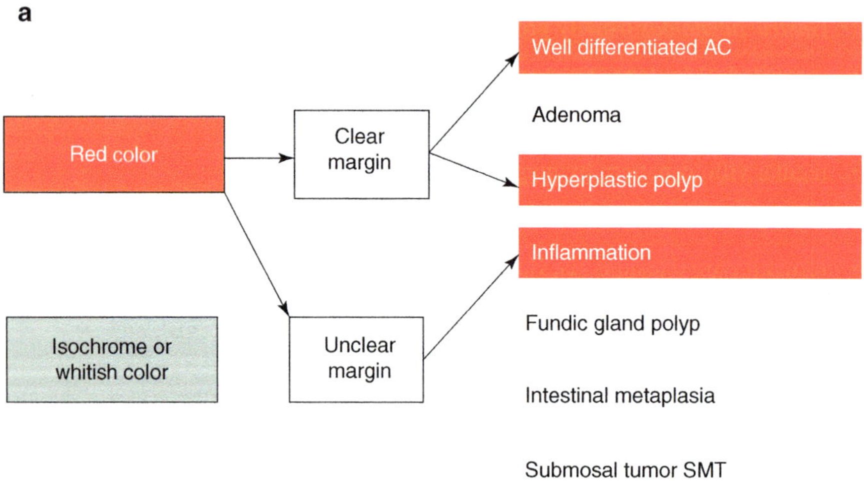

Fig. 9.2 Standard WLI Algorithms. (**a**) Differential diagnosis of reddish protuberant gastric lesions

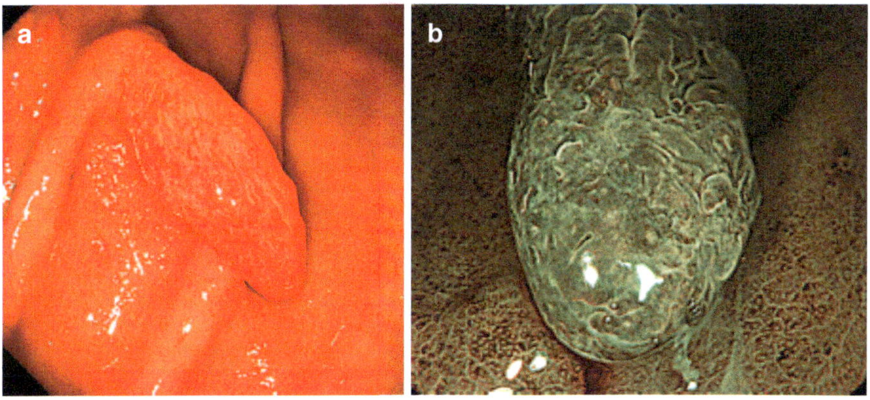

Fig. 9.3 Inflammatory polyp 0-Ip in fundic gland corpus (**a**) WLI, (**b**) magnifying NBI (40x)

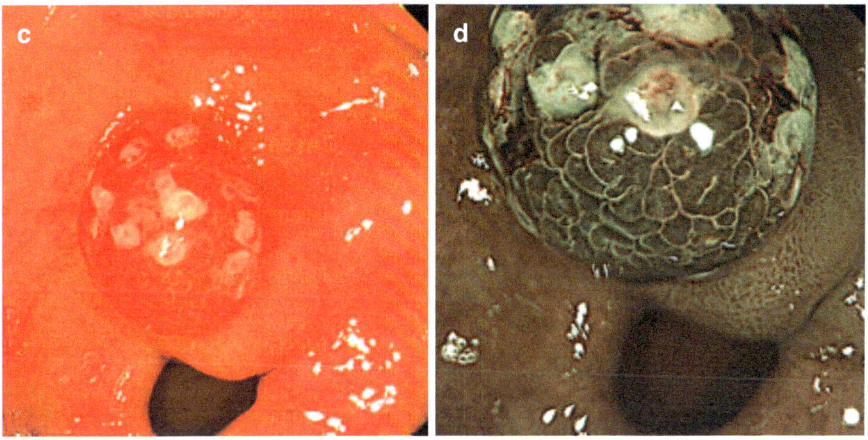

Fig. 9.3 (continued) (**c**) Hyperplastic polyp (reddish on WLI) (**d**) on NBI (20x), distinct pyloric type glands

Whitish protuberant lesion with clear margins supports the diagnosis of fundic gland polyp (Fig. 9.3e, f), adenoma (Fig. 9.4a–k) or less likely well differentiated adenocarcinoma (WDAC) (Fig. 9.6c). Whitish or isochrome protuberant lesions with uncertain margin most likely represent intestinal metaplasia (Fig. 9.1i–l) or submucosal tumor [16] (Fig. 9.3g, h, algorithm in Fig. 9.2b).

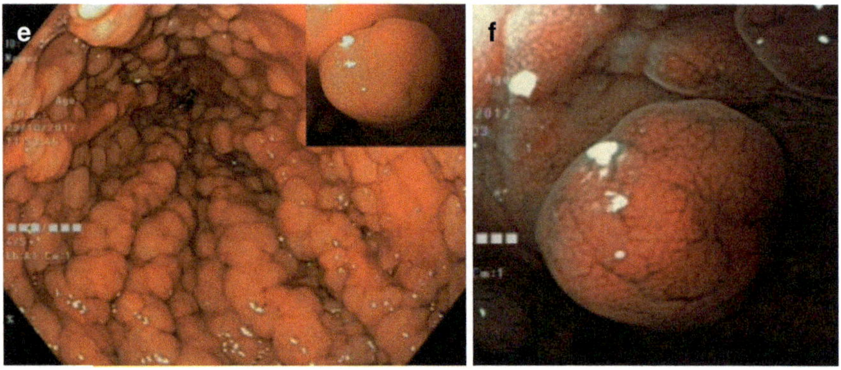

Fig. 9.3 (continued) (**e**) Multiple fundic gland polyps, FAP patient, WLI (insert 20x) (**f**) Fundic gland polyp, NBI (20x)

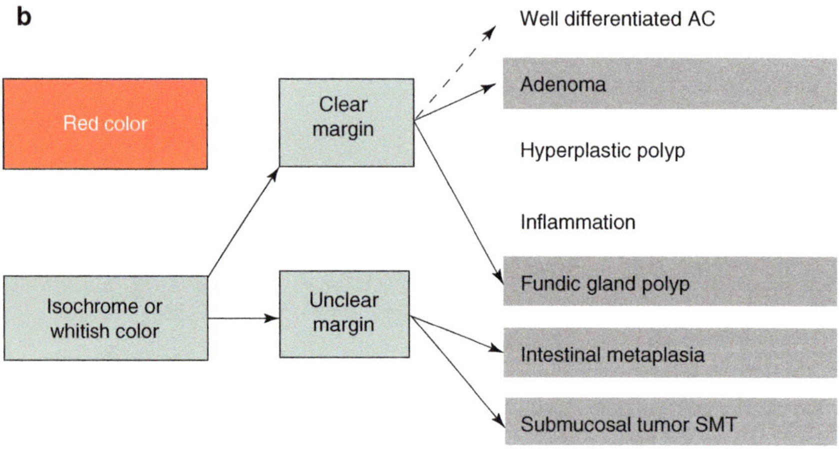

Fig. 9.2 (continued) Standard WLI Algorithms (**b**) Differential diagnosis of whitish (isochrome) protuberant gastric lesion type 0-Is or 0-IIa

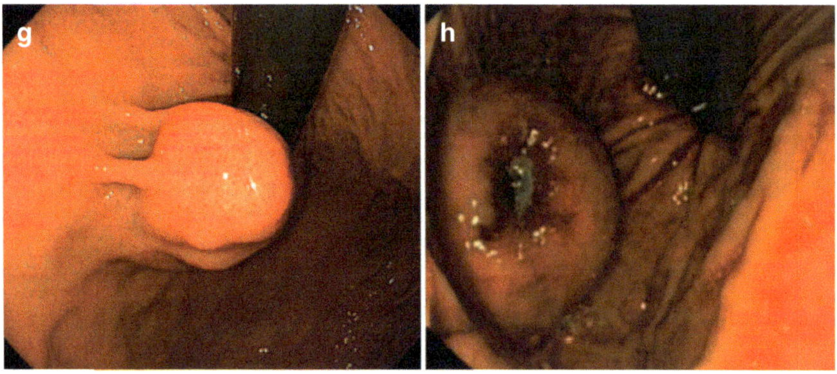

Fig. 9.3 (continued) (**g**) Submucosal gastric tumor – bridging folds and regular fundic type mucosa, (**h**) Submucosal gastroinhtestinal stromal tumor (GIST) with mucosal invasion and ulceration. (diagnosis by EUS & biopsy from ulcer)

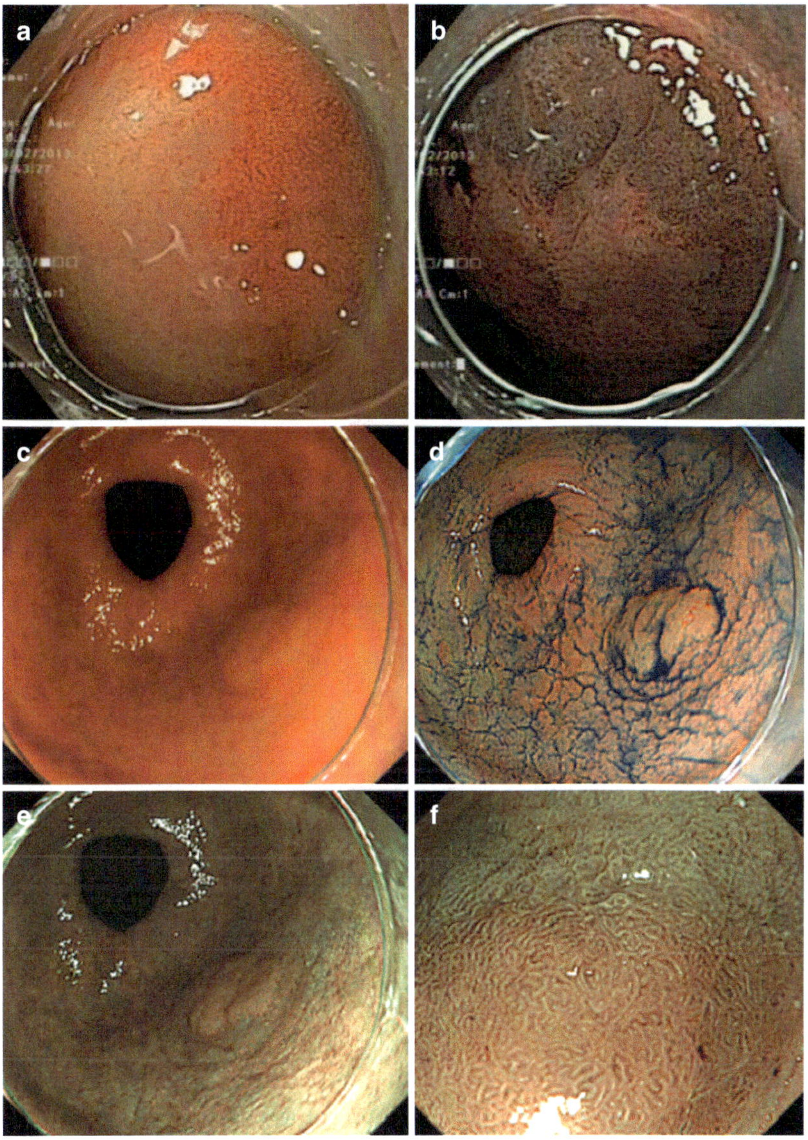

Fig. 9.4 Pyloric type gastric adenomas. (**a**) Clear margin of flat whitish adenoma (0-IIb) vs pyloric type mucosa on WLI, and (**b**) distinct margin of pale adenoma to pyloric type mucosa with chronic gastritis on NBI. (**c**) Pale adenoma (0-IIa) in chronic gastritis (pyloric type mucosa), (**d**) indigo carmin-acetic acid CE, (**e**) standard NBI, (**f**) Villous surface and *even* white opaque zones (i.e. *MCE*, marginal crypt epithelium) of adenoma (top) with clear margin to antrum mucosa (bottom) with SIM (40x magnifying NBI)

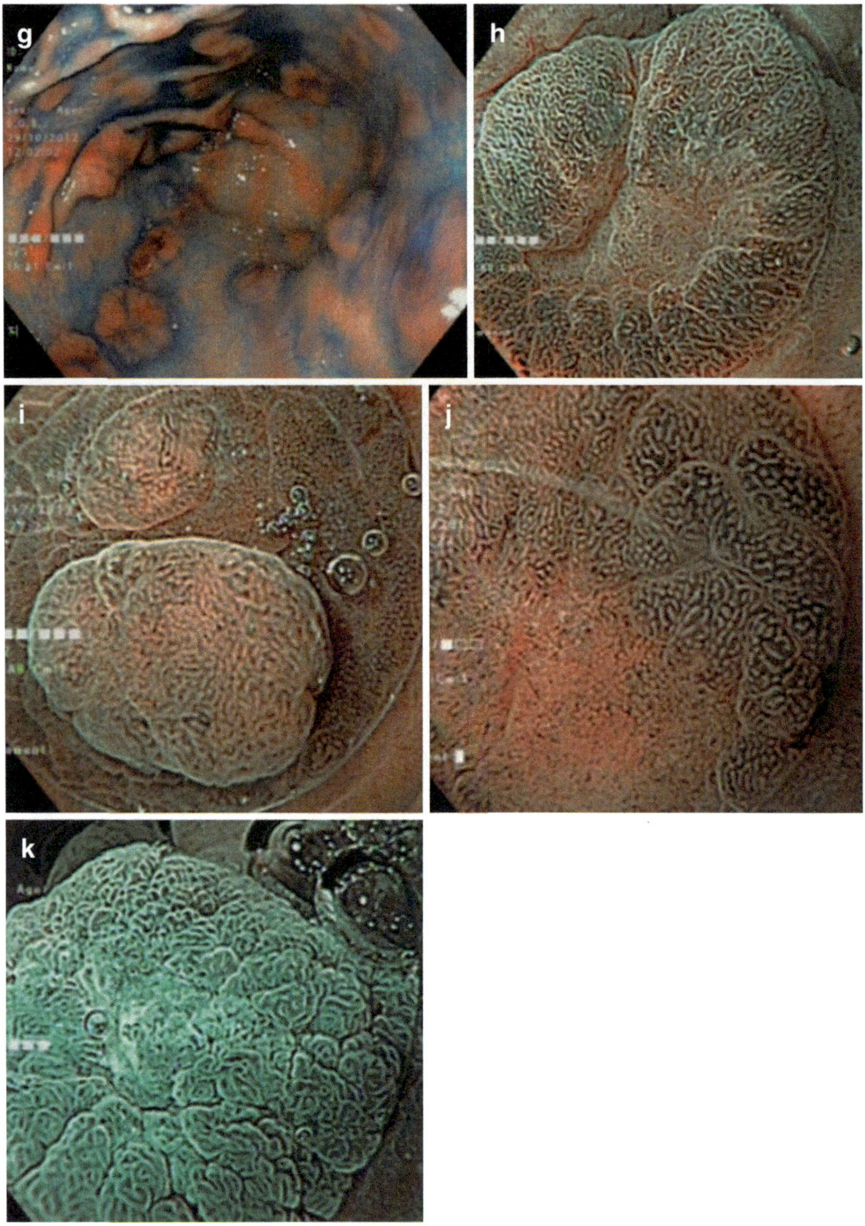

Fig. 9.4 (continued) Patient with FAP (**g**) Multiple adenomas (0-Is, 0-IIa, 0-IIa + c) in antrum, WLI with indigocarmin CE, (**h**) Lesion 0-IIa + c, micrified villous mucosa (gastric adenoma), clear margin and hyperplastic mucosal rim (pyloric type mucosa), M-NBI (60x, under water). (**i**) Protruding lesion 0-IIa with irregular pit/ridge pattern (small gastric adenoma) within fundic-type gastric mucosa (pits). (**j**) Micrified fundic pit pattern with clear margin of *gastric adenoma*, and (**k**) surface enhancement by acetic acid [same as (**j**)]

9.3.2 Differential Diagnosis of Depressed Lesions on WLI Endoscopy

Reddish depressed lesions with clear margins more likely reveal well differentiated adenocarcinoma (WDAC) (Figs. 9.5d and 9.6d, g) or rarley angiodysplasia (Fig. 9.5a, b). Red lesions with uncertain margins usually are erosions or seldom MALT lymphoma (Fig. 9.5e, f), and very seldom PDAC or adenoma (Fig. 9.2c).

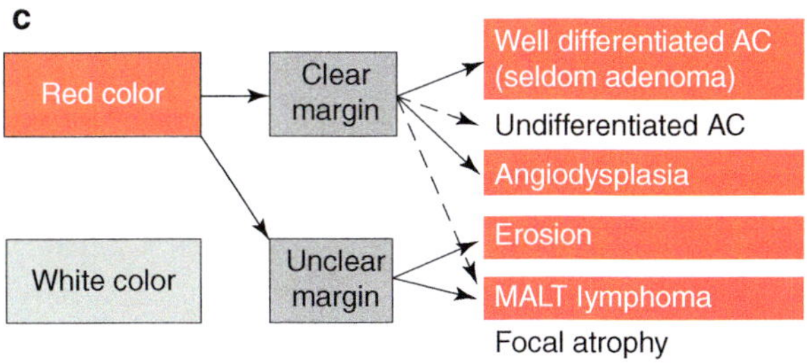

Fig. 9.2 (continued) (**c**) Standard WLI Algorithm. Differential diagnosis of reddish depressed lesions type 0-IIc

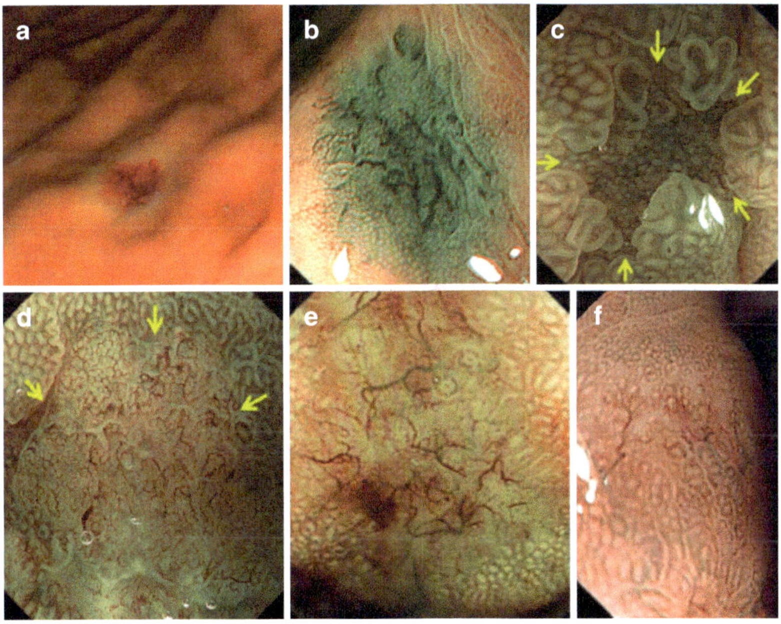

Fig. 9.5 (**a**, **b**) Angiodysplasia in gastric corpus (pit-like SP), ordinary WLI, and M-NBI (40x). (**c**, **d**) Depressed lesions 0-IIc (3–3.2 mm), M-NBI 100x, demarcation line (arrows), (**c**) focal atrophy in chronic gastritis with regular fundic SP (pits) and VP (honey comb-like subepithelial capillary network, SCN). (**d**) depressed differentiated early gastric cancer with clear margin (DL), uncertain surface and irregular microvascular patterns, from [14] with permission by John Wiley and Sons/Digestive Endoscopy. (**e**) mucosal lymphoma with loss of surface structure, unclear margins, and tree-like abnormal blood vessels (M-NBI, 80x) in gastric corpus [WLI: multiple slightly reddish lesions 0-IIa and 0-Is; biopsy: mantle cell lymphoma]. (**f**) same, in partial remission after six courses of chemotherapy. (**e** and **f** From Nonaka et al. [17], with permission of Thieme)

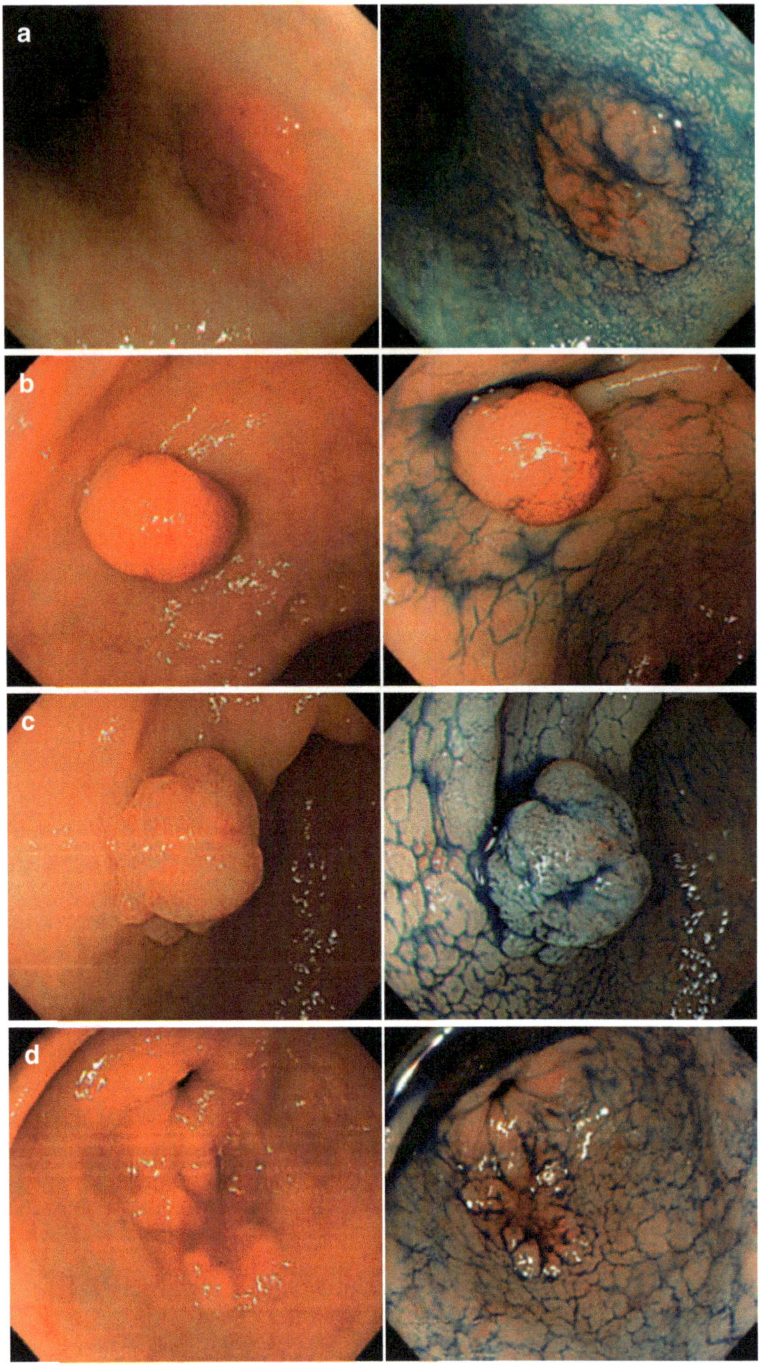

Fig. 9.6 (**a**–**d**) *Signs for intramucosal extension of differentiated AC. Intramucosal* extension of cancer (adenocarcinoma AC) is common in distinct *homogeneous protuberant* lesions (**a**) type 0-IIa, (**b**) type 0-Is smoothly homogenous, (**c**) 0-Is smoothly lobulated, and (**d**) reddish depressed-type 0-IIc. *Left panel*, standard WLI; *right panel*, acetic acid-indigo carmine CE (AIM)

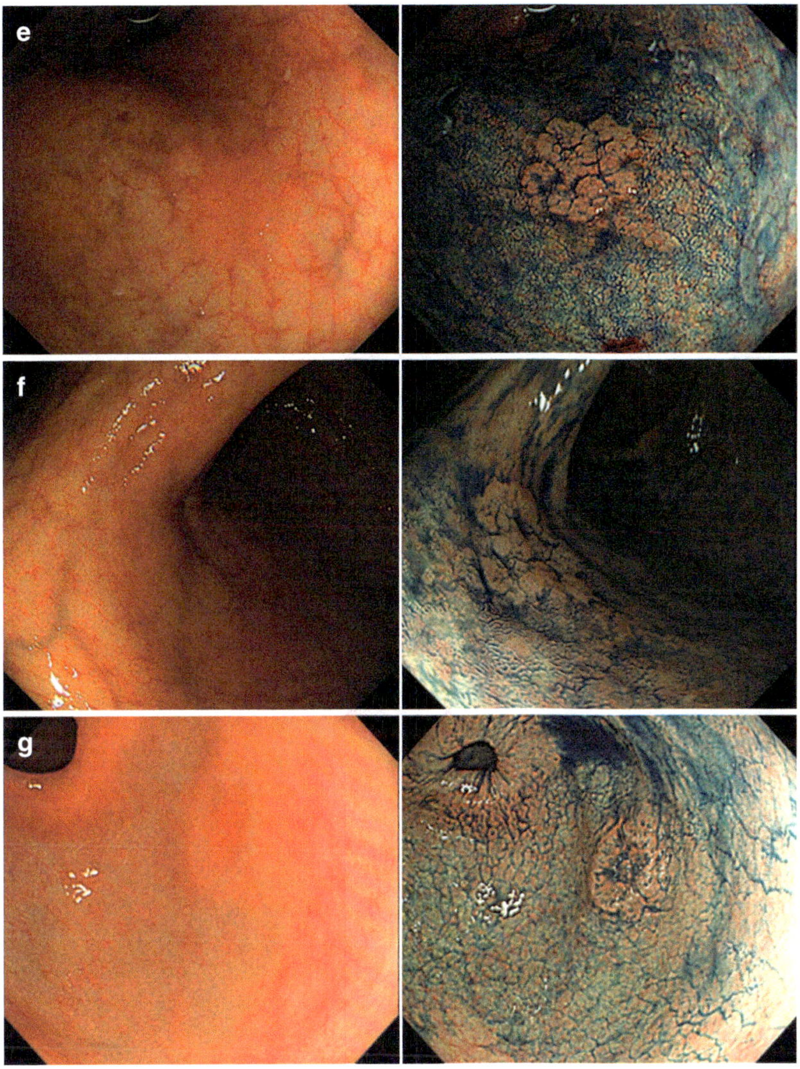

Fig. 9.6 (continued) (**e–g**) *Flat types of well-differentiated gastric adenocarcinoma* (WDAC). Standard WLI (*left*) shows *reddish* lesions, indigo carmine CE (*right*) reveals macroscopic type and lateral margins of WDAC: (**e**) type 0-IIa, (**f**) type 0-IIb, (**g**) type 0-IIc. Types IIa and IIb have low probability of submucosal invasion; type IIc carries substantial risk of sm invasion (in particular when >2 cm). M-NBI analysis of microvascular pattern is mandatory for flat types of early gastric cancer

Pale (whitish) flat or depressed lesions with clear margins are highly suspicious of gastric cancer, typically un–/or poorly differentiated (*PDAC*) (Fig. 9.8), rarely well-differentiated adenocarcinoma (*WDAC*) (Fig. 9.7a–e) or adenoma, but may reveal focal atrophy (Fig. 9.5c) or MALT lymphoma on histology (Fig. 9.5e, f). Pale depressed lesions with unclear margins may represent focal atrophy, rarely undifferentiated AC [14–17] (algorithm Fig. 9.2d). Magnifying endoscopic analysis is useful for differential diagnosis (see below).

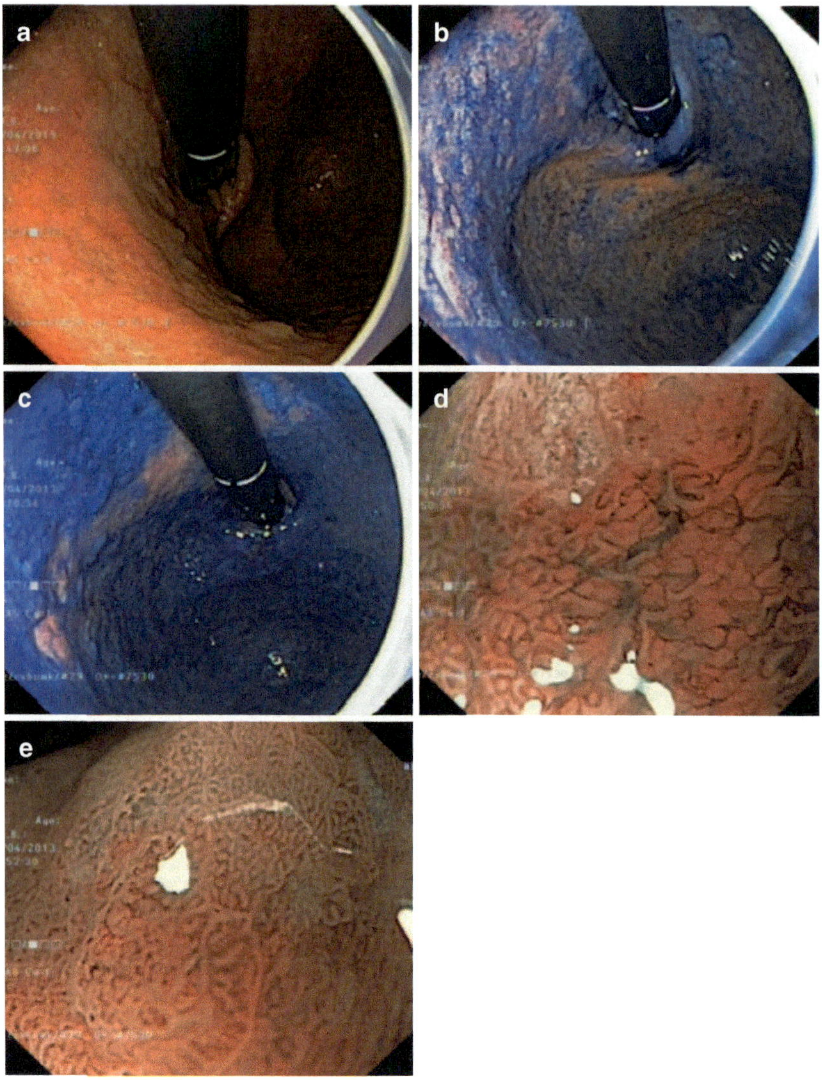

Fig. 9.7 (**a**–**e**) *Signs for intramucosal extension of differentiated AC. Intramucosal* extension of cancer (WDAC, HGIN) is common in *distinct homogeneous* lesions type 0-IIb. (**a**) Pale lesion 0-IIb in chronic Helicobacter-induced gastritis, WLI, (**b**) indigo carmine CE only, (**c**) acetic acid-indigo carmine CE (AIM), (**d**) center with irregular network VP (M-NBI, 80-fold); (**e**) clear margin (*left*, HGIN). ESD en bloc: WDAC (G1 pT0m1), resection R 0

Note Pale *lesion 0-IIb* (HGIN) in chronic Helicobacter-induced gastritis: Lateral extension is *obscured by indigo carmine only* (**b**), but *revealed by AIM-CE* (**c**). Magnifying endoscopic analysis is mandatory.

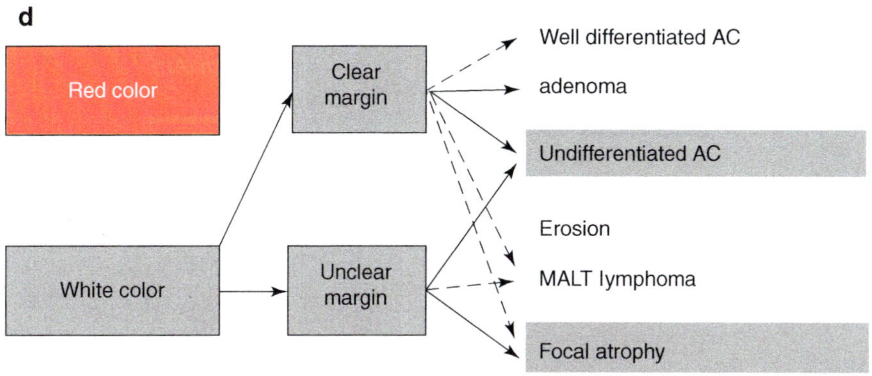

Fig. 9.2 (continued) (**d**) Standard WLI Algorithm. Differential diagnosis of pale flat or depressed lesions type 0-IIc

9.4 Diagnosis of Extension of Early Gastric Cancer on WLI

9.4.1 Information on Invasion Depth from Shape of Lesion

Intra*mucosal extension* of cancer is common in distinct *homogeneous* lesions of flat type, protuberant type and depressed type with *structured areal surface* pattern (Fig. 9.2e (*a–i*) for principles; Figs. 9.6 and 9.7a–e). Flat neoplastic *lesions type 0-IIa* or *IIb* most likely are intramucosal when the surface is smooth, fine granular with structured areal pattern on WLI and indigo carmine CE. *Flat depressed lesions 0-IIc* with *smooth reddish* surface and regular micrified surface pattern or irregular surface structure usually are intramucosal or superficially submucosa-invasive AC, most likely differentiated AC (Figs. 9.5d and 9.6g).

Massive submucosal invasion is heralded with >80% likelihood by the combination of *elevation or depression/ulceration* and *loss of areal pattern* (by destroyed MM layer) in early cancer lesions (Figs. 9.2e (*f–i*) and 9.7f–l), such as [18]:

- depression or ulcer in 0-Is or 0-IIa lesions,
- elevation with amorphous pit pattern in 0-IIc lesion,
- irregular protuberance, bulging area, or nodule in 0-IIc lesion,
- ulceration in 0-IIc lesion (0-IIc + III),
- irregular expansive protuberance in sessile 0-Is or 0-IIa lesion.

The most suspicious areas of the lesion usually loose structured areal pattern and show amorphous, non-structured surface in presence of massive sm-invasion.

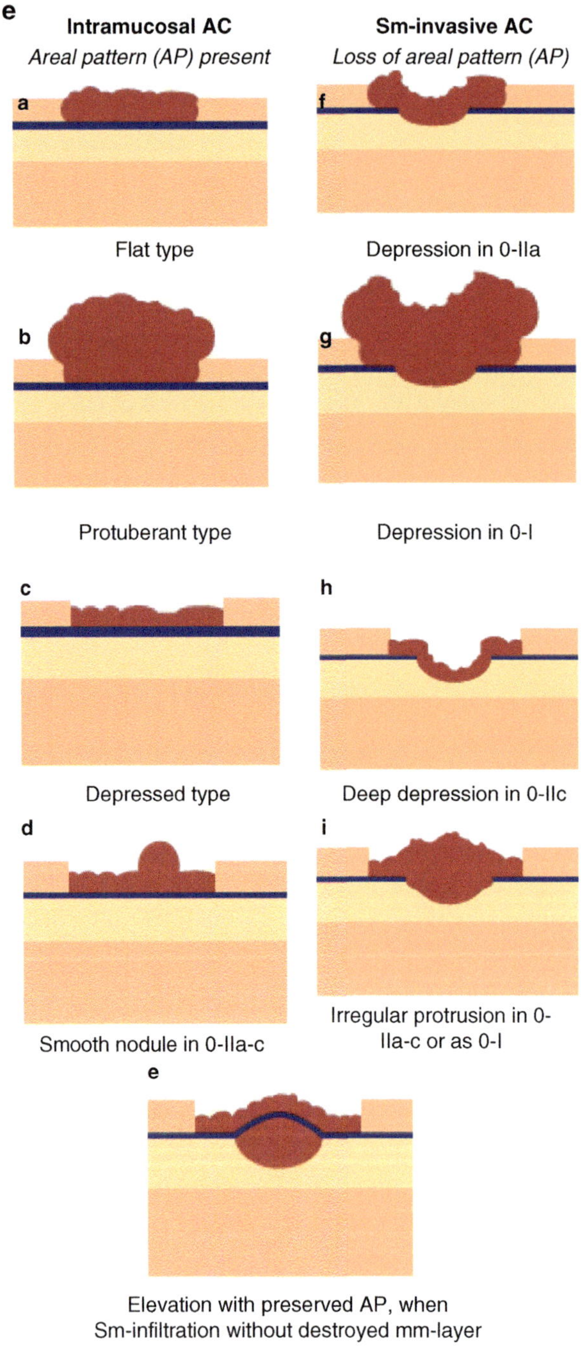

Fig. 9.2 (continued) (**e**)(*a–i*) Standard WLI & CE Signs for mucosal vs. sm invasive WDAC: Mucosal AC T1a presents regular surface with preserved areal pattern (***a–d***). Mucosal areal pattern becomes destroyed in case of coherent sm invasive growth (***f–i***) indicated by *irregular elevation* or *depression*. Discontinuous sm infiltration sometimes preserves mm-layer and areal pattern of AC (***e***), but distinct elevation in AC type 0-IIc remains suspicious for sm-infiltration of AC. Reprinted from Oyama et al. [16], with permission by NANKODO Ltd., Tokyo, JP.)

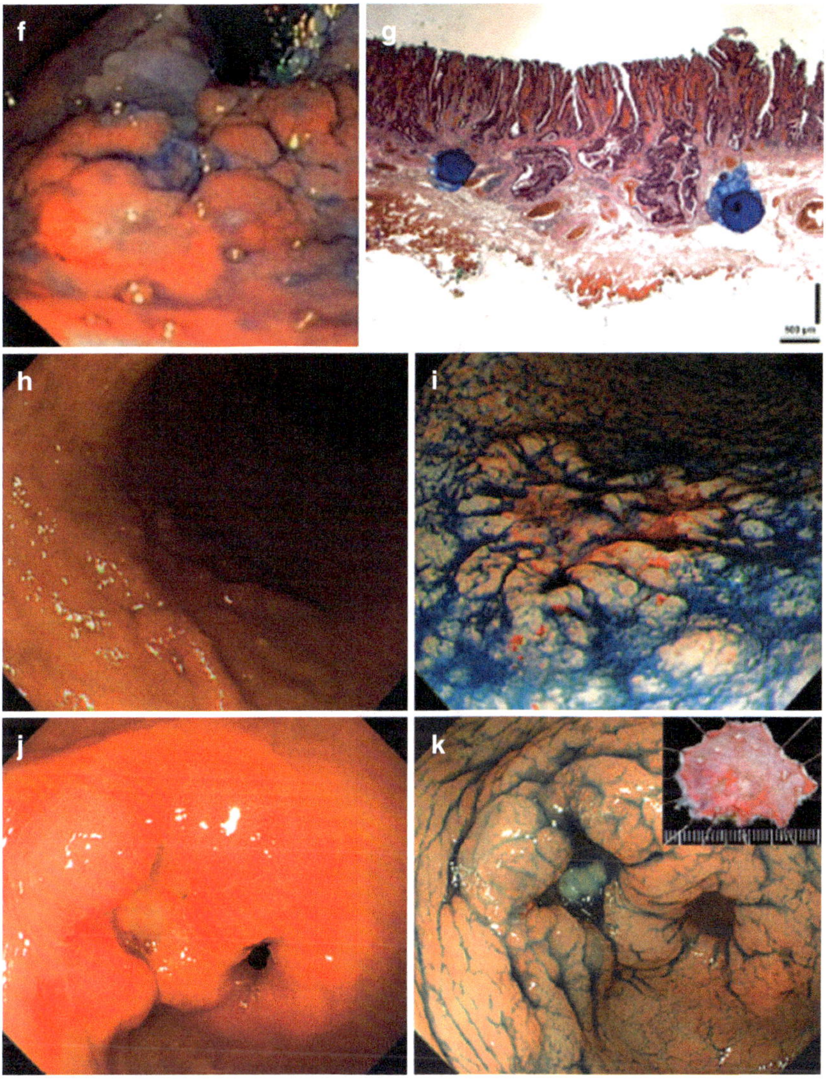

Fig. 9.7 (continued) (**f–k**) *Indirect signs of massive submucosal invasion* of differentiated AC: (**f**) depression in 0-IIa + IIc lesion at gastric cardia (**g**) AC G2. 560 μm sm2-invasion, HE stain 100-fold); (**h**, **i**) Elevation with loss of regular surface structure (amorphous surface pattern) in 0-IIc cancer; (**j**, **k**) Ulcer in depressed 0-IIc lesion (0-IIc + III) ((**j**) WLI; (**k**) IC-CE). Similar significance as (**f**) conveys ulcer with amorphous surface structure in sessile 0-Is lesion

9.4.2 Information on Invasion Depth by Shape of Mucosal Folds

Another clue to *depth of invasion* of early gastric cancer is alteration of form of gastric mucosal folds.

Intramucosal cancer (T1a) commonly shows *rigidity, narrowing, tapering or sharp break* of mucosal folds in a lesion (Fig. 9.2f(*a–c*)). *Submucosal invasion* of

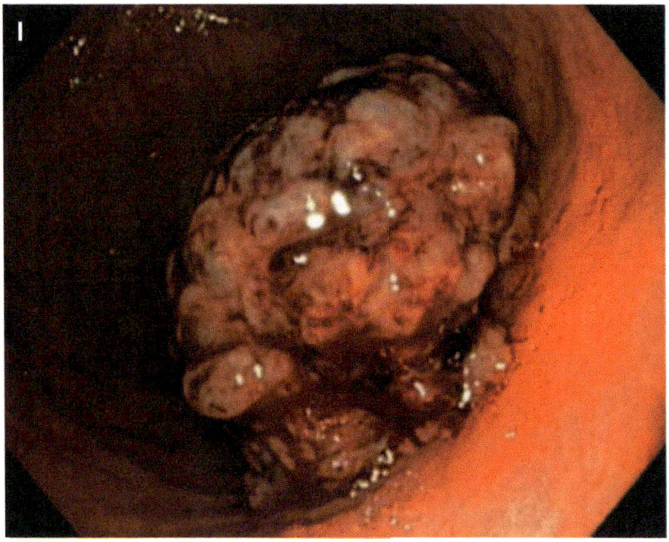

Fig. 9.7 (continued) (**l**) *Indirect signs of massive submucosal invasion* (probability >80%) of differentiated AC: (**l**) irregular protuberance, expansive nodular growth, "fullness of the stalk" in 0-Is or 0-II

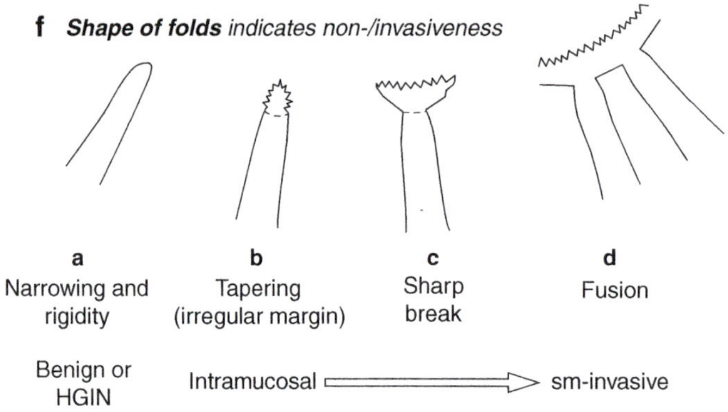

Fig. 9.2 (continued) (**f**) (*a–d*) Standard WLI Signs: Mucosal folds at flat depressed or ulcerated gastric lesions (0-IIc, III). Information on likely vertical extension of early gastric AC gained from shape of folds: (*a*) at benign ulcer or intramucosal AC (EP, LPM), (*b*) intramucosal AC (EP, LPM), (*c*) slightly sm-invasive AC (MM, sm1), (*d*) deeply sm-invasive AC (≥sm2). (Modified from Oyama [16].)

cancer is indicated by *thickening of the fold at the break*, and even more by *fusion of folds at the lesion* (Figs. 9.2f(*c,d*), 9.7m and 9.8e, f)

Submucosal protuberant lesions *without mucosal invasion* show *bridging folds* from mucosal level to the roof of the lesion)(Fig. 9.3g). Invasive SM tumors, however, may exhibit *mucosal* invasion and ulceration (Fig. 9.3h).

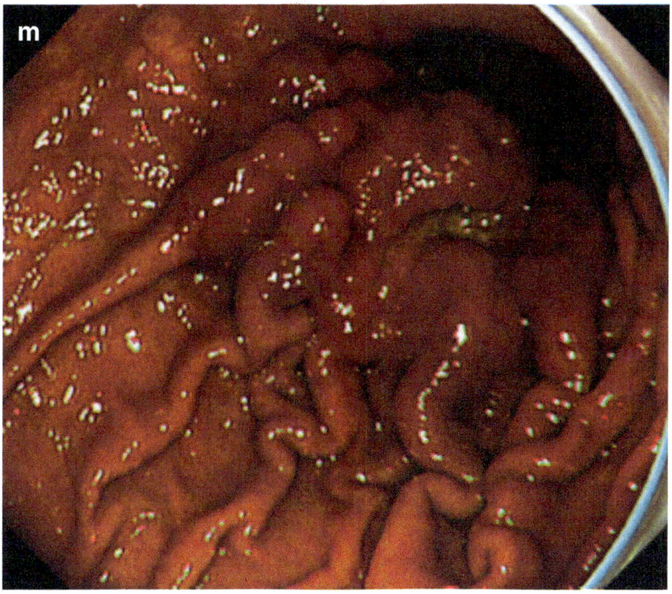

Fig. 9.7 (continued) (**m**) *Infiltrating undifferentiated adenocarcinoma* often shows *thick and irregular folds*, some *folds with fusion* in the center of the lesion, an alteration highly suspicious for *massive sm invasion*

9.4.3 Diagnosis of Lateral Extension of Mucosal Early Gastric Cancer

Well differentiated adenocarcinoma (*WDAC*) typically presents on standard WLI as flat reddish lesion 0-IIb, protruding 0-IIa or depressed 0-IIc, with clear margins in chronic gastritis (Fig. 9.6e–g). By contrast, *undifferentiated adenocarcinoma* typically shows a whitish depressed lesion 0-IIc with clear margin in fundic gland area (Fig. 9.8a–g). Chromoendoscopy with indigo carmine improves detection of the margin of depressed lesions in normal gastric mucosa or the margin of whitish, flat-protruded lesions in chronic gastritis (Fig. 9.6e, f). But it may obscure flat lesion 0-IIb in a background of chronic nodular gastritis. Chromoendoscopy using a freshly prepared mixture of 0.6% acetic acid with 0.4% indigocarmine (*AIM)* accentuates structural differences in epithelial microsurface of whitish flat lesions 0-IIb in gastric mucosa, because acetic acid fixates surface mucins that are contrast visualized by indigo carmine [19]. By contrast, indigo carmine alone does not accentuate this difference of surface structure (Figs. 9.7a–e and 9.8f, g).

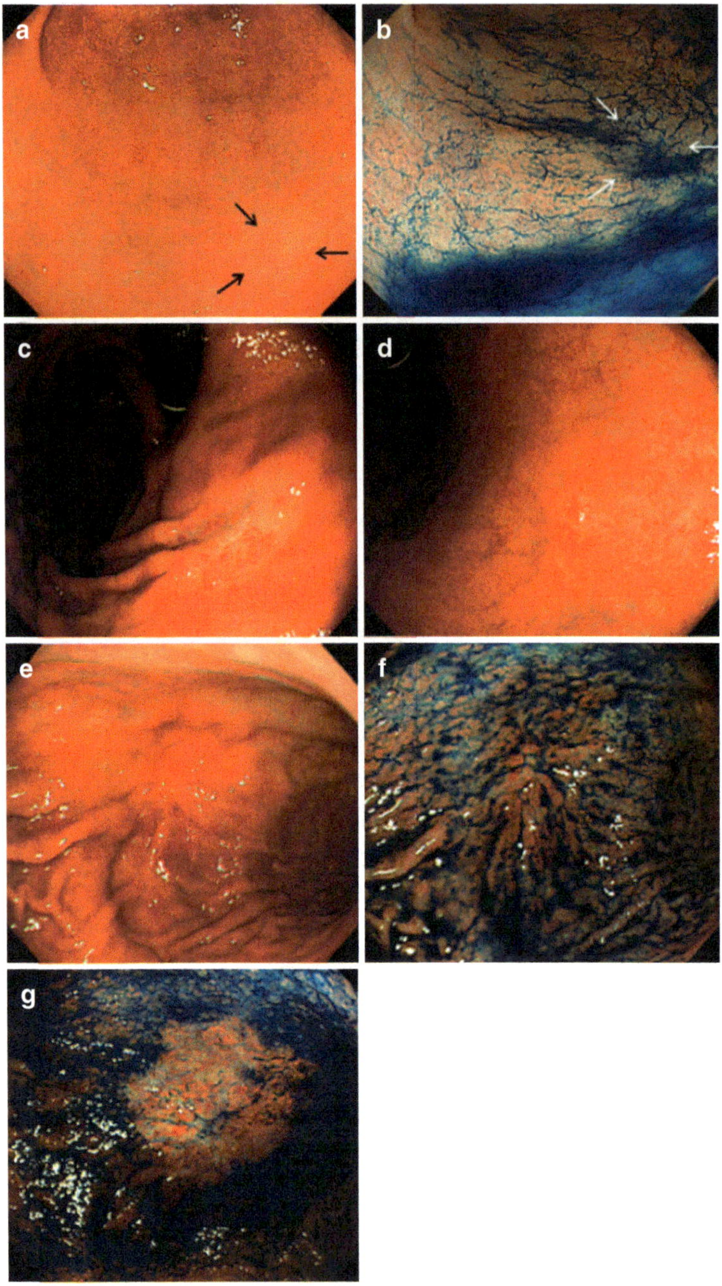

Fig. 9.8 (**a**–**g**) Poorly differentiated cancer *PDAC type 0-IIb* in pyloric-type mucosa. (**a**) PDAC lesion 0-IIb (*arrows*) on WLI, (**b**) indigo carmine CE, *white arrows* mark the lesion. (**c**, **d**) Typical PDAC in fundic gland mucosa. Whitish lesion 0-IIc with clear margin. WLI in (**c**) slight insufflation, (**d**) full insufflation. (**e**–**g**) *PDAC type 0-IIb + c*: (**e**) Isochrome-whitish lesion 0-IIb + c in major curvature with break and some fusion of folds, typical for sm-invasive PDAC in chronic gastritis, WLI. (**f**) Indigo carmine obscures, (**g**) AIM truly reveals lateral PDAC extension

9.5 Analysis of Gastric Adenocarcinoma with Magnified NBI and Surface Enhanced Endoscopy

Suspicious lesions must be observed with magnifying endoscopy (ME, ≥60-fold magnification), native in NBI mode for VP, and after surface enhancement with acetic acid for SP, – and analysed according to the actual JGES guideline (Fig. 9.9a) [8]. Magnification (60- to 100-fold) with ME nearly matches that used on light microscopy and allows analysis of microsurface structure (SP) and microvascular architecture (VP). Characteristics of intestinal-type Early Gastric AC are the presence of a clear demarcation line (DL) between cancerous and non-cancerous mucosa and the presence of an irregular SP and/or irregular VP of the lesion within the DL (diagnostic accuracy 95%). By contrast diffuse type PDAC may exhibit regular SP without DL when spreading in subepithelial LPM and in SM [4, 15].

You have to analyze VP and SP separately. There are two basic SP in stomach – villous in antrum and aboral corpus, and pit-like in corpus and fundus. Altered SP shows surface structure of the cancer, whereas irregular VP presents changes in vessel running caused by the cancer. Both correlate with histological type as well as tumor category (T1a, T1b) of EGC. However, combined interpretation of surface and vessel changes allows to predict the likely histological type of early gastric cancer [4, 8, 13, 15].

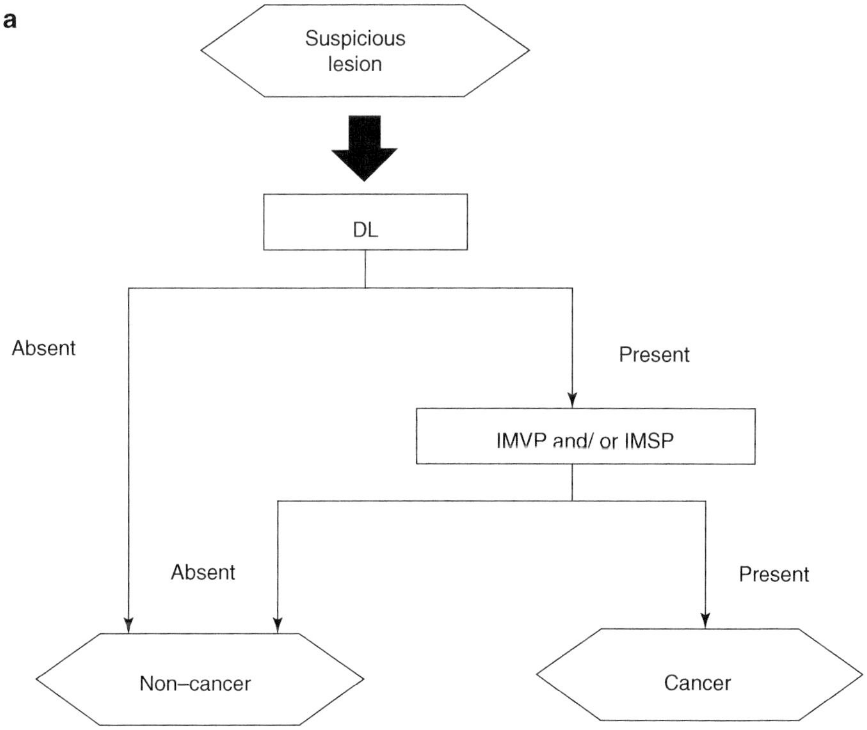

Fig. 9.9 (**a**) Magnifying Endoscopy Diagnostic Algorithm for Gastric cancer (MESDA-G). DL, demarcation line; IMVP, irregular microvascular pattern; IMSP, irregular microsurface pattern. (From Muto et al. [8], reprinted with permission of John Wiley & Sons)

9.5.1 Villous Patterns

Villous pattern means protruded structural components like fingers. The shape and size of non-neoplastic villi is regular and uniform, with enough space between them. The width of white zone (i.e. marginal epithelium) also is even and uniform (Fig. 9.10a).

On the other hand, the shape of ***cancerous villi*** is irregular and uneven. The number of villi became crowded, the density higher, and width of white zone became uneven (Fig 9.10b). Well differentiated adenocarcinoma (*WDAC*) entirely shows dense, micrified villous pattern. However, *fusion of villi* (i.e. destruction by invasive growth) in highly irregular villous pattern is frequent in moderately differentiated adenocarcinoma (*MDAC*) and likely predicts MDAC (Fig. 9.10c, d). WDAC and MDAC lesions show sharp demarcation of SP from non-neoplastic mucosa.

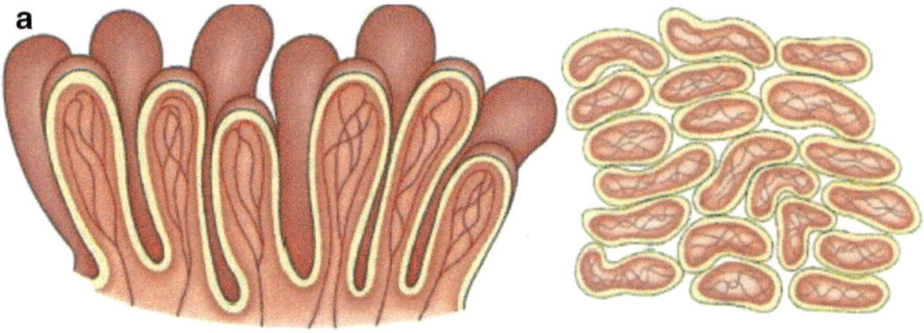

Fig. 9.10 (**a**) Schematic drawing of villous structure of normal pyloric type gastric mucosa which shows subepithelial capillaries (SEC) in mucosal lamina propria (LPM) and a white zone (WZ) of marginal epithelium on the villi (left). The perpendicular view (right) during M-NBI endoscopy projects the SEC in a helix spiral like fashion surrounded by epithelial white zone. Shapes, sizes, VP (SEC), and WZ of normal villi are quite uniform and even. (Reprinted from Oyama [16], with permission of Nankodo Co., Ltd. Tokyo, JP.)

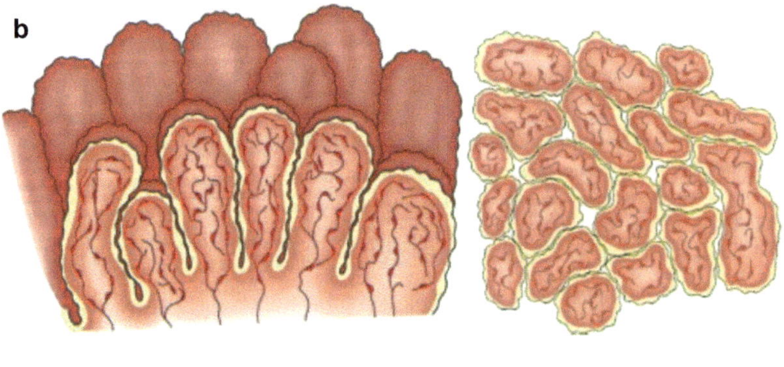

Fig. 9.10 (continued) (**b**) Schematic graphics of ***neoplastic villi*** showing high density (crowding) of villi, uneven distribution of villous sizes and shapes, uneven width of white zones, and irregular capillary pattern (sizes, densitiy, caliber, tortuosity). (Reprinted from Oyama [16], with permission of Nankodo Co., Ltd. Tokyo, JP.)

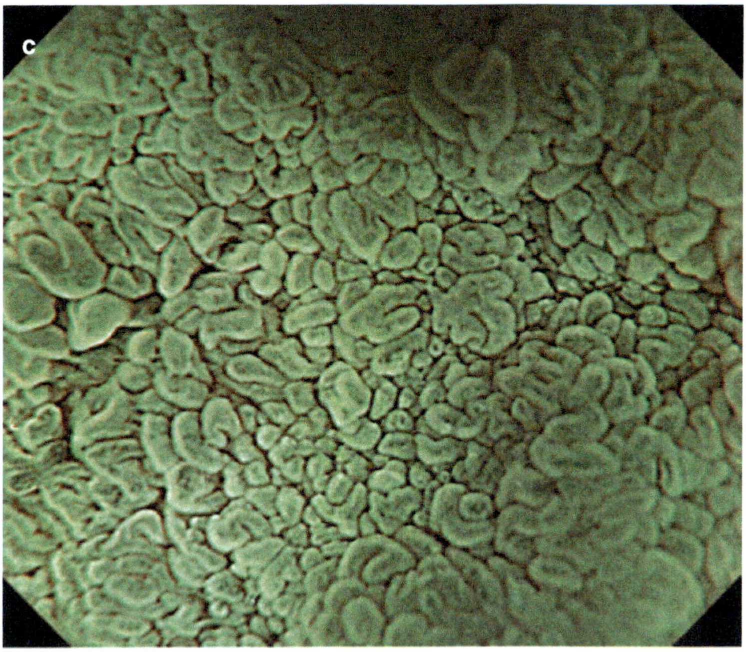

Fig. 9.10 (continued) (**c**) Surface pattern of moderately differentiated adenocarcinoma (MDAC) showing dense villous surface pattern with wide variation of villous sizes and shapes caused by fusion of villi, on M-NBI (100×) after acetic acid surface enhancement

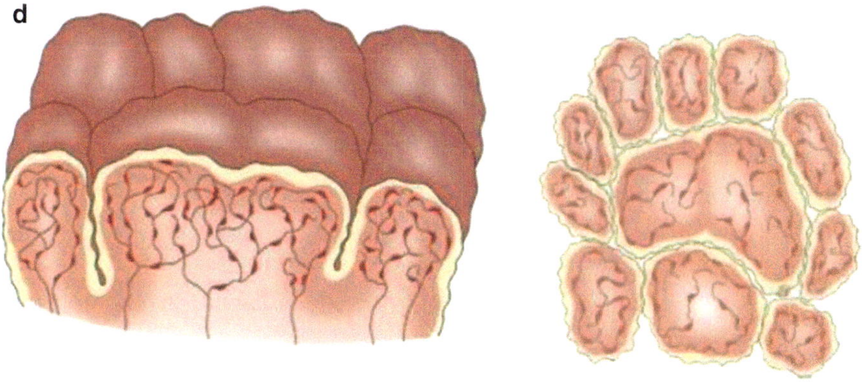

Fig. 9.10 (continued) (**d**) Graphics of fusion of villi in MDAC. Due to fusion of villi, sizes and shape of villi vary and VP of villi became irregular. (Reprinted from Oyama [16], with permission of Nankodo Co., Ltd. Tokyo, JP.)

Key Points for villous pattern

- Shape
- Size
- Density
- Width of white zone

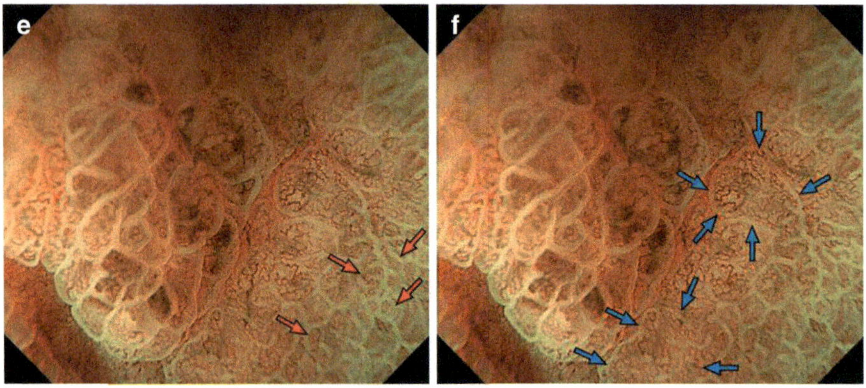

Fig. 9.10 (continued) (**e**, **f**) Fusion of villi. (M-NBI) (**e**) irregularly shaped, variable size villi (red arrows); (**f**) fusion of villi is noted (blue arrows) with longer running, irregular non-spiral VP. (Reprinted from Oyama [16], with permission of Nankodo Co., Ltd. Tokyo, JP.)

9.5.2 Pit Patterns

Pit means a small hole-like structure coated with glandular epithelium (MCE, marginal crypt epithelium). The shape of non-neoplastic pit is round, and surrounded by network of regular subepithlial capillaries (SEC). Pit should be seen as a black circle. However, the size of hole is too small to identify it by moderate magnified view. And, the light reflexed by MCE of the pit gland looks white. Therefore, non-neoplastic pits in fundic mucosa look like white round dots of even sizes surrounded by regular SEC network (Fig. 9.10g).

Structure of neoplastic pits. The shape and size of cancerous pit is irregular and uneven, neoplastic pits are densely packed (Fig. 9.10h, i). And, irregular microvessels are observed in interstitium between the pits (Fig. 9.10j).

Key Points for pit pattern
- Shape
- Size
- Density

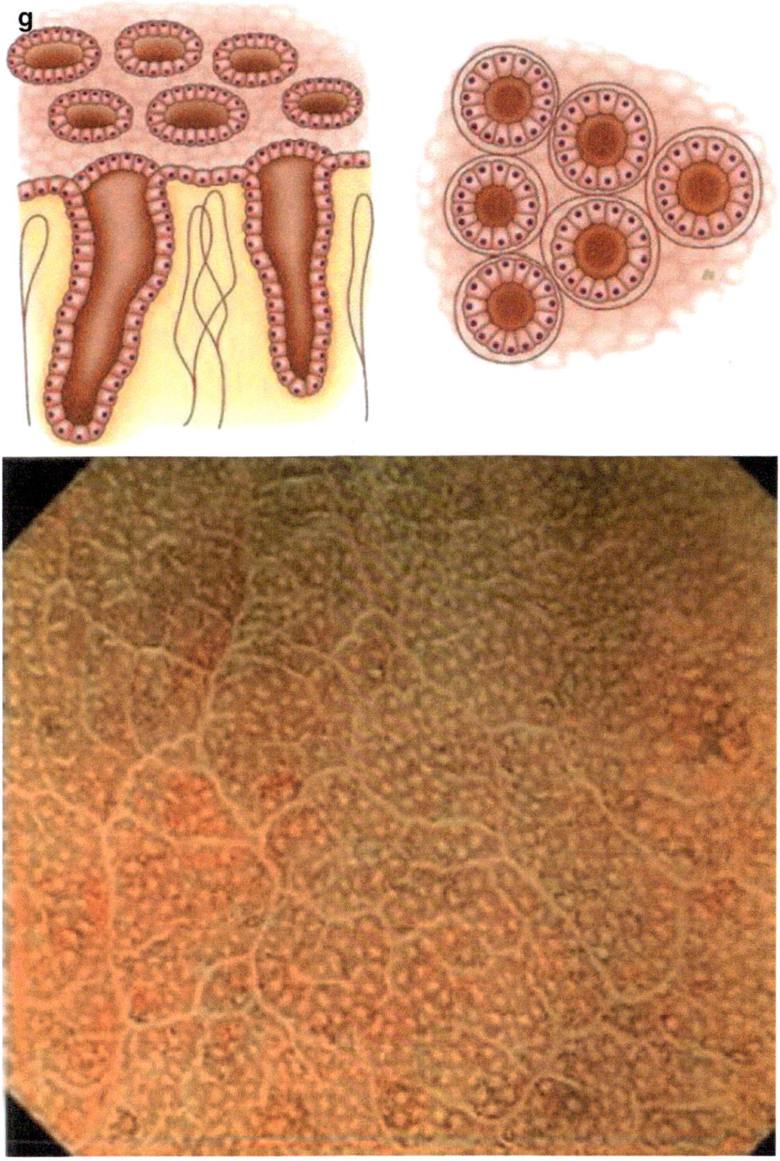

Fig. 9.10 (continued) (**g**) Structure of non-neoplastic pit. The shape of non-neoplastic pit is regular round and surrounded by regular network of microvessels. (Reprinted from Oyama [16], with permission of Nankodo Co., Ltd. Tokyo, JP.)

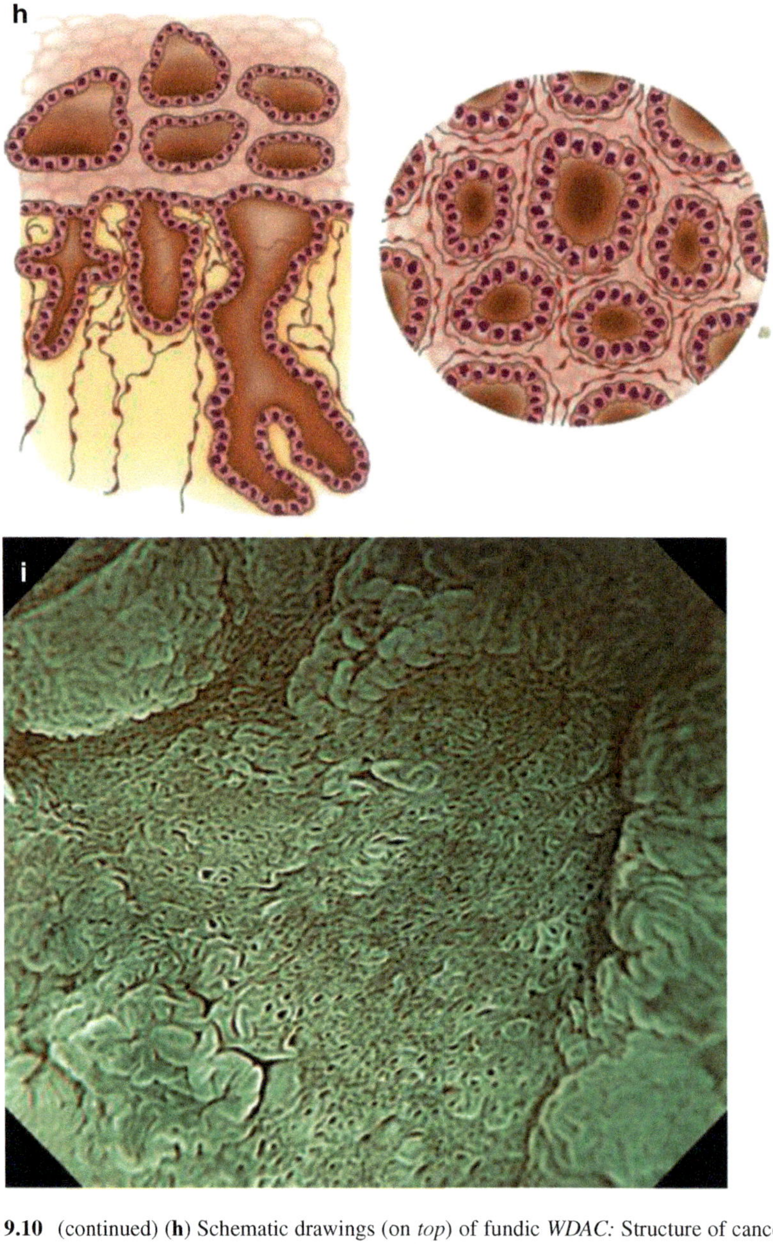

Fig. 9.10 (continued) (**h**) Schematic drawings (on *top*) of fundic *WDAC:* Structure of cancerous pits is irregular and uneven, and irregular capillaries (irreg. network) are present between pits. (Reprinted from Oyama [16], with permission of Nankodo Co., Ltd. Tokyo, JP.) (**i**) Small WDAC type 0-IIc showing micrified, dense pit surface pattern and sharp margins on M-NBI (100×) after acetic acid surface enhancement, in fundic mucosa

9.5.3 Vascular Patterns

Caliber change, *tortuosity* and *network* are the important points to observe on capillaries. Caliber change means the change of diameter. When the diameter of microvessels abruptly became twofold thicker or thinner, they were judged to have caliber change. Network means closed running of microvessels. When the basic structure was pit, capillaries run around pit and make network VP. Nakayoshi proposed that network pattern is evidence of *WDAC* [13] (Fig. 9.10j).

On the other hand, poorly differentiated adenocarcinoma (*PDAC*) spreads throughout parenchyma destroying glandular structures and microvessels. Therefore, microvessels can't make network, but run with complex branching and severe tortuosity. Nakayoshi named these irregular microvessels as corkscrew [13]. But, the shape is different from corkscrew. Therefore, the author uses the term of *"Non-network"* to describe such *irregular microvessels* [4] (Fig. 9.10k).

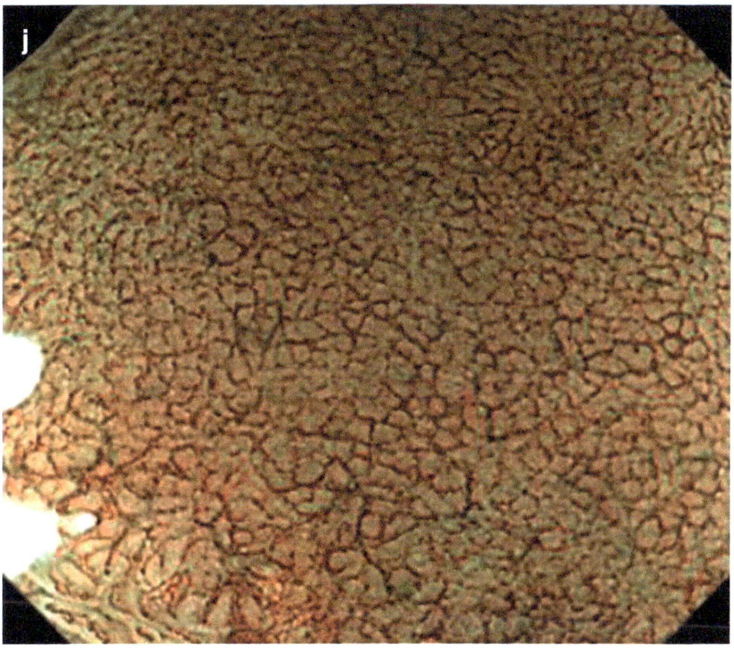

Fig. 9.10 (continued) (**j**) Slightly irregular, dense network VP of WDAC on M-NBI (100×)

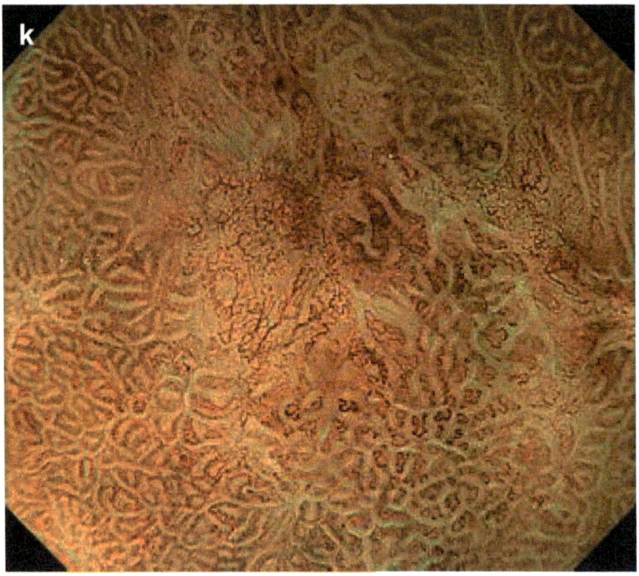

Fig. 9.10 (continued) (**k**) Non-network VP of undifferentiated AC type 0-IIc (signet ring C) on M-NBI

Key Points for vascular patterns

- Tortuosity
- Caliber change
- Network vs. Non-network VP | Short spiral vs. long-running VP

9.5.4 Relationship Between Surface Pattern and Vascular Pattern

Villous structure, when preserved in gastric AC (Fig. 9.10b), displays SEC in villi only for short distance (only *short spirals*), with irregular caliber, without complex branching or augmented tortuosity. This type of *short*, irregular spiral VP suggests villous SP and supports diagnosis of WDAC. However, fusion of some villi leads to very irregular, *variably sized villous* SP with *long* running, irregular capillaries within fused villi (*moderate atypia* with complex branching, tortuosity, caliber changes) (Fig. 9.10d, f). This moderate vessel atypia indicates MDAC, when fused villi are confirmed after acetic acid enhancement (Fig. 9.10c).

Pit-like structure allows capillaries to run longer in ME projection, and display running irregularities and caliber changes in the basic network structure (Fig. 9.10h). Therefore, when basic *network* VP structure is preserved, we can postulate *pit-like* SP structure even in presence of unclear surface pattern after acetic acid enhancement. This allows endoscopic prediction of *WDAC*. By contrast, *MDAC* forms irregular branching of pit-like glands and irregular cell complexes, i.e. uncertain pit-like SP, and therefore vascular structures show complex, destroyed network structure, and severe irregularity and caliber change (*moderate to severe vascular atypia*). – then sometimes, distinction between MDAC (preserved irregular SP) vs. PDAC (unclear or absent SP) is difficult. However, presence (WDAC) or absence of network (MDAC, PDAC) is important for prediction of pathological diagnosis [4, 13].

9.5.5 Prediction of Histological Type with Magnified Endoscopy

ME analysis of *surface pattern* helps to predict the most likely histological type of superficial gastric adenocarcinoma (algorithm in Fig. 9.9b).

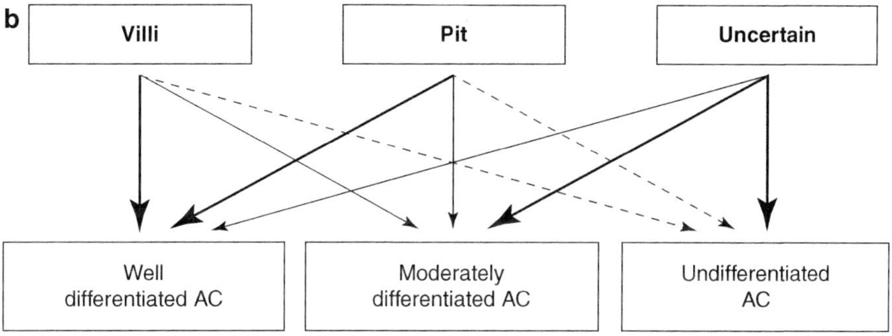

Fig. 9.9 (continued) (**b**) Magnifying Endoscopy Diagnostic Algorithm. Relationship of surface pattern SP with histological type of early gastric cancer. Strength of arrows indicates probability. AC = adenocarcinoma. (Modified from Oyama [16], with permission of Nankodo Co., Ltd. Tokyo, JP.)

Mucosal WDAC shows expansive growth in EP and LPM layer preserving areal pattern and the basic villous or pit-like structure of the native pyloric or fundic type mucosa, with some irregularity of SP (micrification, variation in size & shape, dense placement). WDAC displays distinct irregular villous SP with short irregular helical VP, or pit-like irregular SP (shape, density, size) with irregular network VP (without atypia) (Figs. 9.9c, d and 9.10b, h–j).

MDAC shows longer running vessels with areas of non-network VP and fusion of villi (Fig. 9.10c, f) or rarified pits or unclear SP after surface enhancement. Even fused villiform structures have complex non-network capillary patterns (Fig. 9.10d–f).

Altered villi (SP) and altered vessels (*VP*) – interpreted together – allow tentative diagnosis of pathological type of early gastric cancer in antrum and distal corpus (algorithm in Fig. 9.9c).

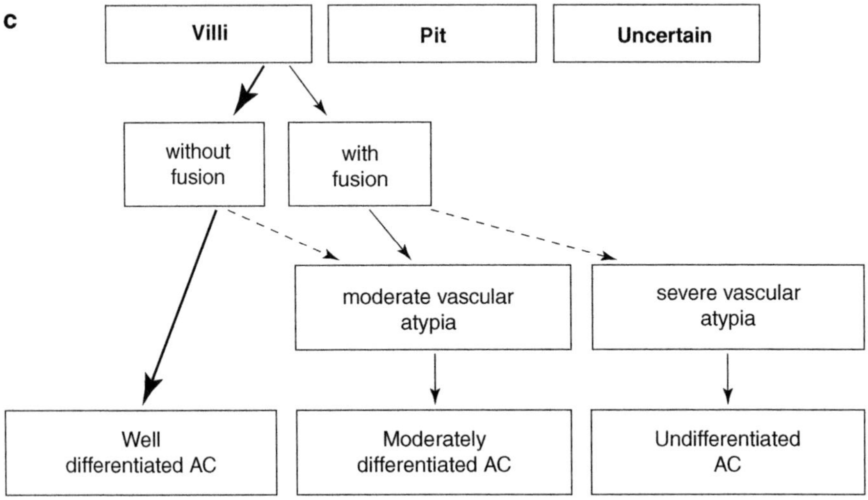

Fig. 9.9 (continued) (**c**) Magnifying Endoscopic Algorithm. Relationship of villous pattern with histological type of AC. (Reprinted from Oyama [16], with permission of Nankodo Co., Ltd. Tokyo, JP.)

Altered pit pattern bears diagnostic relationship with *pathological grading* of early gastric cancer in corpus-fundus region (Figs 9.9d and 9.10h–k). Scrutiny for presence or absence of network VP on M-NBI and presence or absence of irregular pit SP after acetic acid surface enhancement is essential for accurate prediction of histological type of AC (Fig. 9.10j, k).

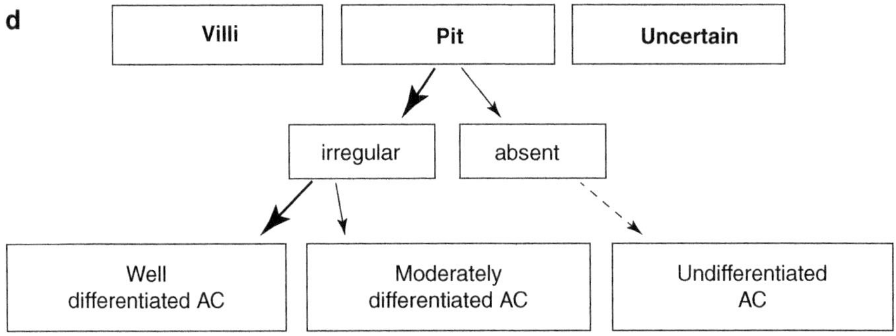

Fig. 9.9 (continued) (**d**) Magnifying Diagnostic Algorithm. Relationship of pit pattern with grading of gastric AC. (Reprinted from Oyama [16], with permission of Nankodo Co., Ltd. Tokyo, JP.)

e

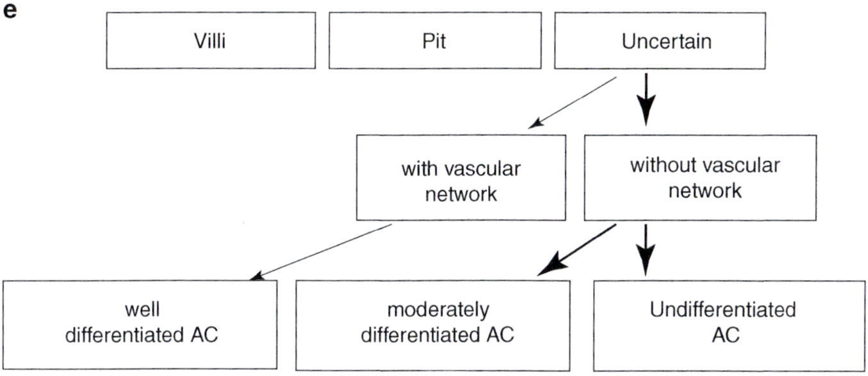

Fig. 9.9 (continued) (**e**) Magnifying Endoscopic Algorithm. Relationship of uncertain surface pattern and histologic grading of AC. (Reprinted from Oyama [16], with permission of Nankodo Co., Ltd. Tokyo, JP.) (see below)

Early PDAC (confined to M or SM layer) presents in most cases uncertain or absent SP and pronounced non-network VP (corkscrew-like)(Fig. 9.10l). However, when diffusely spreading within mucosal LPM layer below the neck of pit-like glands, and in SM, PDAC may show preserved pit-like SP and unclear margin without demarcation line. In such cases with small, flat whitish lesions, diagnosis of PDAC must be confirmed with targeted biopsy and cancer-free status of margins with quadrant biopsies 1 cm beyond the suspected margin.

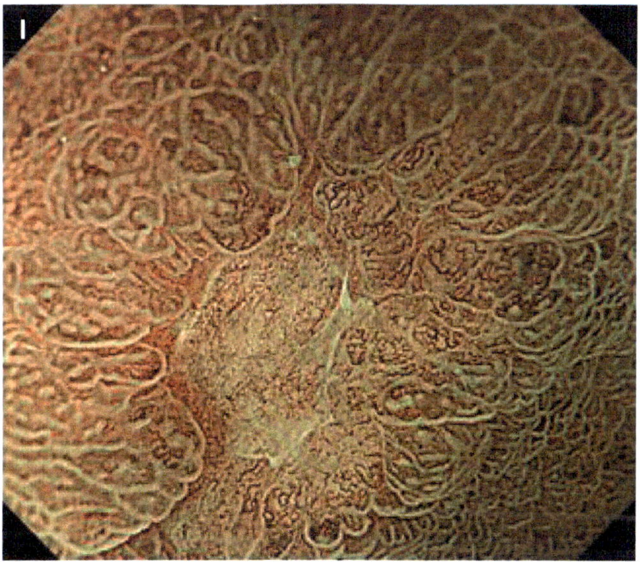

Fig. 9.10 (continued) (**l**) *Uncertain* (absent) surface pattern with *non-network VP* and clear margins to fundic-type gastric mucosa are typical for minute *moderately or undifferentiated AC*

Uncertain surface pattern. When the surface pattern is uncertain, WDAC, MDAC and PDAC should be distinguished (Fig. 9.9e). NBI-observation of VP and of SP with acetic acid is useful (Fig. 9.10f, j, m, n).

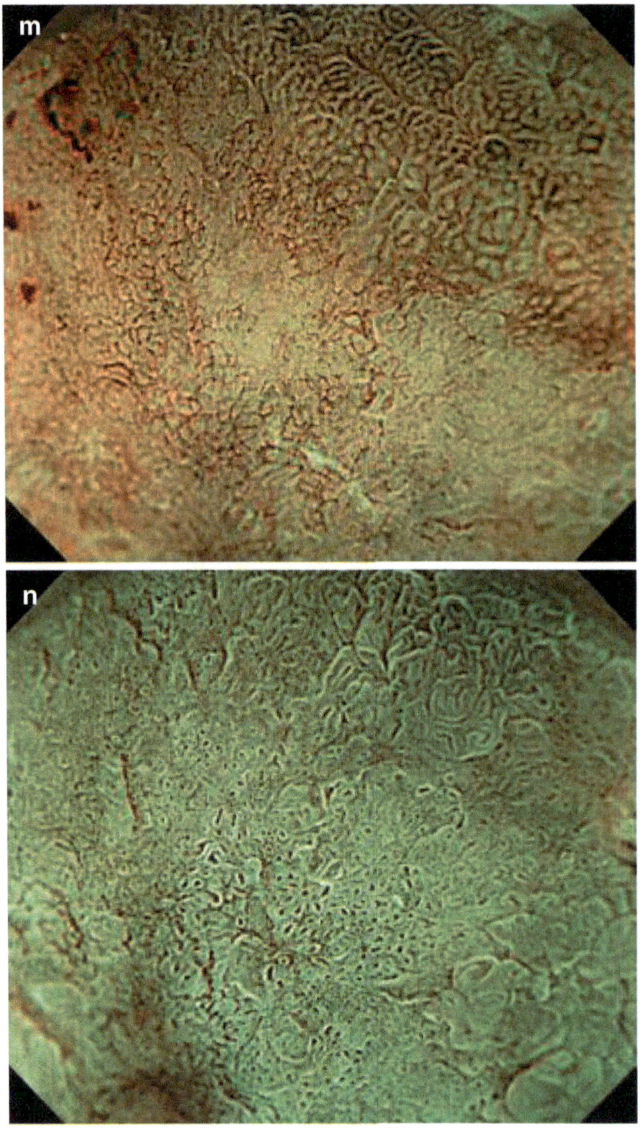

Fig. 9.10 (continued) **(m, n)** *Acetic acid surface enhancement may change the endoscopic grading*: (**m**) On M-NBI only, uncertain SP and non-network vascular pattern indicates MDAC or PDAC. (**n**) Acetic acid spreading clearly reveals irregular pit SP, typical for *well-differentiated AC* in fundic-type mucosa. M-NBI (100×) (*top*, **m**) and with acetic acid surface enhancement (*bottom*, **n**)

9.6 Endoscopic Diagnosis of HGIN or Superficially sm-Invasive Versus Deeply sm-Invasive Carcinoma

The endoscopic key analysis is to define the lateral margins as well as to distinguish superficially vs. deeply sm-invasive (SM2–3) early cancer. A depth predicting score of >3 points indicates SM2–3 invasion of non-protruding differentiated early gastric cancer based on scoring for margin elevation and tumor size >3 cm (2 points ea.), remarkable redness and uneven surface (1 point ea.) [20].

Note Predictors of deep submucosal invasion (≥sm-2) [4, 9, 13, 20]

- Lesions of 0-subtypes IIa-c with *amorphous* SP
- *Irregular VP, dense (density↑)* or *sparse (density↓)*
- Size >2 cm of lesions type 0-IIc
- *Expansive nodule(s)*, fold(s), or elevation(s) in protuberant or flat lesions
- *Depression or ulceration* in flat lesion (0-IIa-c) with irregular SP and VP

9.7 Endoscopic Resection of Early Gastric Neoplasias

The general rule for endoscopic treatment of early gastric cancer is complete en-bloc resection. Clearly, snare-EMR achieves complete en-bloc resection in nearly 100% of lesions 0-IIa or IIb of size ≤20 mm and lesions 0-IIc of size ≤10 mm – *classical* indication criteria for resection with EMR techniques (compare Fig. 3.1).

ESD has been developed for gastric neoplasias too large for EMR by snaring techniques. For lesions larger than 20 mm (IIa,b) or 10 mm (IIc), the *expanded* criteria for *ESD* (Table 3.2) represent constellations with nearly zero percent risk of established lymph node metastasis – provided the resected specimen *does not* show any high risk criteria such as high grading (G3 or G4), lymphovascular invasion (L1 or V1), cancer cell budding (Bd2; Bd3) at invasion front, or submucosal invasion exceeding 500 μm below mucularis mucosae [21]. In addition, clinical staging with endoscopic ultrasound or CT scan must be negative for suspicious regional lymph nodes. Guideline criteria for EMR/ESD, expanded criteria for ESD, and guideline criteria for surgical resection are summarized in Table 9.1 [21–23]. The probability of established lymph node metastasis is *zero percent* [interval of confidence 0 to <3%] for *Classical Criteria* and the *Expanded Criteria* [21, 22, 24–26].

Table 9.1 Classical Criteria for Endoscopic Resection/Expanded Criteria for Endoscopic Submucosal Dissection[e]. (Modified from [23] based on [25, 29])

Depth / Histology	Mucosal Cancer				Submucosal Cancer	
	No Ulceration		Ulcerated		SM1	SM2
	≤ 20 mm	> 20 mm	≤ 30 mm	> 30 mm	≤ 30 mm	any size
Intestinal	a	b	b	d	b	d
Diffuse	c	d	d	d	d	d

[a]**Guideline criteria for EMR or ESD**
[b]Expanded criteria for ESD
[c]Consider surgery when type 0-IIc with size 11- ≤20 mm
[d]Surgery (gastrectomy + lymph node dissection)
[e]consistent with current guidelines [22, 26]

Note Outcome of ESD for early gastric cancer is favourable [24, 27, 28]:

Disease-specific 5-year overall survival	99%
Bleeding	8%
Perforation	0–6%
Local recurrence	0–2%

9.8 Cases: Gastric Neoplastic Lesions

Case 1: Pale Lesion Type 0-IIc (~ 1 cm) Located at Distal Corpus
Surveillance endoscopy for chronic atrophic gastritis type B (Helicobacter pylori induced) pointed out a small pale lesion 0-IIc in 56 y.o. woman (Fig. 9.11).

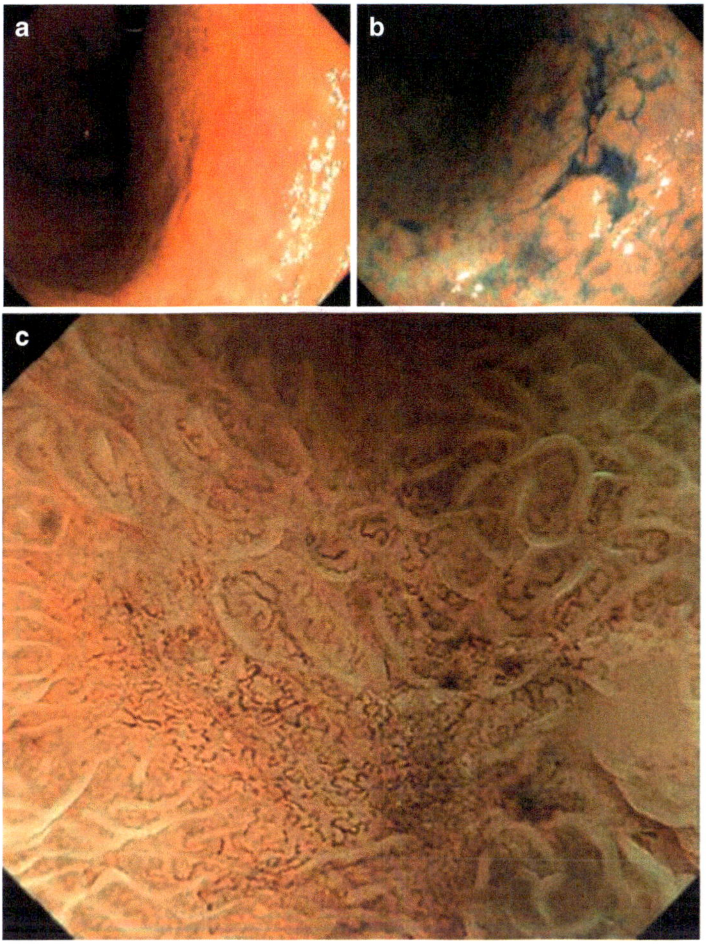

Fig. 9.11 (**a**) Small (<1 cm) pale lesion 0-IIc (WLI), (**b**) indigo carmine CE demonstrates the margins. (**c**) Magnifying NBI shows a tiny spot that exhibits highly irregular CP (*non-network*) and *absent surface pattern*. ESD en-bloc: Small signet ring cancer 0-IIc, pT1a(M), sig., 8 × 4 mm, ly0, v0, no ulcer. R0, curatively resected (compare Table 3.2)

Note Analysis of vascular pattern and surface structure is essential.

Case 2: Reddish Lesion Type 0-IIa + b Located at the Gastric Antrum

Gastroscopy was performed for epigastralgia in an 86 y.o. woman. Small gastric lesion was pointed out at the anterior wall of upper gastric body and evaluated (Fig. 9.12).

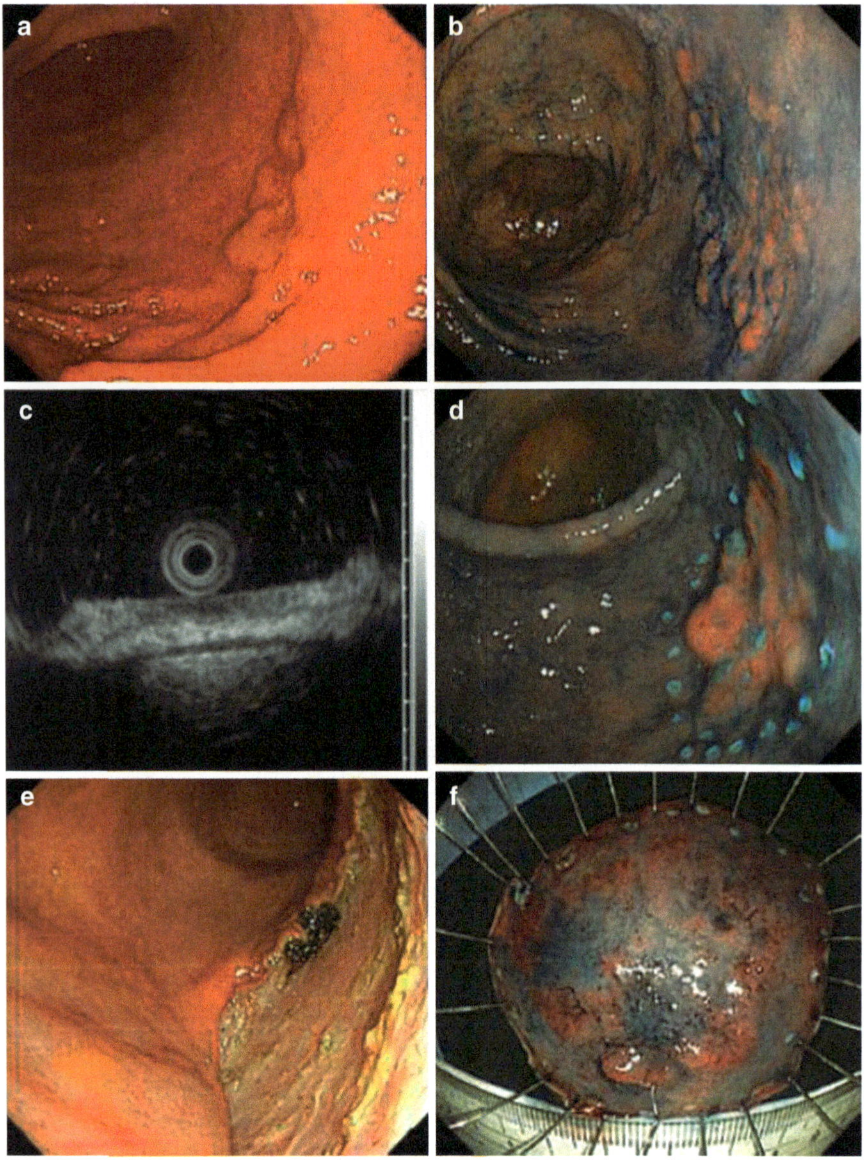

Fig. 9.12 (**a**) Reddish lesion 0-IIa + b, WLI. (**b**) On full insufflation, the lesion 0-IIa evenly distended (AID+), and distinct lateral margins were visible on indigo carmine CE. (**c**) Hr-EUS (20 MHz) showed continuous white sm echo band. (**d**) Lesion 0-IIa + b, safety margin marked (indigo carmine CE). (**e**) Resection bed after ESD using dual knife. (**f**) Specimen (indigo carmine) mounted with pins for pathological work-up: *adenocarcinoma, intestinal type*, pT1aM, tub2, 42 × 33 mm in size, ly0, v0. Curatively resected R0 (guideline criteria see Tables 9.1 and 3.2)

Note Lesion 0-IIa + b, AID, and intact sm echo suggested intramucosal cancer.

Case 3: Reddish Lesion Type 0-IIa + c (1.5 cm), at Upper Corpus

In a 86 y.o. female, gastroscopy was performed for evaluation of epigastralgia. A gastric lesion 0-IIa + c was pointed out at anterior wall of upper gastric body (Fig. 9.13).

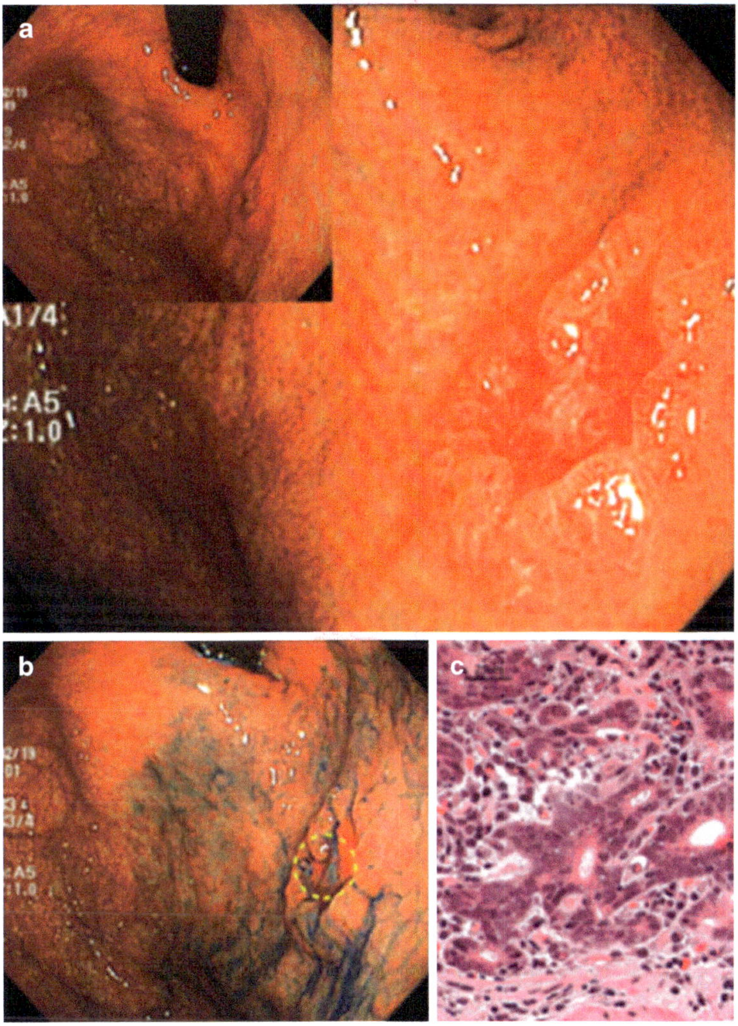

Fig. 9.13 (**a**) Reddish lesion 0-IIa+c in upper part of gastric corpus, WLI, (**b**) Indigo carmine CE. (**c**) Targeted biopsy from area 0-IIc showed moderately differentiated adenocarcinoma, intestinal type (HE). Probability of SM invasion was considered high

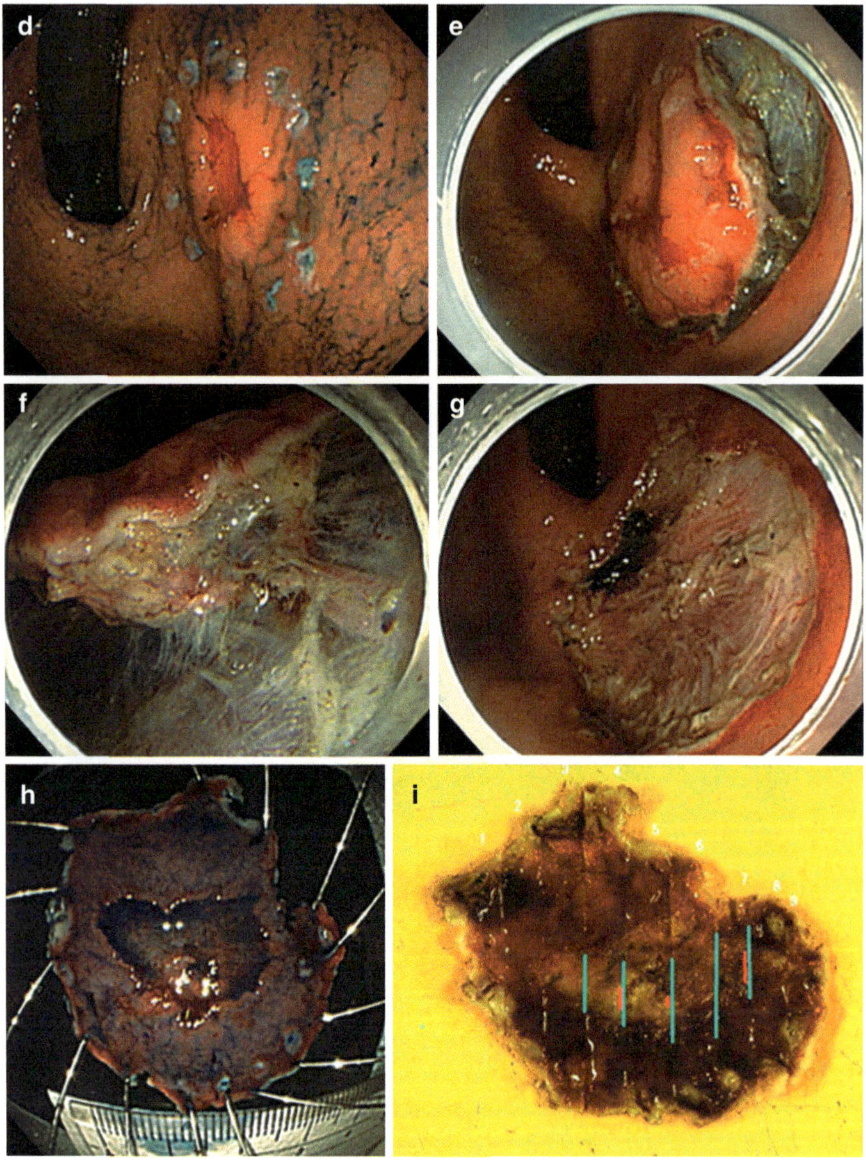

Fig. 9.13 (continued) (**d–g**) ESD using dual knife was conducted en bloc as a palliative therapy. (**h**) The specimen was pinned, photodocumented (suspicious area in 0-IIc marked), and forwarded for histological evaluation (in serial sections). (**i**) *Specimen with histological mapping*: *cyan line* markings reflect intramucosal extension of cancer, *red line* markings indicate sm invasion. Histology: moderately *differentiated* adenocarcinoma G2, pT1b *sm1* (300 μm)

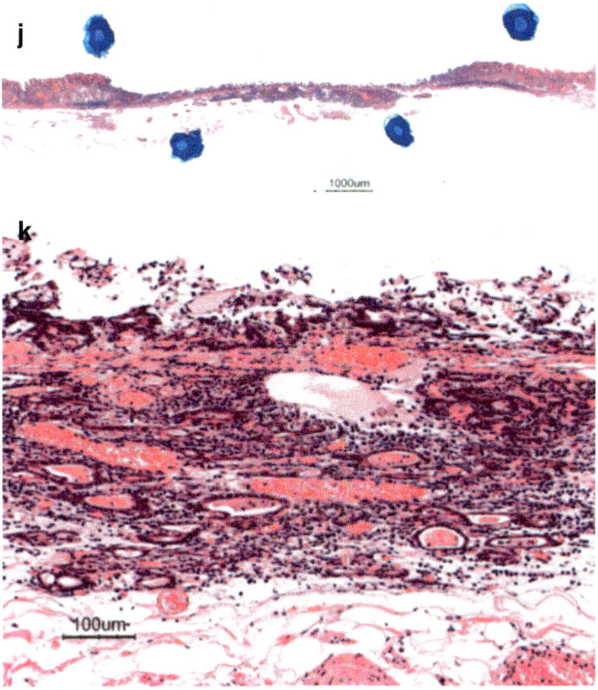

Fig. 9.13 (continued) (**j**, **k**) Histopathology (HE stain) revealed moderately differentiated adenocarcinoma (intestinal type) with (**k**) tiny spots of slight sm1 invasion (HE, 100-fold)

Histopathological diagnosis. p0-IIc, 22 × 10 mm, tub2, sm1(300 μm), ly0, v0, LM(−), VM(−), ul(−), and free margins R0. ESD was curative.

Note ESD was curative according to guideline criteria (see Table 3.2).

- Interdisciplinary cooperation can enhance diagnostic accuracy.

Case 4: Atrophic Gastritis with Tiny Reddish Area Type 0-IIb

A 75 y.o. male underwent an EGD as annual check for atrophic pangastritis. A tiny reddish area at minor curve led to detailed evaluation and ESD (Fig. 9.14a–m).

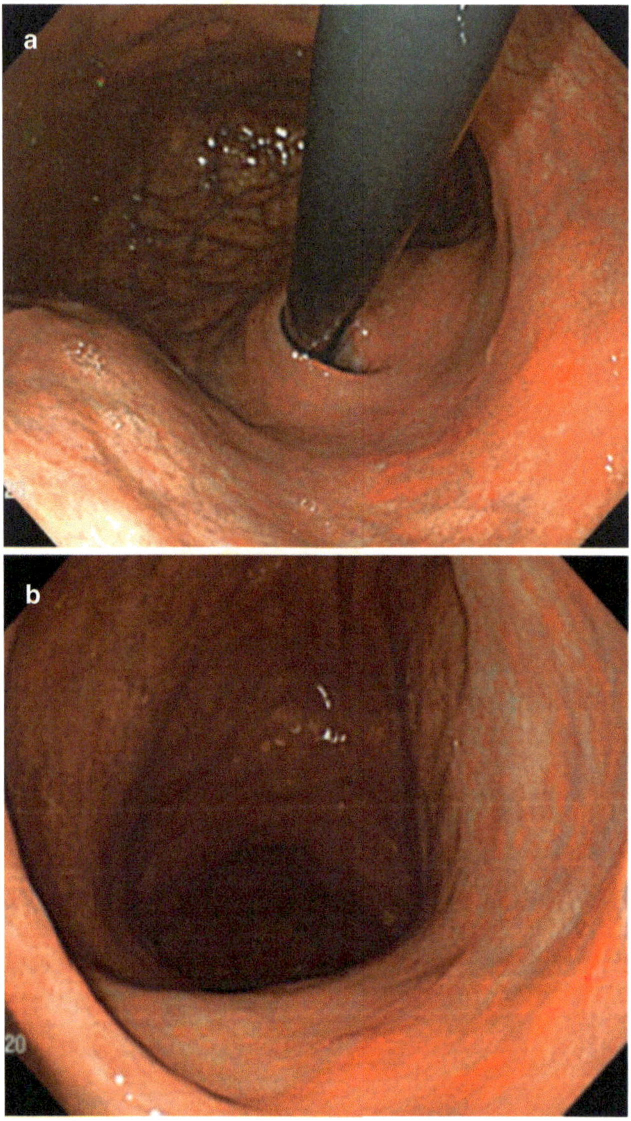

Fig. 9.14 (**a**, **b**) Atrophic pangastritis with tiny *red* spot, (**a**) retroflex view, (**b**) prograde view, standard WLI

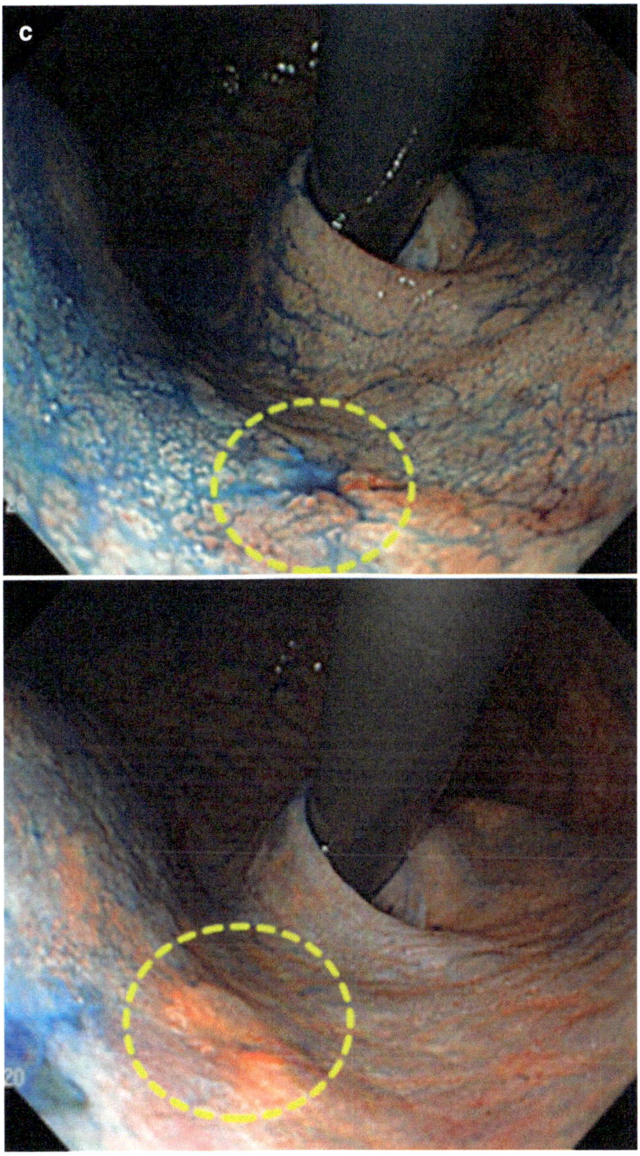

Fig. 9.14 (continued) (**c**) *Lesion no. 1:* Type 0-IIc (yellow circle, upper panel IC = indigo carmine, lower panel AIM = Acetic acid + IC), at minor curve in upper third of gastric body

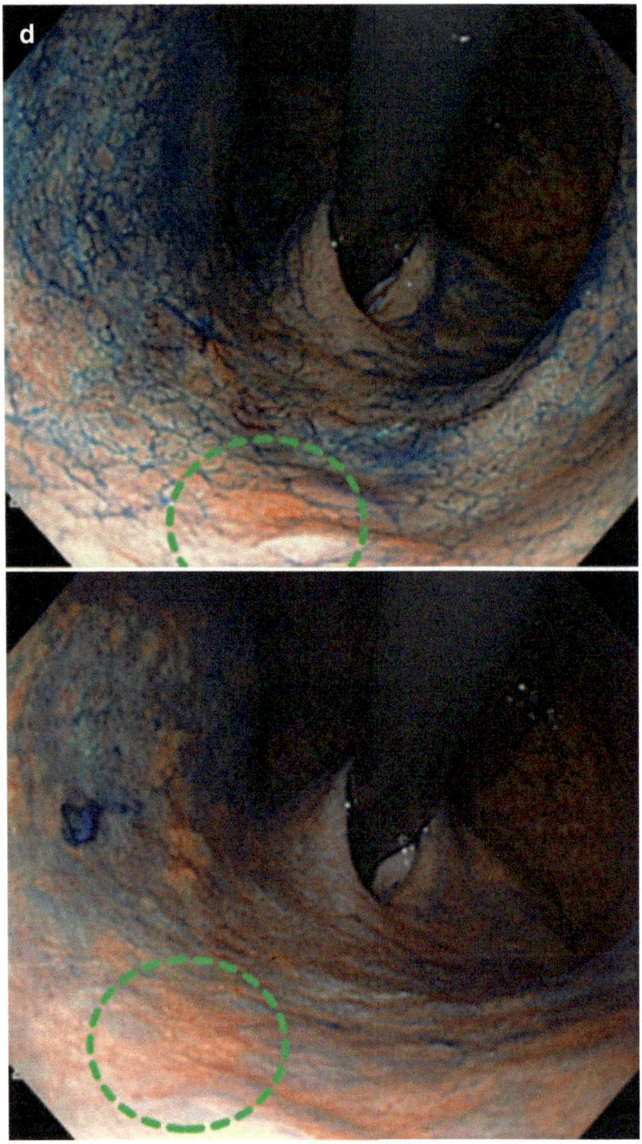

Fig. 9.14 (continued) (**d**) *Lesion no. 2*: type 0-IIb (*green circle*, upper panel IC, lower panel AIM). Targeted biopsies revealed histology shown in (**e**, **f**)

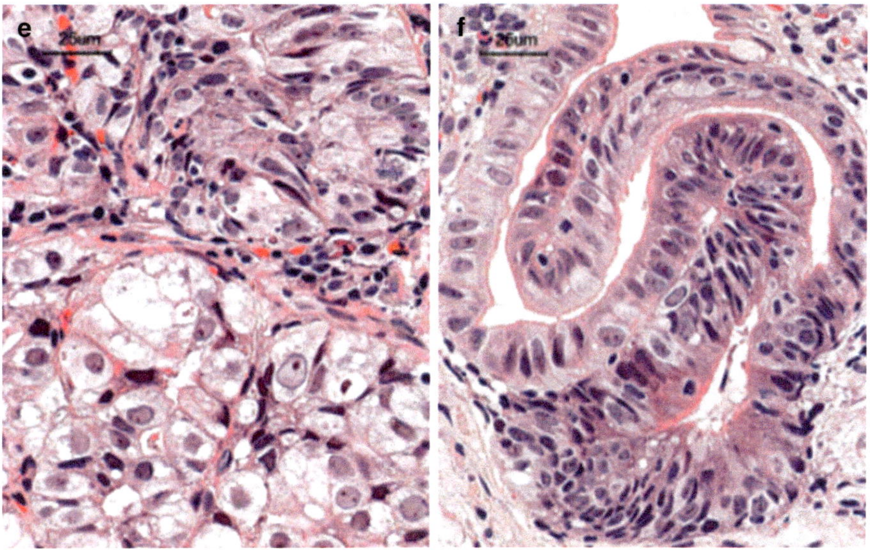

Fig. 9.14 (continued) (**e**) mucosal adenocarcinoma G1-G2 for lesion #1 and (**f**) atypical glands of unclear significance for #2 ⇒ ESD combined for both lesions

Clinical diagnosis.
Lesion 1: c0-IIc,5 mm, well to mod. differentiated adenocarc., m
Lesion 2: c0-IIc, 5 mm, well-differentiated adenocarcinoma, m.

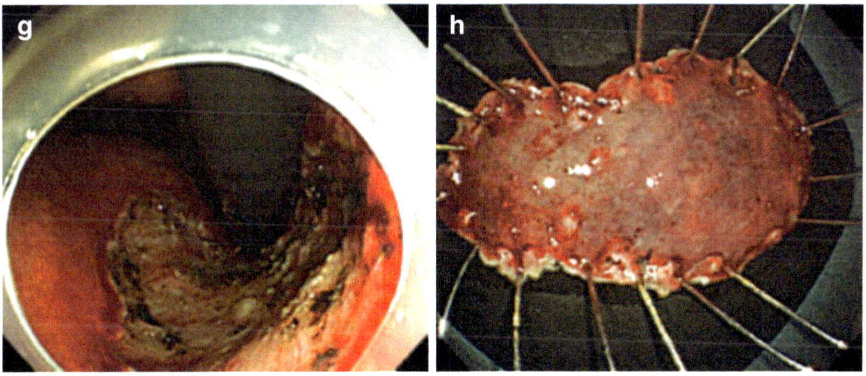

Fig. 9.14 (continued) (**g**) ESD resection bed. (**h**) ESD with *curative* intention included both lesions with safety margin

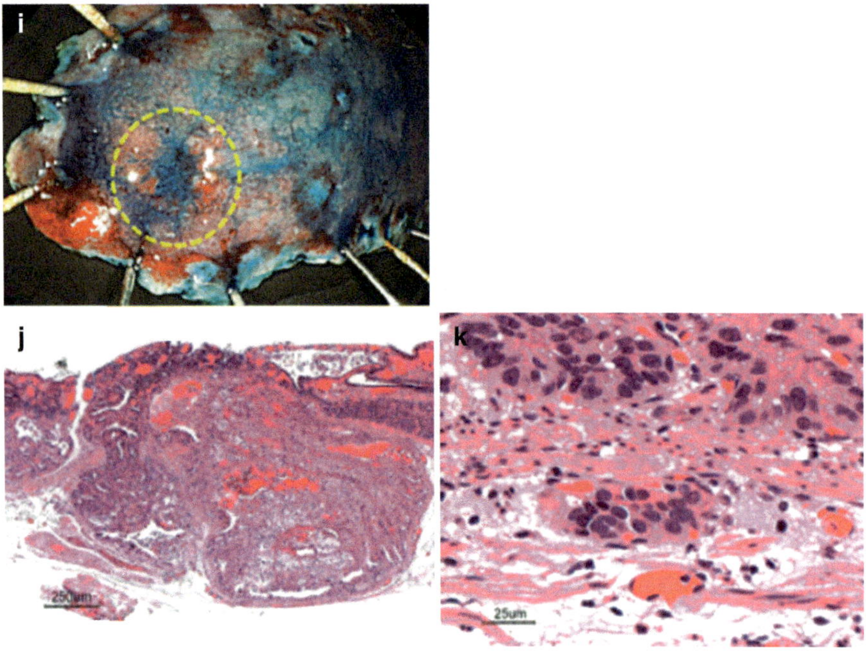

Fig. 9.14 (continued) (**i**–**k**) *Lesion 1* (*yellow circle*): WDAC, 0-IIc 4 × 3 mm, G2 (tub2 > tub1), **sm2,** ly0, ***v1***

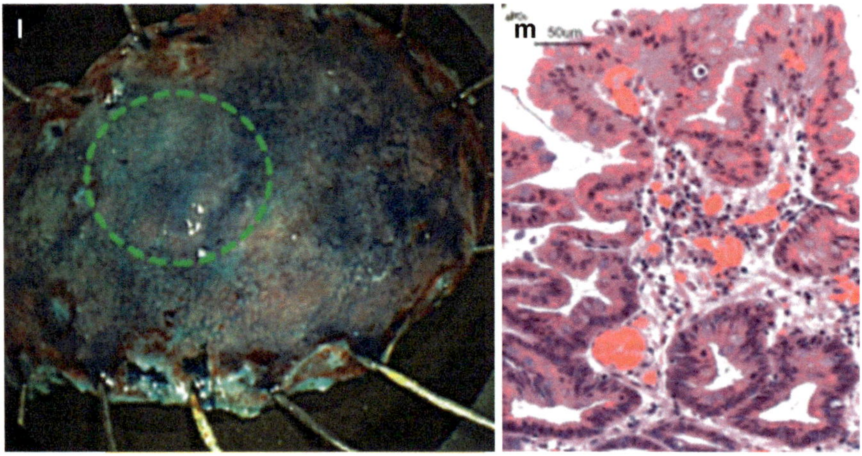

Fig. 9.14 (continued) (**l**) *Lesion 2* (*dotted green circle*): *p0-IIc*, 6 × 5 mm, (**m**) *adenoma*, LM(−), VM(−), resected R0.
For cure of WDAC p**v1**, proximal gastrectomy was conducted: residual tumor (−), pN0 (0/26)

Note Be vigilant for color change (red/pale/variegated) on standard WLI!

- Precise histopathological evaluation of mucosal cancer is mandatory.
- Interdisciplinary cancer panel decision has to follow guideline criteria.

Case 5: Small Lesion 0-IIa Located at the Middle Gastric Body.
This patient underwent surveillance gastroscopy for atrophic pangastritis (Fig. 9.15).

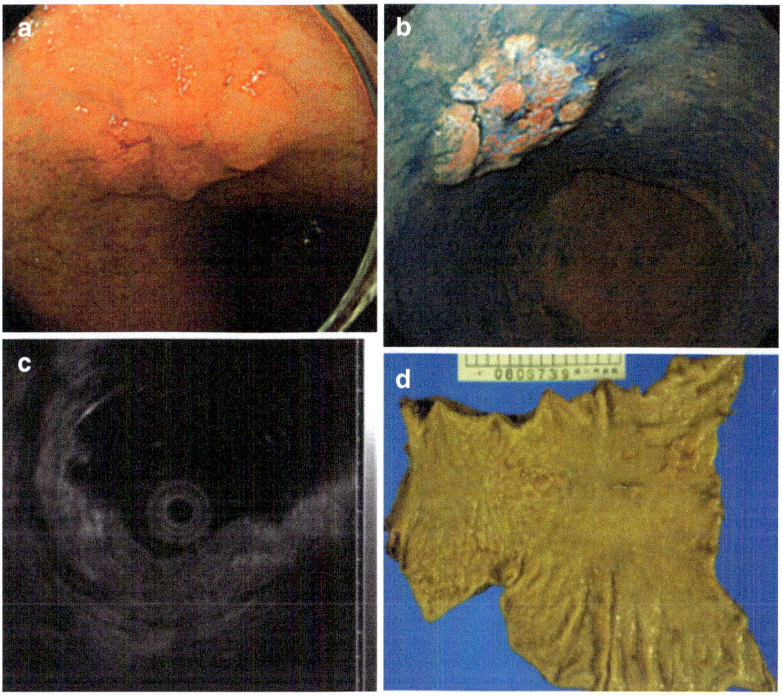

Fig. 9.15 (**a**) Lesion type 0-IIa, 2 cm (WLI), (**b**) indigo carmine CE showed type 0-IIa + IIc. (**c**) Miniprobe hr-EUS (20 MHz) indicates deeper sm-invasive cancer (breaks of hyperechoic sm layer). (**d**) Gastrectomy specimen yielded differentiated adenocarcinoma G2 (tub2 > tub1), pT1b *sm2, ly1*, v0, pPM0, pDM0, 0-IIa + IIc, 22 × 15 mm

Note High-resolution radial EUS (20 MHz) may guide decision for resective strategy and is recommended for centers involved in ESD.

Case 6: Suspect Lesion 0-IIa + c Located in minor side of Prepyloric Antrum
This 75 years old man (ASA II, stable coronary heart disease) was referred for small prepyloric ulcer-like lesion (0-IIa + c) prolapsing into the duodenal bulb, slowly progressive under PPI for 4 months. Unsuccessful ESD attempt 2 months ago, then referred for ESD of suspected early gastric cancer (Fig. 9.16).

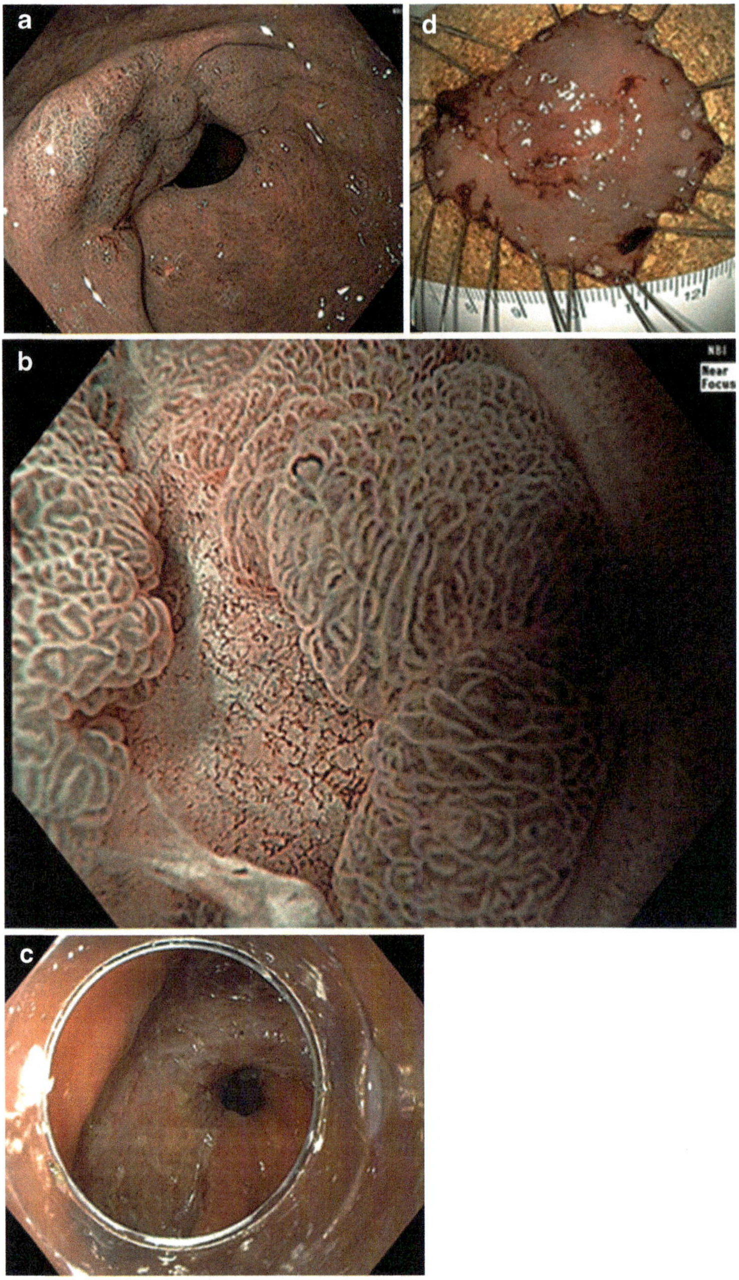

Fig. 9.16 (**a**) The Lesion 0-IIa + c is located before and direct at the pylorus in minor antral curve, and shows at the dorsal side & into pylorus a scar from attempted ESD. The IIa part is covered with regular antral mucosa. (**b**) In depressed areal (10 × 5 mm) unclear SP with slightly irregular fine structured network VP. *Diagnosis*: network VP = pit structure SP → W*ell Differentiated AC*. (**c**) Resection bed. ESD en-bloc (prograde approach, hook knife, starting at aboral pyloric side, then oral side for dissection). (**d**) specimen (4.5 × 3.7 cm). *Histology*: *WDAC (*1.7 × 1.0 cm*)*, G1, pT1a-m2, L0, V0, resection R0, curative

Note Diagnosis of WDAC from such nice network pattern is highly accurate. Prolapsing lesions at pylorus can be very challenging for ESD.

Acknowledgments The contribution of cases by Dr. Hans P. Allgaier/Freiburg, Germany and some images and histology by Dr. Tobias Kiesslich and Dr. Daniel Neureiter/Salzburg, Austria, is gratefully acknowledged.

References

1. Hamashima C, et al. The Japanese guidelines for gastric cancer screening. Jpn J Clin Oncol. 2008;38:259–67.
2. Hirota WK, et al. ASGE guideline: the role of endoscopy in the surveillance of premalignant conditions of the upper GI tract. Gastrointest Endosc. 2006;63:570–80.
3. Shimodate Y, et al. Gastric superficial neoplasia: high miss rate but slow progression. Endosc Int Open. 2017;5:E722–6.
4. Oyama T. Diagnosis of gastric adenocarcinoma with magnified endoscopy. In: Oyama T, editor. Endoscopic diagnosis of superficial gastric cancer for ESD: Springer Japan; 2016. p. 39–51.
5. Leung WK, et al. Screening for gastric cancer in Asia: current evidence and practice. Lancet Oncol. 2008;9:279–87.
6. Yao K, et al. Development of an e-learning system for teaching endoscopists how to diagnose early gastric cancer: basic principles for improving early detection. Gastric Cancer. 2017;20:28–38.
7. Lambert R. The Paris endoscopic classification of superficial neoplastic lesions: esophagus, stomach, and colon: November 30 to December 1, 2002. Gastrointest Endosc. 2003;58:S3–43.
8. Muto M, et al. Magnifying endoscopy simple diagnostic algorithm for early gastric cancer (MESDA-G). Dig Endosc. 2016;28:379–93.
9. Yagi K, et al. Magnifying endoscopy with narrow band imaging for early differentiated gastric adenocarcinoma. Dig Endosc. 2008;20:115–22.
10. Yagi K, et al. Characteristic endoscopic and magnified endoscopic findings in the normal stomach without Helicobacter pylori infection. J Gastroenterol Hepatol. 2002;17:39–45.
11. Kawamura M, et al. Magnifying endoscopic findings of the surface structure of non-cancerous mucosa surrounding differentiated and undifferentiated gastric carcinoma. Dig Endosc. 2011;23:37–42.
12. Tanaka K, et al. Features of early gastric cancer and gastric adenoma by enhanced-magnification endoscopy. J Gastroenterol. 2006;41:332–8.
13. Nakayoshi T, et al. Magnifying endoscopy combined with narrow band imaging system for early gastric cancer: correlation of vascular pattern with histopathology (including video). Endoscopy. 2004;36:1080–4.
14. Yao K, et al. Detection and characterization of early gastric cancer for curative endoscopic submucosal dissection. Dig Endosc. 2013;25(Suppl 1):44–54.
15. Okada K, et al. Diagnosis of undifferentiated type early gastric cancers by magnification endoscopy with narrow-band imaging. J Gastroenterol Hepatol. 2011;26:1262–9.
16. Oyama T. Endoscopic diagnosis of gastric adenocarcinoma for ESD. Tokyo: Nankodo Co., Ltd; 2010.
17. Nonaka K, et al. Magnifying endoscopic observation of mantle cell lymphoma in the stomach using the narrow-band imaging system. Endoscopy. 2010;42(Suppl 2):E94–5.
18. Tomori A, et al. Diagnosis of invasion depth. In: Oyama T, editor. Endoscopic diagnosos of superficial gastric cancer for ESD: Springer Japan; 2016. p. 17–27.

19. Sakai Y, et al. Chromoendoscopy with indigo carmine dye added to acetic acid in the diagnosis of gastric neoplasia: a prospective comparative study. Gastrointest Endosc. 2008;68:635–41.
20. Abe S, et al. Depth-predicting score for differentiated early gastric cancer. Gastric Cancer. 2011;14:35–40.
21. Gotoda T, et al. Endoscopic submucosal dissection of early gastric cancer. J Gastroenterol. 2006;41:929–42.
22. Ono H, et al. Guidelines for endoscopic submucosal dissection and endoscopic mucosal resection for early gastric cancer. Dig Endosc. 2016;28:3–15.
23. Soetikno R, et al. Endoscopic mucosal resection for early cancers of the upper gastrointestinal tract. J Clin Oncol. 2005;23:4490–8.
24. Abe S, et al. Short- and long-term outcomes of endoscopic submucosal dissection for undifferentiated early gastric cancer. Endoscopy. 2013;45:703–7.
25. Gotoda T, et al. Incidence of lymph node metastasis from early gastric cancer: estimation with a large number of cases at two large centers. Gastric Cancer. 2000;3:219–25.
26. Japanese Gastric Cancer Association. Japanese gastric cancer treatment guidelines 2014 (ver. 4). Gastric Cancer. 2017;20:1–19.
27. Gotoda T, et al. Endoscopic resection of early gastric cancer treated by guideline and expanded National Cancer Centre criteria. Br J Surg. 2010;97:868–71.
28. Sekiguchi M, et al. Favorable long-term outcomes of endoscopic submucosal dissection for locally recurrent early gastric cancer after endoscopic resection. Endoscopy. 2013;45:708–13.
29. Hirasawa T, et al. Incidence of lymph node metastasis and the feasibility of endoscopic resection for undifferentiated-type early gastric cancer. Gastric Cancer. 2009;12:148–52.

Chapter 10
Duodenum and Small Bowel: Mucosal Neoplasias

Motohiko Kato, Naohisa Yahagi, and Thierry Ponchon

The incidence of adenoma is highest in the duodenum and decreases progressively throughout the small intestine. The incidence of adenocarcinomas increased by 26% (to 7.3 per million) in the United States in the 30 years from 1973 to 2004, and the incidence of neuroendocrine tumours (NETs) increased fourfold (to 9.3 per million) in the duodenum and small intestine. Overall, 37% of malignancies were NETs; 37%, adenocarcinomas; 17%, malignant lymphomas; and 8.4%, gastrointestinal stromal tumours (GIST). Malignant tumours were most frequently adenocarcinomas in the duodenum and jejunum, but NETs in the ileum [1]. There is also an adenoma-carcinoma sequence for small bowel adenomas and a high association (50–65%) with colonic adenomas [2–4].

Small intestinal (mainly duodenal) and ampullary adenomas arise during the lifetime of nearly all individuals with familial adenomatous polyposis (FAP) and are a leading cause of cancer death in colectomized FAP patients [5].

10.1 Incidence and Risk of Malignant Transformation of Small Bowel Adenomas

Sporadic non-ampullary duodenal adenomas and small bowel adenomas are incidental findings. In upper GI endoscopies, duodenal polyps are observed with a prevalence of 1.5–4.5%, and sporadic non-ampullary duodenal adenomas are seen

M. Kato · N. Yahagi (✉)
Division of Research and Development for Minimally Invasive Treatment, Cancer Center, Keio University School of Medicine, Shinjuku-ku, Tokyo, Japan
e-mail: yahagi-tky@umin.ac.jp

T. Ponchon
Department of Digestive Diseases, Hôpital Eduard Herriot, Lyon, France

F. Berr et al. (eds.), *Atlas of Early Neoplasias of the Gastrointestinal Tract*,
https://doi.org/10.1007/978-3-030-01114-7_10

in 0.1–0.3% [6]. Adenomas are present in 68% of duodenal non-ampullary protruding lesions and in 84% of larger lesions (diameter > 20 mm) [2]. Colonoscopy is indicated in the light of high association with colonic adenomas. The risk of synchronous small bowel adenomas seems increased with sporadic duodenal adenomas and may justify capsule endoscopy [3]. The natural history of sporadic duodenal adenomas has barely been studied. A recent follow-up of 43 such adenomas with low-grade intraepithelial neoplasia (LGIN) indicated that 21% progress to high grade (HGIN) within a median span of 14 months, and 5% progress to intraepithelial cancer, supporting an adenoma-carcinoma sequence for the small intestine. Risk factors for malignant transformation were size >20 mm and HGIN at first biopsy [4].

High-risk individuals. Surveillance strategies have been proposed for small bowel adenomas in *FAP* [8] and for small bowel polyps in Peutz-Jeghers syndrome (*PJS*) [7]. In FAP, the lifetime risk is nearly 100% for duodenal adenomatosis and approximately 5–10% for duodenal adenocarcinoma [8]. Little is known about small bowel involvement in Lynch syndrome (hereditary nonpolyposis colorectal cancer, *HNPCC*), but autosomal recessive *MUTYH*-associated polyposis (*MAP*) carries a 20% risk of duodenal adenomas and a 4% lifetime risk for duodenal cancer [9].

FAP duodenal adenomatosis bears substantial *risk of malignant transformation* that is best estimated with the *modified Spigelman score* (Table 10.1), based on scoring for number, size, and histology (tubular, tubulovillous, villous) of adenomas, and the presence of dysplasia [8, 10]. A high initial Spigelman score (>7 points) is a risk factor for transformation to HGIN [8]. Duodenal adenomas in Spigelman stage II and III should undergo endoscopic resection, whereas advanced duodenal polyposis (Spigelman stage IV) may be treated with duodenopancreatectomy [11], at substantial perioperative risk; alternatively, downstaging of the score may be attempted with multiple endoscopic resections, depending on the patient's preference and alert surveillance of papilla and duodenum [10–12].

Table 10.1 Modified Spigelman Score [5]

					Staging of duodenal FAP	
Number (A)	Size (mm) (B)	Histology (C)	Dysplasia (D)	Score points	Stage	Σ score points
<10	<5	Tubular	Low-grade	1	0	0
10–20	5–10	Tubulovillous	Low-grade	2	I	1–4
>20	>10	Villous	High-grade	3	II	5–6
Score = sum of points for criteria A to D.					III	7–8
					IV	9–12

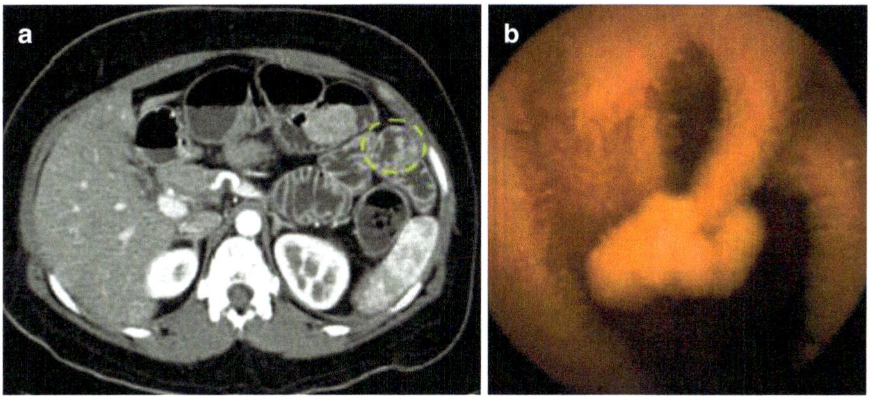

Fig. 10.1 (**a**) Computerized enteroclysis tomography of jejunal polyp type 0-Ip (*circle*). (**b**) Wireless capsule endoscopy image of jejunal polyp type 0-Ip

Note In patients with FAP and duodenal adenomatosis, we recommend the following:

- Endoscopic surveillance (and resection) for ampullary and non-ampullary lesions [13]
- Downstaging of Spigelman stage II and III by cold snaring of multiple small adenomas
- Endoscopic mucosal resection (EMR) for larger adenomas (>15 mm), but resection en bloc for advanced adenoma (HGIN), performed by an endoscopist highly experienced in endoscopic submucosal dissection (ESD)

Hamartomatous polyps in PJS harbour a low risk of malignant conversion [7, 14]. However, the risk of complications (e.g., small bowel invagination) increases with polyp size. Therefore, polypectomy or EMR is recommended during double-balloon enteroscopy [15]. In PJS, the extent of small bowel polyposis is usually diagnosed with CT enteroclysis or entero-MR imaging (to avoid radiation exposure) and wireless capsule endoscopy (Fig. 10.1).

10.2 Ampullary Adenomas

Peri-ampullary or ampullary adenomas involving the major duodenal papilla are usually diagnosed because of symptoms or parameters of cholestasis or pancreatitis. These neoplasias occur sporadically or genetically (in FAP). In both conditions, cancerous transformation is more frequent than for non-ampullary adenomas and ranges from 26% to 65% [16].

Evaluation of adenoma *versus* adenocarcinoma relies mainly on macroscopic signs of malignancy—such as firmness, ulceration, and friability—and targeted biopsy. The extent and local spread of tumour, including lymph node involvement, is best staged with 7.5-MHz endoscopic ultrasound (EUS) as well as with endoscopic retrograde cholangiopancreatography (ERCP) and intraductal ultrasound (IDUS, 20 MHz) to map the extent and intramural invasion of the tumour as well as extension in the bile duct and pancreatic duct. Duodenoscopic imaging of microsurface and microvascular structure has not been analysed systematically in ampullary neoplasias, but a demarcation line around irregular villous and/or microvascular areas suggests adenoma or early cancer [11–13]. Endoscopic snare papillectomy is preferred for adenoma or focal differentiated adenocarcinoma with inconspicuous regional lymph nodes and without evidence of submucosal invasion, extending for less than 10 mm into the bile duct [17]. Staging of pT category in en bloc specimens reveals whether resection was curative. More advanced ampullary cancer requires surgical en bloc resection [16].

10.3 Endoscopic Analysis of Small Intestinal Lesions

The standardized approach for non-ampullary duodenal lesions uses a prograde viewing high-definition (HD) endoscope with magnifying narrow-band imaging (M-NBI) (80-fold), with the patient in left lateral or dorsal decubitus position, application of butyl scopolamine to inhibit peristalsis, and white-light imaging (WLI)–guided inspection, with or without indigo carmine chromoendoscopy (CE) and M-NBI [13, 18].

Normal mucosa shows a regular microsurface pattern (MSP) of villous intestinal columnar epithelium with light blue crest, which is a finding of brush border (confirmed by CD10 immunohistochemistry) [19] (Fig. 10.2a, b).

Gastric metaplasia, a frequent non-neoplastic finding, is presented as a reddish nodule by WLI. Magnified endoscopy with image-enhanced endoscopy reveals a regular microsurface and microvascular pattern without a clear demarcation line (Fig. 10.2c, d).

10.3.1 Differential Diagnosis of Non-neoplastic Versus Neoplastic Non-ampullary Mucosal Lesions in the Small Bowel

Protruding lesions in the small bowel, especially the duodenum, have a wide differential diagnosis and may require capsule endoscopy and double-balloon enteroscopy for the lesions located beyond the ligament of Treitz [15]. Endoscopic analysis of the lesions usually needs confirmation by targeted biopsy, except for flat or depressed lesions scheduled for endoscopic resection, and occasionally further workup with high-resolution EUS (20 MHz) or (for submucosal tumours type 0-Is/Isp) linear array EUS (7.5 MHz) and fine needle-puncture biopsy. Neuroendocrine tumours of size larger than 10 mm require scintigraphic and radiological staging.

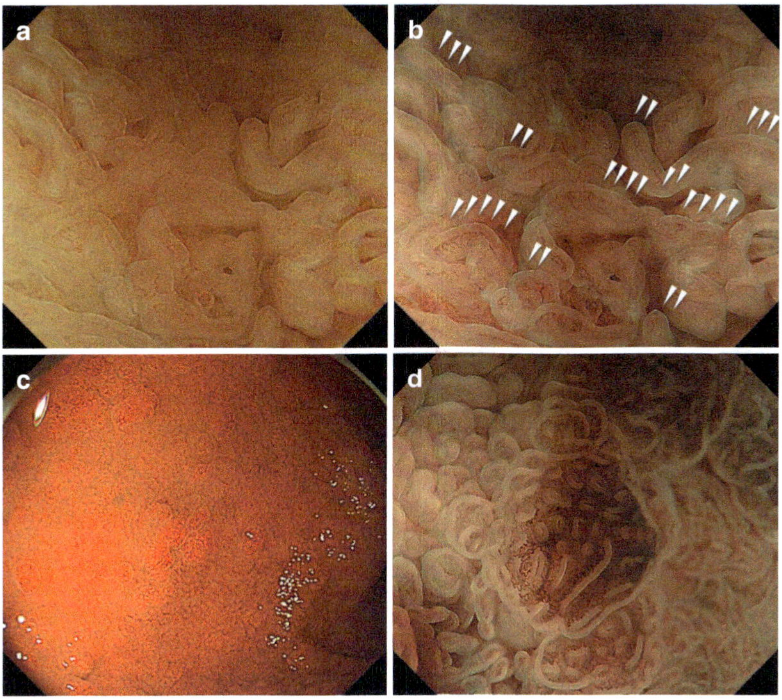

Fig. 10.2 Endoscopic findings of non-neoplastic duodenal mucosa (**a**, **b**) and gastric metaplasia (**c**, **d**); villous microstructure with light blue crest (LBC) is observed. (**a**) Magnifying WLI (80× magnification) and (**b**) M-NBI (80×). *Arrowheads* reveal LBC. (**c**) Gastric metaplasia is found as a reddish nodule on the bulbs. (**d**) M-NBI (80×) reveals regular tubular microstructure with increased regular vessels

Table 10.2 Differential Diagnosis and Management of Sporadic Non-ampullary Protuberant (0-Isp or 0-IIa) Duodenal Lesions [6]

Classification	Histology	Management	Surveillance
Epithelial Lesion	Gastric metaplasia	None	None
	Adenoma −/+ HGIN[a]	Endoscopic resection	6–12 months
	Carcinoma T1b[a]	Surgical resection	Stage-dependent
Submucosal Lesion	Inflammatory fibroid ~	? Endoscopic resection[b]	None
	Lipoma (symptomatic)	? Resection (endo/surg.)[b]	None
	Leiomyoma	? Resection (surg)	None
	NET	Resection (endo/surg.)	Stage-dependent
	GIST	Resection (surg.)	Stage-dependent
Hamartoma	Brunner's gland ~	? Endoscopic resection[b]	None
	Peutz-Jeghers ~	Endoscopic resection[b]	See PJ syndrome
Lymphoma	MALT or T cell ~[a]	Biopsy	Stage-dependent

GIST gastrointestinal stromal tumours, *HGIN* high-grade intraepithelial neoplasia, *MALT* mucosa-associated lymphoid tissue, *NET* neuroendocrine tumours,~ as classified

[a]May also show lesions type 0-IIb, 0-IIc, and 0-III

[b]Resection only for clearly symptomatic, large lesions (0-Ip, Isp)

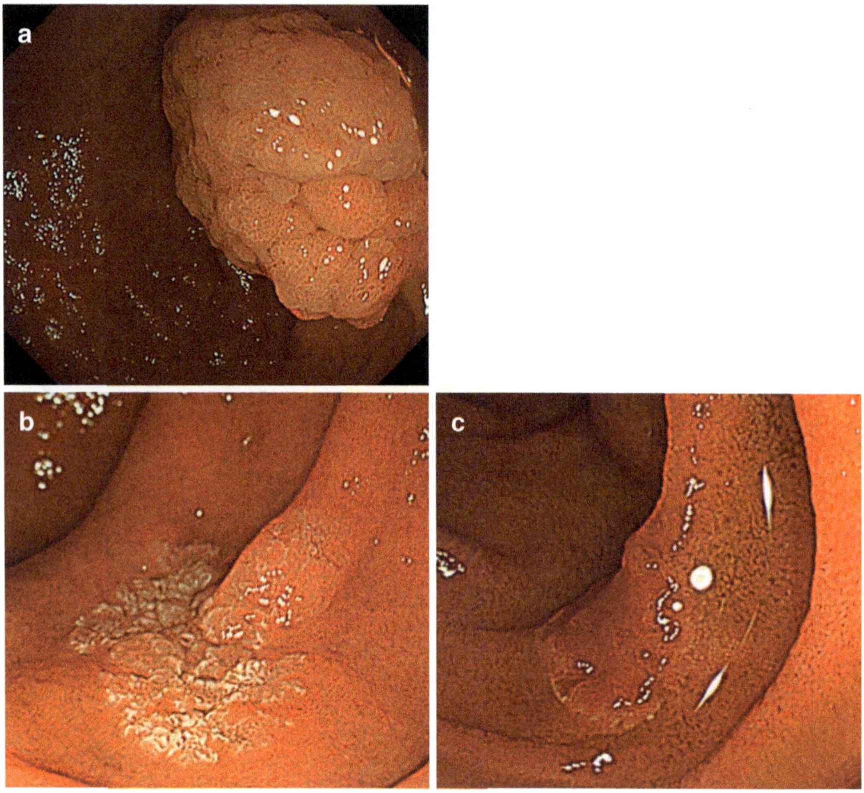

Fig. 10.3 Typical WLI findings of duodenal epithelial neoplasia. (**a**) Protrusion (Paris 0-I) with villous surface. (**b**) Slight elevation (Paris IIa) with whitish color. (**c**) Reddish depression (Paris IIc). All these lesions have a clear border separating them from surrounding mucosa

The differential diagnosis and management recommendations for protruding duodenal lesions [6] are listed in Table 10.2.

Diagnosis of duodenal epithelial neoplasia by WLI is basically decided on the basis of the presence or absence of a clearly localized border. Typically, duodenal adenoma reveals three macroscopic findings: protrusion (Paris 0-I) with villous surface, slight elevation (Paris 0-IIa) with whitish color, and reddish depression (Paris 0-IIc) (Fig. 10.3).

Using magnified endoscopy with image enhanced endoscopy (m-IEE), duodenal epithelial neoplasia reveals tubular/villous microstructure, and white opaque substance (WOS) is observed, especially in a whitish lesion. WOS has been reported to be an accumulation of fat droplets within the epithelium [20, 21] (Fig. 10.4).

In FAP, non-ampullary adenomas present the same morphology, but usually there are multiple duodenal lesions [5, 8, 22] (Fig. 10.5, Table 10.1). In a prospective study of progression of duodenal polyposis based on the modified Spigelman score, the estimated cumulative risk for stage IV duodenal polyposis was 43% at age 60 years and 50% at age 70 years [8]. The rate of advanced adenocarcinoma was 36% within a median of 8 (4–10) years for Spigelman stage IV disease [5].

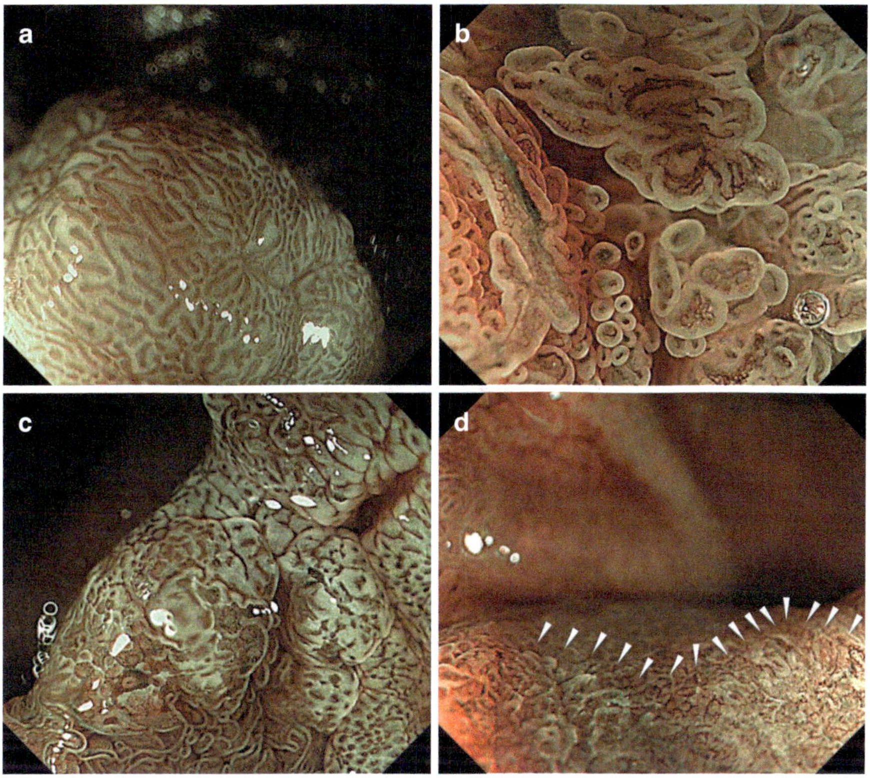

Fig. 10.4 Magnified NBI findings of duodenal epithelial neoplasia. (**a**) Tubular microstructural pattern. (**b**) Villous microstructural pattern. (**c**) Diffuse white opaque substance (WOS). (**d**) Reticular/granular WOS pattern (*arrowheads*)

10.3.2 Differential Diagnosis Between Adenoma and Adenocarcinoma in the Duodenum

A depressed and reddish area in a whitish elevated area on WLI would be a predictor of histology with cytological/structural atypia [23].

Some studies have mentioned magnified endoscopy with electronic image-enhanced endoscopy (NBI etc.) or chromoendoscopy as a useful tool for the differential diagnosis between adenoma and adenocarcinoma. These studies suggested that an irregular microsurface or microvascular pattern, in addition to a clear demarcation line, is useful as a predictor of adenocarcinoma [24–26]. However, most of these studies are retrospective studies with a limited number of cases, and there is not yet an established diagnostic system using these modalities for diffential diagnosis between adenoma and adenocarcinoma or between noninvasive and invasive cancer.

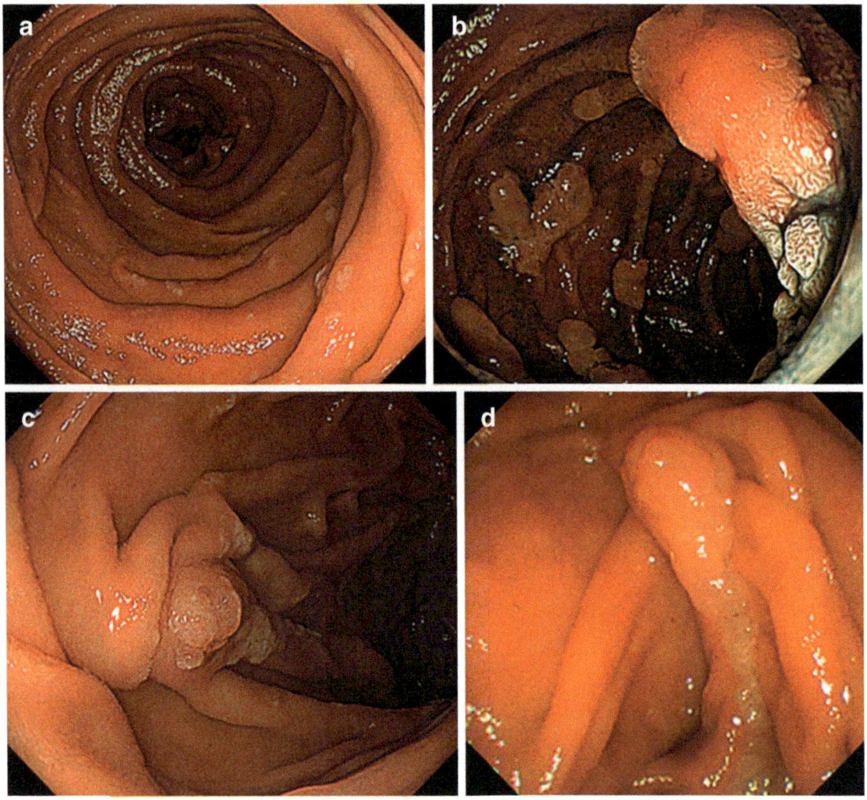

Fig. 10.5 Duodenal adenomatosis in familial adenomatous polyposis (FAP). (**a**) Multiple small nodules 0-IIa (WLI). (**b**) Flat, elevated type 0-IIa (WLI + indigocarmine). (**c**) Ampullary adenomas detected by forward-viewing scope and (**d**) side-viewing endoscope

Pathological diagnosis using biopsy specimens is also difficult. Additional biopsies did not significantly improve the accuracy beyond that of the endoscopic diagnosis [23, 27]. Moreover, preoperative biopsy may cause submucosal fibrosis, making endoscopic treatment difficult [27] (Fig. 10.6). Therefore. preoperative biopsies should be avoided, especially for flat or depressed lesions scheduled for endoscopic resection.

10.4 Endoscopic Resection of Duodenal Neoplasias

Because of its abundant submucosal vessels, thin muscular wall, and restricted manoeuverability of the endoscope, the duodenum is considered one of the most difficult locations for endoscopic resection using snare polypectomy or EMR, even in piecemeal fashion [28–31]. The EMR technique for mucosal lesions in the duodenum demands special expertise and precautions [29, 32]. Rates of

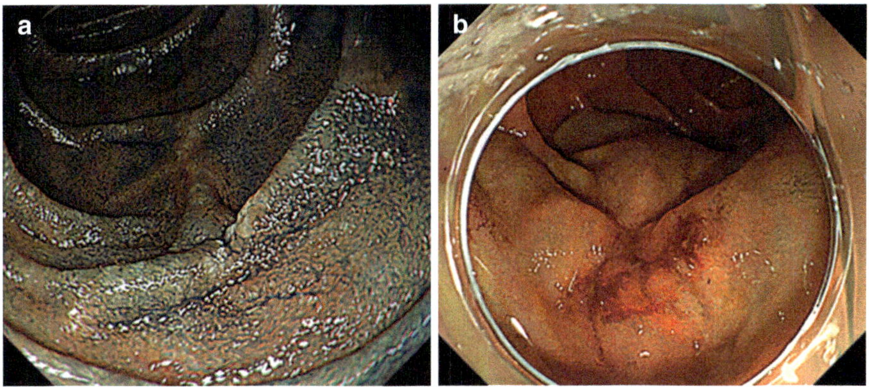

Fig. 10.6 Submucosal fibrosis caused by biopsy. (**a**) Fold convergence is seen on the site of a previous biopsy. (**b**) Remarkable non-lifting sign was observed after submucosal injection

complications for EMR of duodenal non-ampullary adenomas were relatively low in a recent case series, with perforations in 1.6%, delayed bleeding in 10%, and morbidity in 11.5% of procedures, with no mortality [30]. EMR does leave behind larger ulcerations or coagulation marks, which can pose a high risk for delayed bleeding and perforation. Pre-emptive closure of the resection ulcer with endoclipping prevents delayed ulceration in the presence of pancreatobiliary secretion [29, 31]. The rate of local recurrence has been high following EMR, in particular piecemeal EMR (up to 33%), but there was no recurrence after ESD en bloc [29, 31–36].

Recently, some novel kinds of endoscopic procedures—cold polypectomy and underwater EMR—have been proposed for duodenal epithelial neoplasia. Cold polypectomy has spread widely as a treatment for diminutive colorectal polyp, and because of its favorable outcomes in colorectal polyps [37], it might be a treatment option for duodenal adenomatosis in FAP patients, as discussed below. Underwater EMR (UEMR) is an unique endoscopic resection technique proposed by Binmoeller et al., in which the duodenal lesion is resected by snare without injecting solution into the submucosa after filling water inside the lumen [38]. UEMR would be effective even for lesions with submucosal fibrosis, because it does not require submucosal injection (Fig. 10.7).

Duodenal ESD is very challenging even for experts (perforation rate 7–20%) and is acceptable only in professional ESD centers [30, 32, 39]. Nevertheless, in first case series, ESD has been feasible for duodenal mucosal neoplasias, though with considerable rates of perforation and delayed bleeding (5%, up to 22% within 12 h); most were managed by endoscopic intervention. The pocket-creation method [39] and water pressure method [40] are new techniques to facilitate safe submucosal dissection, especially in the duodenum. Laparoscopic and endoscopic cooperative resective surgery (laparoscopic reinforcement after ESD) prevents postoperative complications [41]. Moreover, recent advances in endoscopic technique have made it possible to close even a large mucosal defect after ESD without laparoscopic

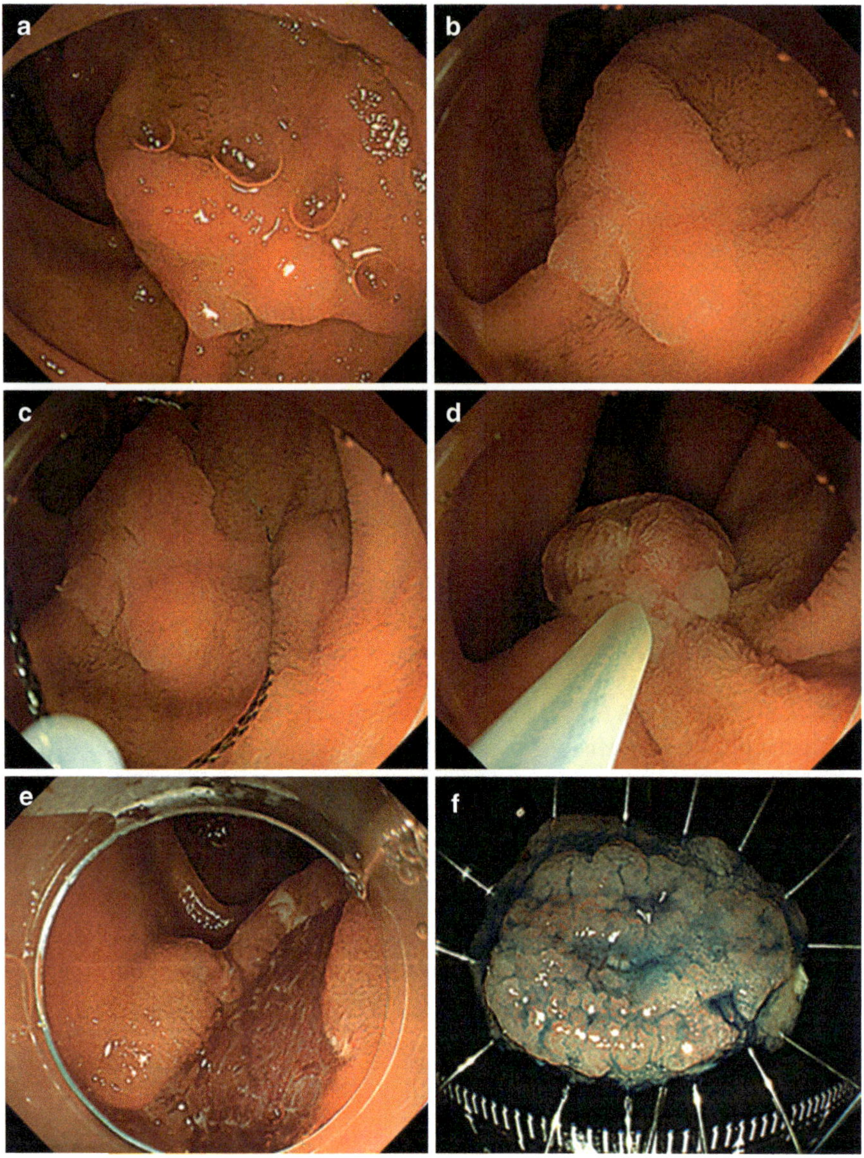

Fig. 10.7 Underwater EMR for a dudodenal adenoma. A sessile duodenal lesion 22 mm in diameter is seen on the lateral wall of the inferior duodenal angle (**a**). After filling normal saline into the lumen (**b**), the lesion was captured by a snare (**c**, **d**). The lesion was resected without perforation (**e**). Complete margin free resection was acheived (**f**)

assistance. These techniques could improve the clinical outcomes of duodenal ESD [42, 43] (Fig. 10.8).

Note *Submucosal invasive* cancer in the duodenum or small bowel requires *surgical resection* and *lymphadenectomy* [11, 41].

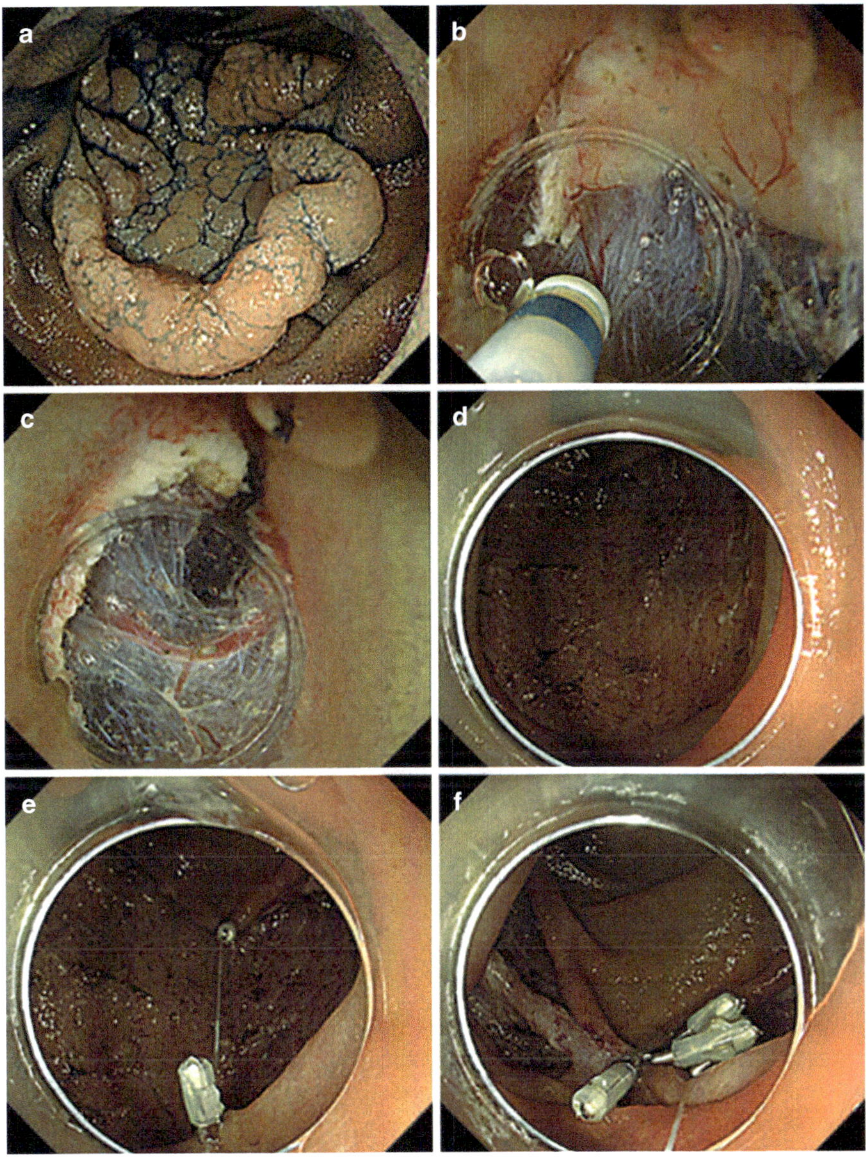

Fig. 10.8 ESD for a large, laterally spreading duodenal adenoma. (**a**) A flat, elevated duodenal lesion (Paris 0-IIa) is seen on the posterior wall of the inferior duodenal angle. (**b**, **c**) Water pressure method with a small-caliber tip hood (Fujifilm Medical, Japan) is useful to go beneath the mucosal flap and obtain good submucosal visualization. (**d**) A large mucosal defect was created by ESD. (**e**) The clip with string is deployed at the distal edge of the large mucosal defect, and a second clip is placed at the opposite side to anchor the string. (**f**) The wound is approximated by pulling the free end of the string; complete closure is achieved by placement of additional clips

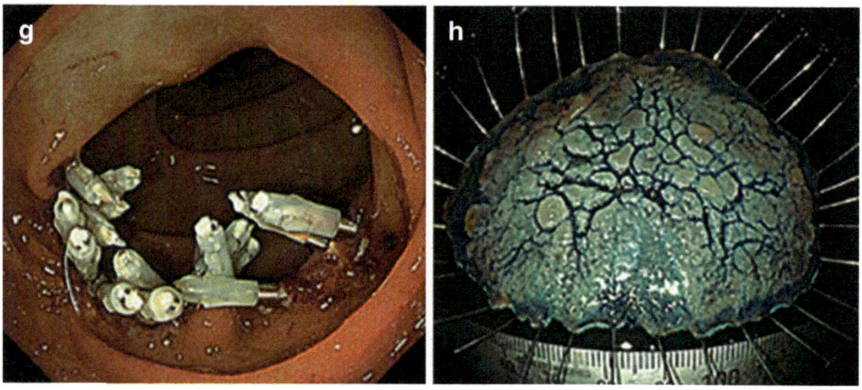

Fig. 10.8 (continued) (**g**) Complete closure was finally accomplished. (**h**) Resected specimen revealed *well-differentiated adenocarcinoma confined within mucosa*. The resected margin was free from tumour

10.4.1 Resection of Adenomas in Familial Adenomatous Polyposis

According to guideline recommendations, progression to severe duodenal adenomatosis (Spigelman stage IV) in FAP marks the indication point for extended surgery involving total duodenectomy and Whipple's hemipancreatectomy, a procedure still rated at 6% mortality [11]. A fraction of 42–50% of FAP patients become eligible for extended duodenectomy and Whipple's hemipancreatectomy, strongly arguing for preventive endoscopic resection of duodenal adenomas [10]. There are encouraging results for EMR and even ESD of sporadic duodenal adenomas with LGIN and few early duodenal carcinomas [25, 30, 38, 44].

Multiple small duodenal adenomas are rapidly removed by cold snaring of the lesions (collected for histology in an aspiration trap), allowing efficient downstaging in the presence of multiple small adenomas [45] (Fig. 10.9). Minute duodenal adenomas are efficiently ablated by argon plasma coagulation (APC); the combination of EMR and APC achieves efficient downstaging in 97% of cases for an extended time (>5 years) [10]. An ESD technique for larger-size duodenal lesions is in progress and will become available in specialized centres involved in the surveillance of FAP patient cohorts [30].

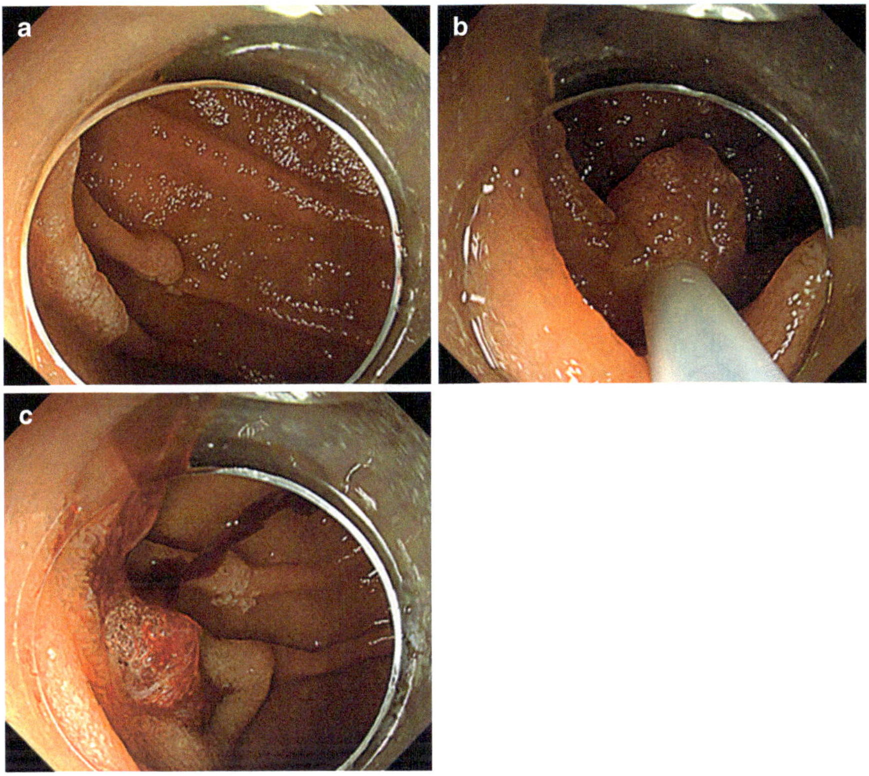

Fig. 10.9 Cold snare polypectomy (CSP) for multiple small nodules of adenomatous lesion in an FAP patient. (**a**) Multiple small lesions in the duodenum. (**b**) In CSP, the lesion is resected mechanically without electric cautery. (**c**) There is no active bleeding or perforation

10.5 Cases of Non-ampullary Duodenal Adenomas

Case 1: Low-grade Duodenal Adenoma, Complete EMR

A 67-year-old woman was referred for endoscopic resection of a 20 × 12-mm sessile adenoma (Paris 0-I) in the posterior wall of the descending part of the duodenum. The lesion crossed one Kerckring fold (Fig. 10.10a, b). Magnified NBI revealed a tubular structure without irregular vessels, with a clear demarcation line from surrounding epithelium (Fig. 10.10c). Underwater EMR of this relatively large lesion was attempted, and complete resection was achieved. Pathological findings (Fig. 10.10f) revealed neoplastic glands without structural/cytological atypia (suggesting low-grade adenoma) and negative horizontal/vertical margins.

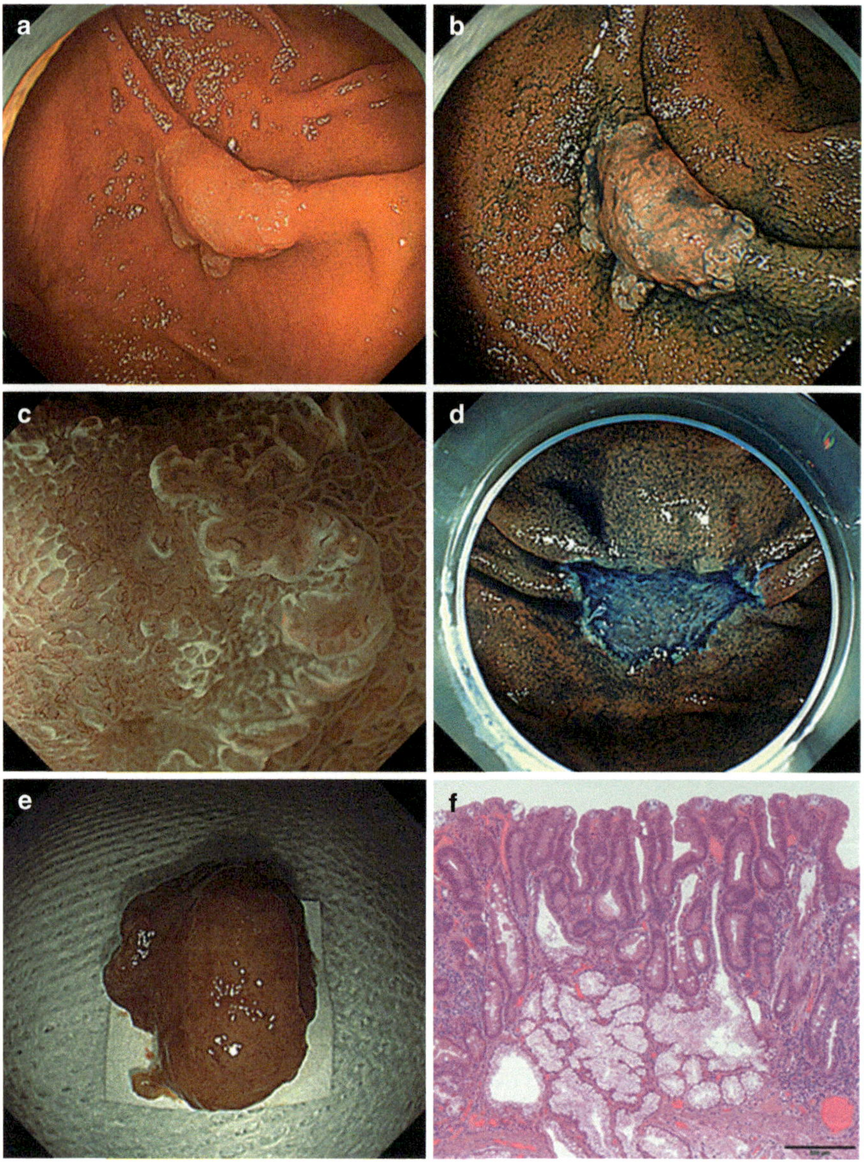

Fig. 10.10 *Case 1*. Sessile duodenal adenoma (20 × 12 mm) type 0-I, seen (**a**) on WLI, (**b**) indigo carmine CE, and (**c**) M-NBI. (**d**) Resection bed and (**e**) en-bloc specimen after EMR, (**f**) Pathological findings (HE) of resected specimen

Case 2: Duodenal Adenocarcinoma with Submucosal Invasion

In a 65-year-old otherwise healthy woman a 30-mm elevated lesion was pointed out on the anterior wall of the duodenal bulbs. There was a remarkable protrusion in the lesion, and its surface revealed a villous structure (c) (M-NBI) in the lesion (Fig. 10.11a, b). The lesion was resected in a single piece by ESD without any complications. Specimen: *Well-differentiated adenocarcinoma* which *invaded beyond the muscularis mucosae*. Distal gastrectomy revealed no lymph node metastasis.

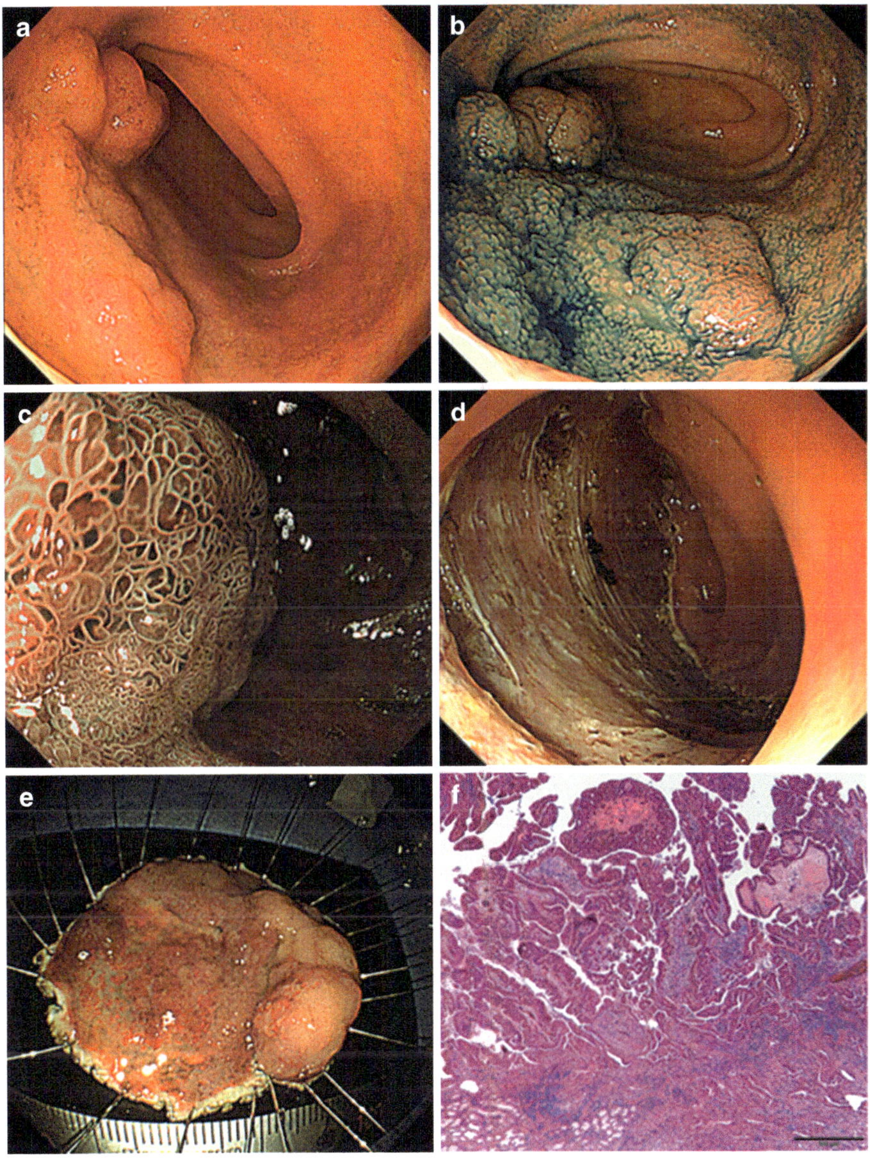

Fig. 10.11 Duodenal lesion (30 mm) type 0-IIa, as seen (**a**) on WLI, (**b**) on indigo carmine CE, and (**c**) on magnified NBI. (**d**) Resection bed and (**e**) specimen after ESD en-bloc. (**f**) Specimen (HE): *Well-differentiated adenocarcinoma*, sm-invasive

References

1. Bilimoria KY, et al. Small bowel cancer in the United States: changes in epidemiology, treatment, and survival over the last 20 years. Ann Surg. 2009;249:63–71.
2. Abbass R, et al. Nonampullary duodenal polyps: characteristics and endoscopic management. Gastrointest Endosc. 2010;71:754–9.
3. Friedrich-Rust M, et al. Early-stage small-bowel adenocarcinoma: a review of local endoscopic therapy. Endoscopy. 2005;37:755–9.
4. Okada K, et al. Sporadic nonampullary duodenal adenoma in the natural history of duodenal cancer: a study of follow-up surveillance. Am J Gastroenterol. 2011;106:357–64.
5. Groves CJ, et al. Duodenal cancer in patients with familial adenomatous polyposis (FAP): results of a 10 year prospective study. Gut. 2002;50:636–41.
6. Culver EL, et al. Sporadic duodenal polyps: classification, investigation, and management. Endoscopy. 2011;43:144–55.
7. Beggs AD, et al. Peutz-Jeghers syndrome: a systematic review and recommendations for management. Gut. 2010;59:975–86.
8. Saurin JC, et al. Surveillance of duodenal adenomas in familial adenomatous polyposis reveals high cumulative risk of advanced disease. J Clin Oncol. 2004;22:493–8.
9. Vogt S, et al. Expanded extracolonic tumor spectrum in MUTYH-associated polyposis. Gastroenterology. 2009;137:1976–85.
10. Moussata D, et al. Endoscopic treatment of severe duodenal polyposis as an alternative to surgery for patients with familial adenomatous polyposis. Gastrointest Endosc. 2014;80:817–25.
11. Parc Y, et al. Surgical management of the duodenal manifestations of familial adenomatous polyposis. Br J Surg. 2011;98:480–4.
12. Sourrouille I, et al. Surveillance of duodenal polyposis in familial adenomatous polyposis: should the Spigelman score be modified? Dis Colon Rectum. 2017;60:1137–46.
13. Kallenberg FGJ, et al. Cap-assisted forward-viewing endoscopy to visualize the ampulla of Vater and the duodenum in patients with familial adenomatous polyposis. Endoscopy. 2017;49:181–5.
14. Belsha D, et al. Effectiveness of double-balloon enteroscopy-facilitated polypectomy in pediatric patients with Peutz-Jeghers syndrome. J Pediatr Gastroenterol Nutr. 2017;65:500–2.
15. Mitsui K, et al. Role of double-balloon endoscopy in the diagnosis of small-bowel tumors: the first Japanese multicenter study. Gastrointest Endosc. 2009;70:498–504.
16. ASGE Standards of Practice Committee, et al. The role of endoscopy in ampullary and duodenal adenomas. Gastrointest Endosc. 2015;82:773–81.
17. Bohnacker S, et al. Endoscopic resection of benign tumors of the duodenal papilla without and with intraductal growth. Gastrointest Endosc. 2005;62:551–60.
18. Mizumoto T, et al. Clinical usefulness of magnifying endoscopy for non-ampullary duodenal tumors. Endosc Int Open. 2017;5:E297–302.
19. Uedo N, et al. A new method of diagnosing gastric intestinal metaplasia: narrow-band imaging with magnifying endoscopy. Endoscopy. 2006;38:819–24.
20. Ueo T, et al. White opaque substance represents an intracytoplasmic accumulation of lipid droplets: immunohistochemical and immunoelectron microscopic investigation of 26 cases. Dig Endosc. 2013;25:147–55.
21. Yao K, et al. White opaque substance within superficial elevated gastric neoplasia as visualized by magnification endoscopy with narrow-band imaging: a new optical sign for differentiating between adenoma and carcinoma. Endoscopy. 2008;68:574–80.
22. Moussata D, et al. Could therapeutic endoscopy be an alternative to surgery for the treatment of advanced duodenal polyposis in patients with familial adenomatous polyposis? Gut. 2009;58(Suppl. II):A62.
23. Kakushima N, et al. Endoscopic and biopsy diagnoses of superficial, nonampullary, duodenal adenocarcinomas. World J Gastroenterol. 2015;21:5560–7.

24. Goda K, et al. Endoscopic diagnosis of superficial non-ampullary duodenal epithelial tumors in Japan: Multicenter case series. Dig Endosc. 2014;26(Suppl 2):23–9.
25. Tsuji S, et al. Preoperative endoscopic diagnosis of superficial non-ampullary duodenal epithelial tumors, including magnifying endoscopy. World J Gastroenterol. 2015;21:11832–41.
26. Yoshimura N, et al. Endoscopic features of nonampullary duodenal tumors with narrow-band imaging. Hepato-Gastroenterology. 2010;57:462–7.
27. Kinoshita S, et al. Accuracy of biopsy for the preoperative diagnosis of superficial nonampullary duodenal adenocarcinoma. Gastrointest Endosc. 2017;86:329–32.
28. Kakushima N, et al. Treatment for superficial non-ampullary duodenal epithelial tumors. World J Gastroenterol. 2014;20:12501–8.
29. Lepilliez V, et al. Endoscopic resection of sporadic duodenal adenomas: an efficient technique with a substantial risk of delayed bleeding. Endoscopy. 2008;40:806–10.
30. Yahagi N, et al. Outcomes of endoscopic resection for superficial duodenal epithelial neoplasia. Gastrointest Endosc. 2018;88:676–82.
31. Yamasaki Y, et al. Current status of endoscopic resection for superficial nonampullary duodenal epithelial tumors. Digestion. 2018;97:45–51.
32. Hoteya S, et al. Endoscopic submucosal dissection and endoscopic mucosal resection for non-ampullary superficial duodenal tumor. Digestion. 2017;95:36–42.
33. Honda T, et al. Endoscopic submucosal dissection for superficial duodenal neoplasms. Dig Endosc. 2009;21:270–4.
34. Jung JH, et al. Endoscopic submucosal dissection for sessile, nonampullary duodenal adenomas. Endoscopy. 2013;45:133–5.
35. Matsumoto S, et al. Endoscopic submucosal dissection for duodenal tumors: a single-center experience. Endoscopy. 2013;45:136–7.
36. Nonaka S, et al. Clinical outcome of endoscopic resection for non-ampullary duodenal tumors. Endoscopy. 2015;47:129–35.
37. Kato M, et al. Validation of treatment algorithm based on the Japan narrow band imaging expert team classification for sub-centimeter colorectal polyps. Endosc Int Open. 2018;6:E934–40.
38. Binmoeller KF, et al. "Underwater" EMR of sporadic laterally spreading nonampullary duodenal adenomas (with video). Gastrointest Endosc. 2013;78:496–502.
39. Miura Y, et al. Duodenal endoscopic submucosal dissection is feasible using the pocket-creation method. Endoscopy. 2018;49:8–14.
40. Yahagi N, et al. Water pressure method for duodenal endoscopic submucosal dissection. Endoscopy. 2017;49:E227–8.
41. Ichikawa D, et al. Laparoscopic and endoscopic co-operative surgery for non-ampullary duodenal tumors. World J Gastroenterol. 2016;22:10424–31.
42. Nishizawa T, et al. Endoscopic string clip suturing method: a prospective pilot study (with video). Gastrointest Endosc. 2018;87:1074–8.
43. Yahagi N, et al. New endoscopic suturing method: string clip suturing method. Gastrointest Endosc. 2016;84:1064–5.
44. Yamamoto Y, et al. Therapeutic outcomes of endoscopic resection for superficial non-ampullary duodenal tumor. Dig Endosc. 2014;26(Suppl 2):50–6.
45. Hamada K, et al. Safety of cold snare polypectomy for duodenal adenomas in familial adenomatous polyposis: a prospective exploratory study. Endoscopy. 2018;50:511–7.

Chapter 11
Colorectum: Mucosal Neoplasias

Andrej Wagner, Tadateru Maehata, Frieder Berr, and Naohisa Yahagi

11.1 Introduction

Most lesions (74%) detected on screening colonoscopy are *protruded-type polyps* (0-I), of which about a third are hyperplastic (non-neoplastic), and the remaining two thirds are neoplastic (i.e., adenomas or carcinomas). The other lesions (24%) are flat (0-II) or laterally spreading tumors (LSTs) [1]. The probability of detecting small and minute neoplasias is much higher for protruded lesions than for flat lesions [1–3], but 50% of colorectal carcinoma (CRC) originates from flat precursors [4].

The importance of flat- and depressed-type lesions, well known in Japan [2, 5], was first proven in Western patients in a prospective study of 1000 routine colonoscopies in Leeds, UK. Apart from 2.5% advanced carcinomas, a total of 327 neoplasias (including 6 early CRC) were detected with 62% polypoid, 36% flat (including 15% LST), and 1.2% depressed-type morphology. High-grade intraepithelial neoplasia (HGIN) or carcinomas were present in 8% of polypoid, 14% of flat, and 75% of depressed-type neoplasias [6]. Therefore, we must know the different lesions and their malignant potential.

A. Wagner
Department of Internal Medicine I, University Hospital, Paracelsus Medical University, Salzburg, Austria

T. Maehata · N. Yahagi
Division of Research and Development for Minimally Invasive Treatment, Cancer Center, Keio University School of Medicine, Shinjuku-ku, Tokyo, Japan
e-mail: yahagi-tky@umin.ac.jp

F. Berr (✉)
Department of Internal Medicine I, Paracelsus Medical University, Salzburg, Austria
e-mail: frieder.berr@pmu.ac.at

F. Berr et al. (eds.), *Atlas of Early Neoplasias of the Gastrointestinal Tract*,
https://doi.org/10.1007/978-3-030-01114-7_11

Furthermore, a recent meta-analysis has shown poor curative endoscopic resection rates outside East Asia, caused by frequent resection of deep submucosal (sm)-invasive early CRC [7]. For curative endoscopic resection, we must be able to distinguish superficial versus deep sm-invasive early CRC by gross morphology and magnifying endoscopic signs of surface and capillary structures.

11.2 Prevalence and Carcinoma Risk of Macroscopic Types of Colorectal Neoplasias

Prevalence of lesions and *risk of cancer* are shown for macroscopic types in Table 11.1a and for LSTs in Table 11.1b. The overall prevalence of these lesions compares well with the adenoma detection rate between 15% (women) and 25%

Table 11.1 (a) Prevalence and cancer risk of colonic mucosal neoplasms [2, 5, 6, 9, 10]

Superficial neoplastic lesion		Prevalence (%)	Cancer risk (%)	Recommended resection
Polypoid 0-Ip/Isp/Is	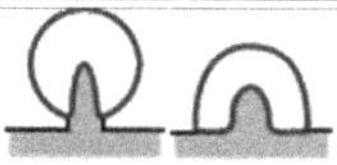	~15–20	1–15	Snaring
Elevated/flat 0-IIa/b		~5	4–6	EMR
Depressed 0-IIc	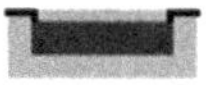	~0.5	30–75	→ En bloc

Table 11.1 (b) Prevalence and cancer risk of laterally spreading tumors [5, 9–13]

Superficial neoplastic lesion			Prevalence[a] (%)	Cancer risk[b] (%)	SMI risk[c] 95% CI	Recommended resection[d]
	% LST[c]					
LST-GH	35	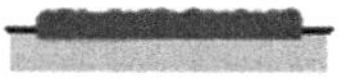	~1.9	0.9	0.1–1.0	→ EMR
LST-GM	26	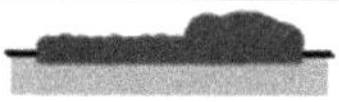	~1.4	40–45[b]	6–15	IEE → En bloc[d]
LST-NG	33	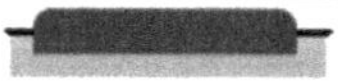	~1.8	20–29[b]	2–8	IEE → En bloc?
LST-NG-PD	5.5	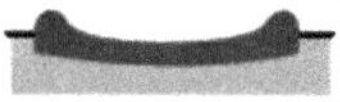	~0.3	70–75[b]	20–43	→ En bloc[d]
All LST			5.4%[a]	37%[c]	8.5%[c]	

GH granular homogenous, *GM* granular, nodular-mixed, *HGD* high-grade dysplasia, *IEE* image-enhanced endoscopy, LST laterally spreading tumor, *NG* non-granular, flat-elevated, *NG-PD* non-granular, pseudo-depressed, *SMI* sm invasion

[a]Prevalence 5% and 5.84% in two CRC screenings [9, 10]; subtype prevalence = 0.054 × %LST

[b]Cancer risk according to Refs. [9, 12, 13]

[c]Data from recent meta-analysis (with unconvincing analysis for LST prevalence of 0.83%) [11]

[d]ESD for large size (>40 mm) LST-GM, for LST-NG, and LST-NG-PD according to [12]

(men), a *benchmark* for screening colonoscopy [8]. The prevalence of non-protruded neoplasias represents their predicted low detection rate—but it's important not to miss them, because of their considerable cancer risk.

11.3 Basic Structure of Colorectal Mucosa and Neoplasias

Colorectal mucosa shows (on standard WLI) smooth surface reflex (of mucin layer) and mildly reddish color with a branching (dendritic) submucosal vascular pattern of collecting venules (Fig. 11.1). Colonic mucosal glands are tubular structures, and the pit-like gland openings form a regular carpet of small round pits—normal *PP type I* [14] (Table 11.2b and Fig. 11.2). Inflammation causes edema and vascular erythema of the mucosal and sm layer, diminished surface reflex (by inhomogeneous mucin layer), and epithelial erosions or submucosal ulcers. Permeation of the dendritic sm vascular pattern is diminished or absent, but the surface shows normal round pits type I or, when chronic, regenerative hyperplasia with stellar pits type II (Fig. 11.2a, b).

Analysis of mucosal neoplasias uses magnifying NBI (M-NBI) and chromoendoscopy (M-CE) with indigo carmine or crystal violet. S. Kudo [14] had characterized on M-CE the surface structure of glands (*pit pattern, PP*) (Fig. 11.2), and Y. Sano [15] illustrated the alterations of capillary pattern (CP) in normal mucosa, hyperplastic and neoplastic mucosal lesions (Table 1.3). The Narrow-Band Imaging International Colorectal Endoscopic (NICE) Classification (Table 1.4) was developed to standardize optical diagnosis with non-magnifying NBI, according to color, vessels, and surface pattern. The NICE classification is a simple and accurate tool to differentiate hyperplastic and adenomatous polyps. However, it is difficult to differentiate HGIEN from submucosal invasive cancer. Therefore, the Japanese NBI Expert Team Classification (JNET) for M-NBI analysis was conceived to predict

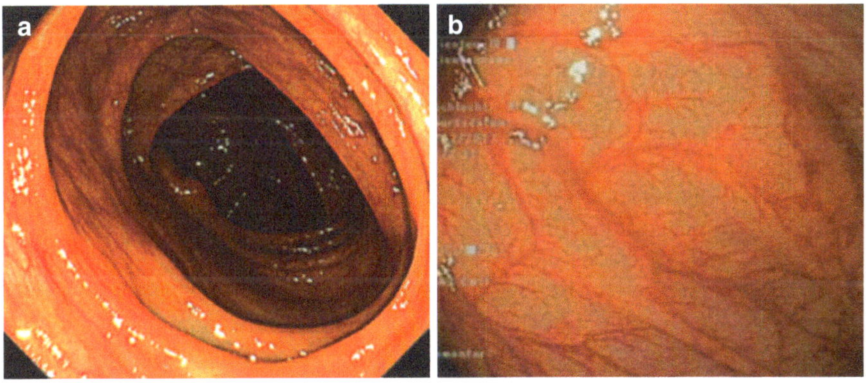

Fig. 11.1 (**a**) Normal ascending colon, WLI. (**b**) Normal ascending colonic mucosa, WLI

Table 11.2 (a) Magnifying NBI classification of colorectal neoplasias by Japan NBI Expert Team (JNET)

JNET	Type 1	Type 2A	Type 2B	Type 3
Vessel type	Invisible [*1]	Regular caliber Regular distribution (meshed/spiral) [*2]	Variable caliber Irregular distribution	Loose vessel areas Interruption of thick vessels
Surface type	Regular dark or white spots similar to normal mucosa	Regular (tubular/ branched/papillary)	Irregular or obscure	Amorphous areas
Likely histology	Hyperplastic polyp / SSA/P	LGIEN	HGIEN/Shallow sm- invasive cancer[*3]	Deep sm- invasive cancer
NBI	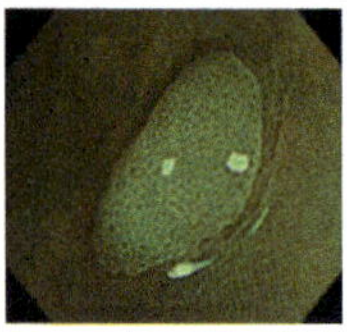	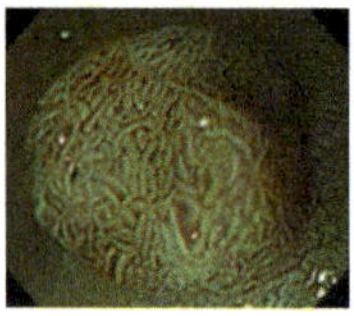	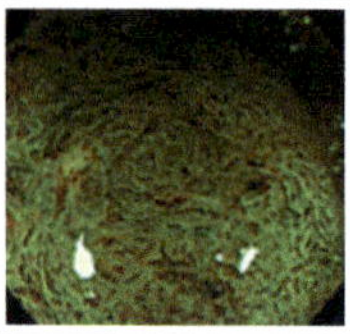	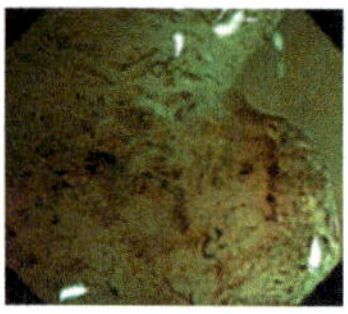

Adapted from Sano [17], with permission of John Wiley and Sons
*1. If visible, the caliber in the lesion is similar to surrounding normal mucosa
*2. Micro-vessels are often distributed in a punctate pattern, and well-ordered reticular or spiral vessels may not be observed in depressed lesions
*3. Deep submucosal invasive cancer may be included
SSA/P sessile serrated adenoma/polyp

the T category of early neoplasias [16, 17] (Table 11.2a). JNET has renamed capillary pattern (CP I/II/IIIA/IIIB) to vessel pattern (V1/2A/2B/3). JNET classification includes vessel and surface pattern and consists of three types: In Type 1 lesions (hyperplastic polyp / SSA/P), the vessel pattern is barely visible (regular network) or invisible and the surface pattern is dark spots or white spots. Type 2 is subdivided into two subtypes: Type 2A lesions, indicating low-grade intraepithelial neoplasia (LGIEN), show regular vessel (caliber, distribution) and surface pattern. Type 2B lesions, indicating HGIEN or superficial submucosa (sm)-invasive cancer, show irregular vessel pattern, such as variable caliber and irregular distribution, and irregular or obscure surface pattern. Type 3 lesions show loose vessel areas, thick-caliber vessels, and amorphous surface, and suggest sm2–3 invasive cancer (specificity 85%) [17, 18].

NICE and *JNET* classifications belong to *minimal standard terminology (MST)* of the World Endoscopy Organization (WEO). However evaluated for sm-invasive cancer on still images, the NICE classification without any magnifying endoscopy yielded inadequate accuracy, and the JNET classification, without exact surface pattern (SP) on crystal violet M-CE, had only moderate accuracy [16, 18]. By contrast, combined vessel pattern (VP) and pit pattern (PP) classifications accurately discriminate mucosal *versus* sm-invasive cancer and educate for both SP and VP diagnosis [14, 15, 19–22]. Endoscopic diagnosis is then summarized as the JNET type. (Compare algorithm Fig. 11.10.)

Table 11.2 (b) Pit pattern type of colonic mucosa [14, 19]

	Type[a]	Description of pits	Histopathological correlates
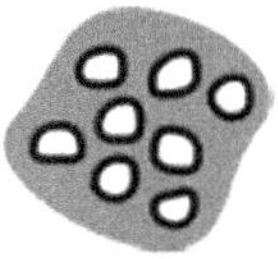	I	Round (uniform pits)	Normal or inflammatory mucosa
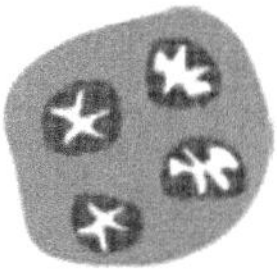	II	Stellar or papillary	Hyperplastic mucosa (hyperplastic polyp or serrated adenoma)
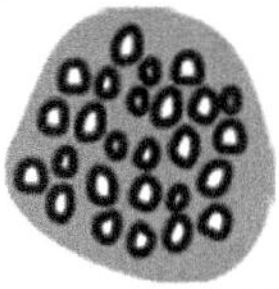	IIIs[b]	Small tubular, round	Adenoma or carcinoma (often depressed type)
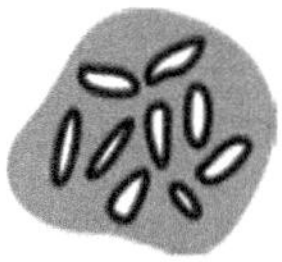	III_L	Large tubular or round	Adenoma (often classical polypoid adenoma)
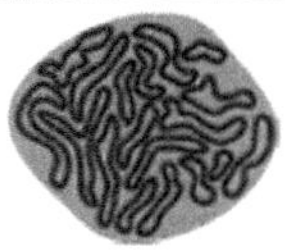	IV[a]	Branching or gyrus-like	Adenoma (often villous)
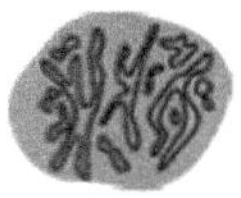	V_I low-grade	Irregular pits with smooth margins	Adenoma (LGIN), early cancer (HGIN, T1 m, or T1 sml)
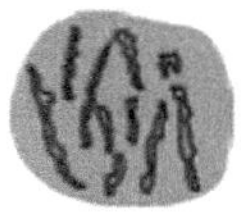	V_I high-grade	Irregular, narrow pits with rough margins	sm-invasive cancer (80% ≥ sm2)
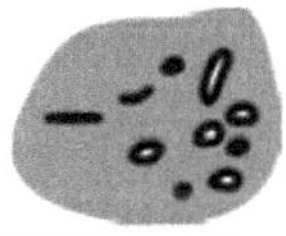	V_N	Nonstructured	sm-invasive cancer (≥sm2)

[a]Patterns: normal (type I), hyperplastic or serrated (type II), neoplastic (types III–V)
[b]IIIs and V show amorphism (i.e., asymmetrical pits irregular in arrangement and sizes, in part destructed) and are highly predictive of malignancy. Type IIIs adenoma probably is the precursor lesion for flat and depressed superficial cancers and carries a high risk of minute mucosal cancer nests; type V areas (Vi high grade, V_N) indicate a high risk of submucosal invasion [5, 14, 19, 20]

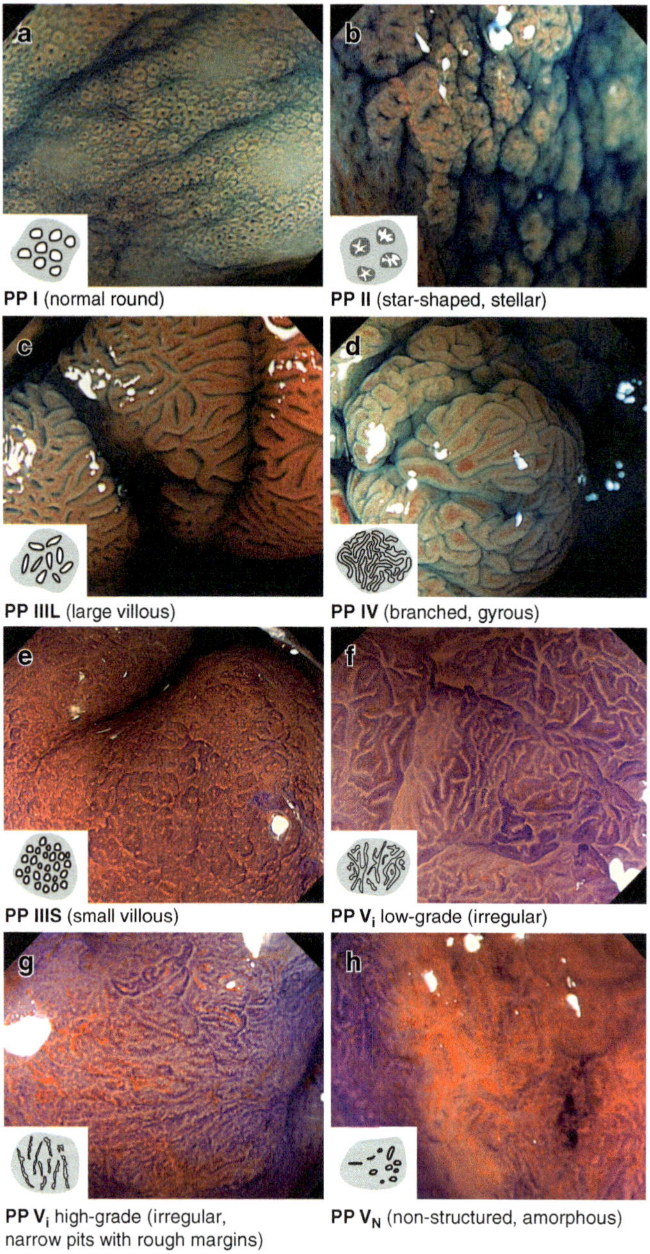

Fig. 11.2 Colonic pit pattern types I–V_N on magnified (~40–80-fold) chromoendoscopy ((**a**–**e**) indigo carmine; (**f**–**g**) crystal violet). (**a**) PP I (normal round). (**b**) PP II (star-shaped, stellar). (**c**) PP IIIL (large villous). (**d**) PP IV (branched, gyrous). (**e**) PP IIIs (small villous). (**f**) PP V_I low-grade irregular. (**g**) PP V_I high-grade irregular (narrow pits with rough margins). (**h**) PP V_N (non-structured, amorphous). (According to Kudo [14, 19]). Compare Table 11.2a for explanation

11.4 Macroscopic Type and Appearance of Colorectal Lesions

11.4.1 Distinction of NICE Types on Standard WLI and CE

Mucosal neoplasias (adenoma, HGIN, adenocarcinoma) are lesions with clear *margins*, *disappearance* of *dendritic submucosal vessel pattern*, and the presence of *neoplastic pit patterns* (PP III–V) with indigo carmine CE or (in cases of serrated adenomas) variants of hyperplastic PP (Fig. 11.3). Delineation of the lateral margins of protruding or flat neoplasia is easy in normal colonic mucosa. A lack of clear margin in the presence of hyperplastic PP favors *hyperplastic* (non-neoplastic) *polyps* (*HP*), most of them in rectosigmoid colon as lesions 0-Is/Isp or 0-IIa (Fig. 11.4a, b). They must not be confused with serrated adenomas, which also exhibit hyperplastic PP, often in the right colon as lesions 0-Is or 0-IIa. (Compare Sect. 11.4.2, below). In addition, several similar protruding lesions (0-Isp, 0-Is, 0-IIa) present normal mucosal surface and submucosal vascular pattern, such as submucosal tumor (*SMT*), rare *hamartoma* (Peutz-Jeghers polyp, juvenile polyp), or *inverted diverticulum*, which is soft and pliable. Reddish or isochrome polypoid or sessile lesions with normal or hyperplastic surface pattern are typical of *inflammatory pseudopolyps* in ulcerative colitis or Crohn's disease (Fig. 11.4c, d), and rarely typical of sm-infiltrating lymphoma or secondary carcinoma originating from other sites or organs (peritoneum, ovary, metastatic cancer).

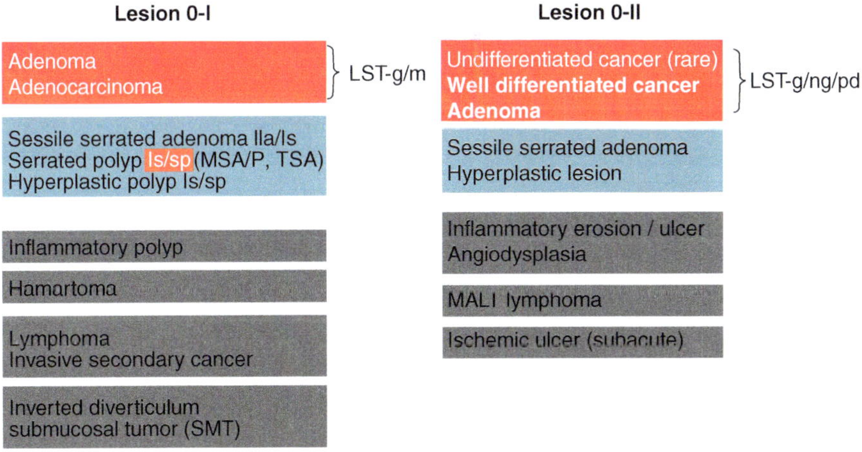

Fig. 11.3 Differential diagnosis of colorectal lesions according to pit pattern on *indigo carmine CE*: neoplastic (*red*), hyperplastic/serrated (*blue*), and normal pit pattern (*grey*). Mucosal neoplasias (adenomatous, serrated, and cancerous) exhibit distinct *sharp margins* on indigo carmine CE or magnifying NBI, in contrast to hyperplastic or inflammatory lesions or diffuse submucosa-infiltrative neoplasias. MSA/P—mixed serrated adenoma/polyp; TSA—traditional serrated adenoma

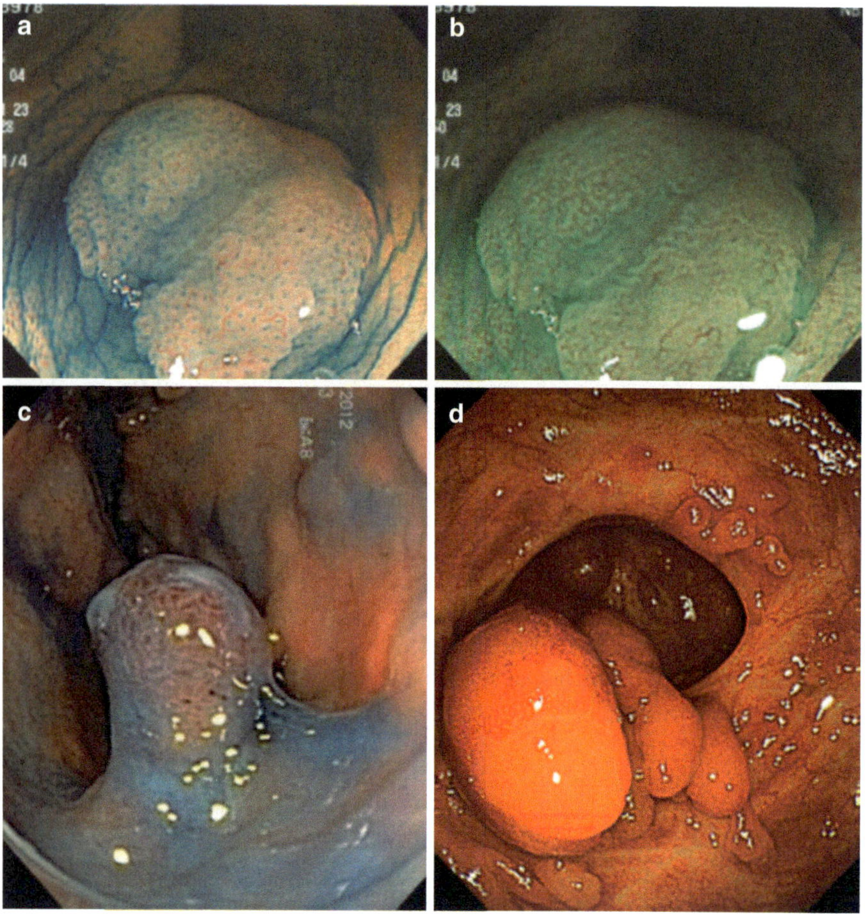

Fig. 11.4 (**a**, **b**) *Sessile hyperplastic polyp*, PP II (stellar) = SP 1 in cecum. (**a**) Indigo carmine CE. (**b**) VP 1 (faint mesh) in cecum, JNET type 1, M-NBI (40×). (**c**) *Nonneoplastic 0-Ip* (chronic inflammatory-regenerative lesion in moderately active ulcerative colitis, PP II), sigmoid colon indigo carmine CE. (**d**) *Nonneoplastic 0-Isp and 0-Is lesion* with unclear margin, in part visible VP 1, PP II (inflammatory-regenerative, moderately active Crohn's disease), sigmoid colon, JNET type 1, WLI

Flat or depressed lesions (*0-IIa–c*, often reddish) with key neoplastic signs (clear margins, neoplastic PP, and disappearance of dendritic sm vascular pattern) are *mucosal neoplasias*. Reddish hyperemic lesions with uncertain margins comprise inflammatory mucosal lesions, such as erosions and inflammatory ulcer (Fig. 11.5), ischemic ulcer, or angiodysplasia. Pale, flat lesions with nearly *normal PP* are typical for mucosal *MALT lymphoma* or subacute *ischemic ulcerations* that show pale or mildly red lesions, but they differ by having a bare proper muscle layer in the center surrounded by a margin of regular mucosa (lack of neoplastic PP) (Fig. 11.6). Pale, flat lesions with the disappearance of the sm vascular pattern and some unclear

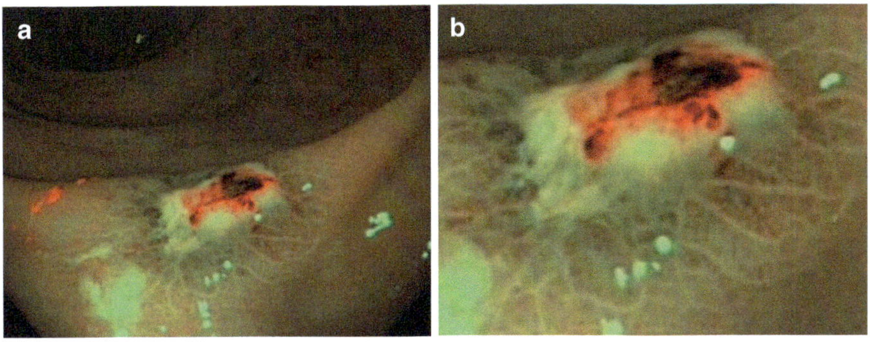

Fig. 11.5 (**a**) Solitary rectal ulcer in an 82-year-old man, on standard NBI. (**b**) VP type 1 (meshed), PP type I, and uncertain margin of fibrin covered ulcer, standard NBI

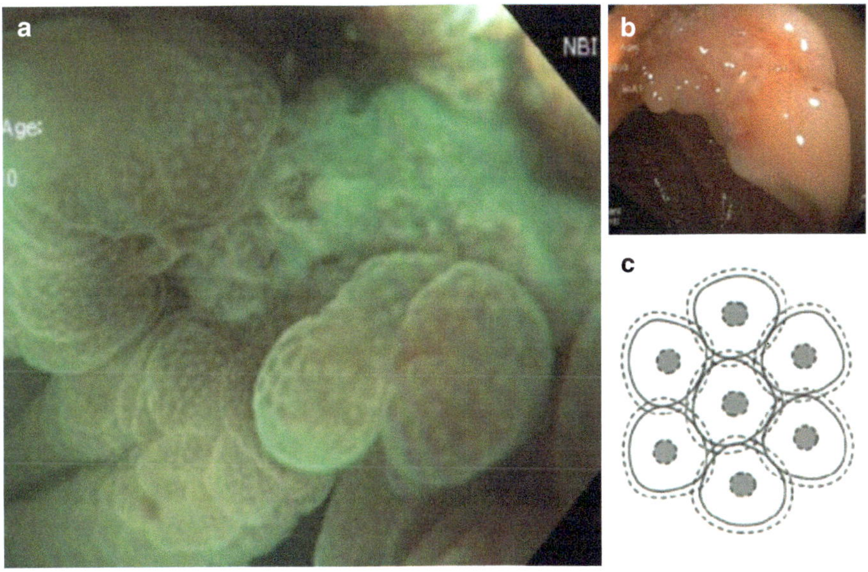

Fig. 11.6 Lesion type 0-III. One of the two ulcers on neighboring haustral folds in the left transverse colon in an 80-year-old woman. (**a**) Typical *subacute ischemic ulcer* with bare ground (proper muscle) and mucosal margins showing normal VP (meshed) and PP I. (**b**) Standard WLI aspect. (**c**) Schema of PP I and VP 1

margins are also compatible with *LST-NG*, but that shows *clear margins* on magnifying NBI.

Flat and *depressed neoplasias* including *LST-NG* and most *LST-granular* types, including *LST-GH*, *LST-GM*, and *LST-G-whole nodular,* show discolored, often pale, areas with clear margins and disappearance of normal sm vascular pattern (Fig. 11.7a–j). They are further distinguished in *classic adenoma, serrated adenomas, HNPCC-associated adenoma*, and *HGIN/intramucosal carcinoma* (*See* Sect. 11.5).

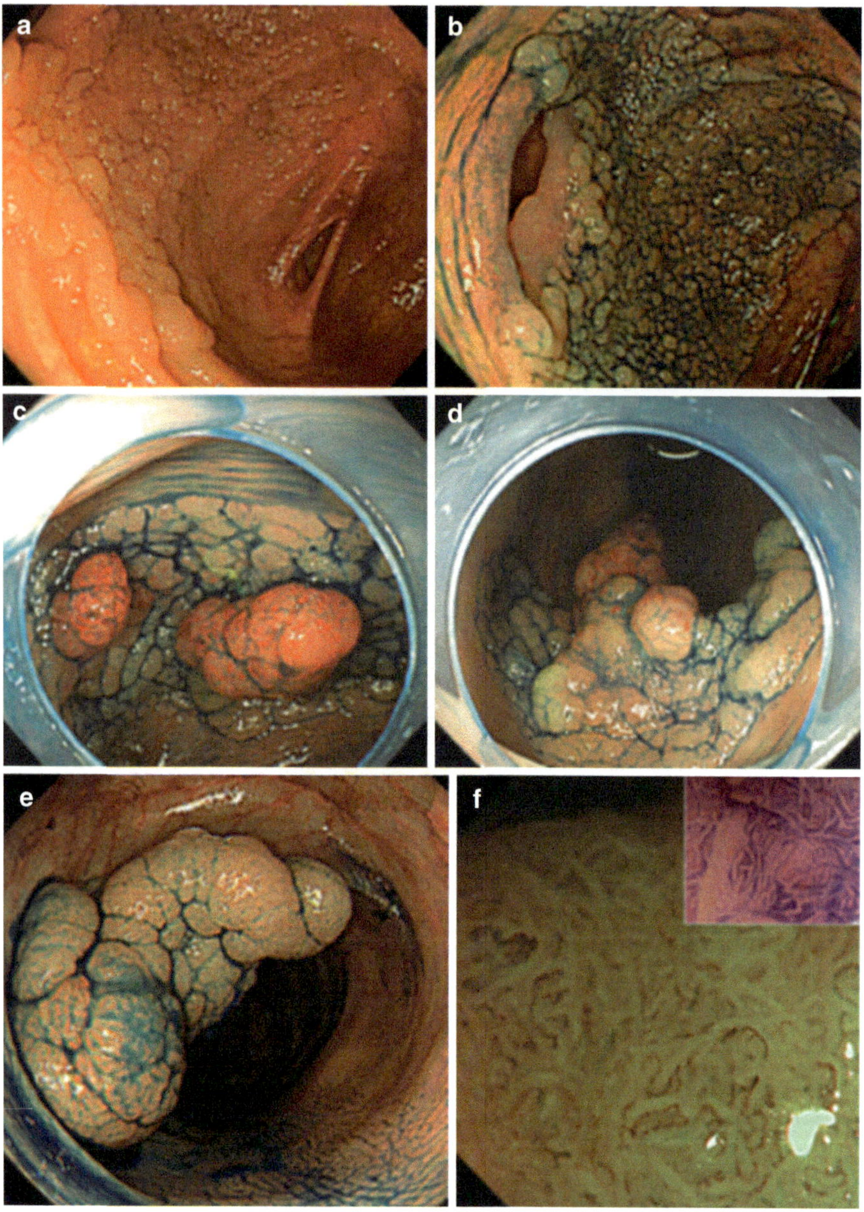

Fig. 11.7 *LST-G*. (**a**, **b**) LST-G granular homogenous type, cecum. (**a**) WLI; (**b**) indigo carmine CE. (**c**, **d**) Rectal LST-GM, granular mixed nodular type, indigo carmine CE, (**c**) prograde view; (**d**) retroflex view. (**e**) LST-G whole nodular. 0-Is + IIa, 30 mm in diameter, transverse colon, indigo carmine CE. (**f**) Same LST-GM as in (**e**) on M-NBI (80×): VP 2B (*insert* with crystal violet CE: PP type $V_{I\ low\ grade}$), *JNET type 2B*. ESD: tubular adenocarcinoma T1a (LPM)

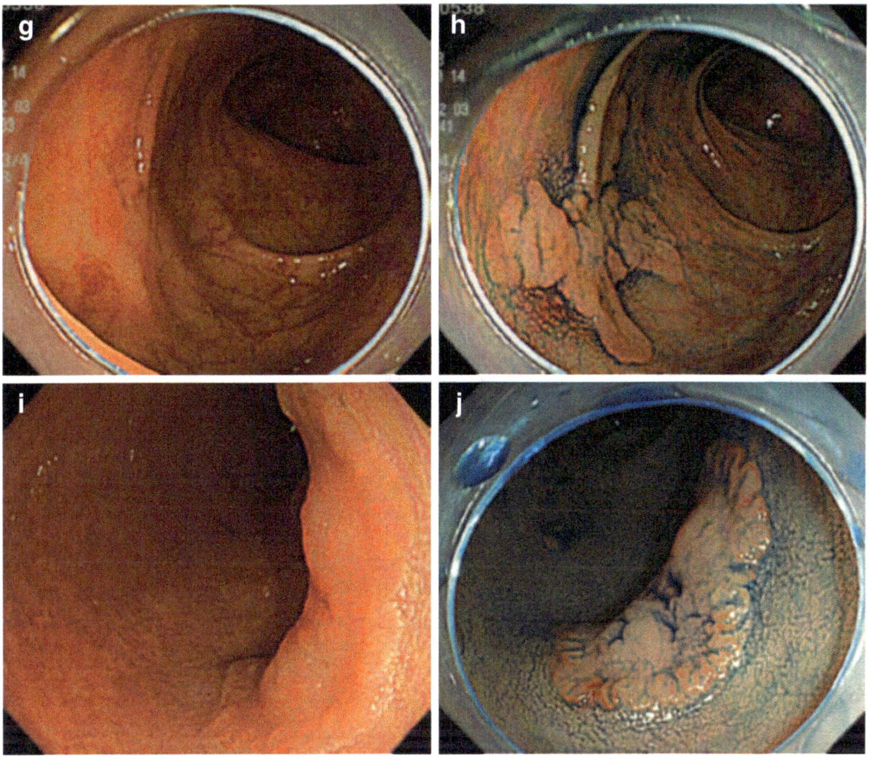

Fig. 11.7 (continued) ESD: tubular adenocarcinoma T1a (LPM) (**g**, **h**) LST-NG flat (0-IIa); WLI and indigo carmine; (**i**, **j**) LST-NGPD (0-IIa + IIc, central protrusion), WLI and indigo carmine CE

Early cancer with invasion into sml often presents mild (0-IIc) or marked (IIc + IIa) surface depression (Fig. 1.2). Depressed neoplasias type 0-IIc display *air-induced deformation* (*AID*) when infiltrating only muscularis mucosae (MM) or superficial sml submucosa layer. (*Compare* Fig. 11.14.)

Most *LST-NG* show normal color and *relatively ill-defined margins*; therefore, only larger LST-NG lesions are easily apparent on WLI endoscopy. LST-NG may be overlooked, unless you pay alert attention to convergent folds, loss of glossy surface reflex, and especially disappearance of dendritic sm vessel pattern. Indigo carmine CE demonstrates the distinct margins of the lesion (Fig. 11.7h, j). Prevalence of LST is highest in the right colon and the rectum. Risk of focal cancer in different LST types [13] is detailed in Table 11.3. The probability of *malignant transformation of LST* increases with *size* of the lesion, especially when >30 mm, and *type*, being high in *LST-GM* and *LST-NG*, and highest in pseudo-depressed *LST-NGPD* (Fig. 11.7i, j). Retrospective analysis (period 1998–2006) of LSTs ≥20 mm in size resected at the National Cancer Center, Tokyo, confirmed sm-invasive cancer in 0.9% of LST-GH, 16% of LST-GM, 23% of LST-NG, and 58% of LST-NGPD, but only in 5% of small size (d < 20 mm) LST-GM or LST-NG [12]. Hence, the NCC

Table 11.3 Characteristics of LST and Lesion 0-IIc (and IIa + c) treated with ESD [13]

		Mean		Percentage of lesion type			
	Lesion	*n*	Size (mm)	Adenoma (%)	T1a[b] (%)	Ca sm1 (%)	Ca ≥sm2[a] (%)
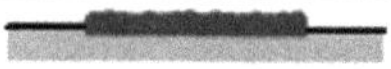	LST-G(H)	57	32	58	42	0	0
	LST-G(M)	86	39	40	42	14	5
	LST-NG(F)	77	22	60	30	7	3
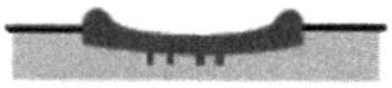	LST-NG(PD)	25	20	28	24	44	4
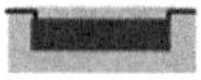	IIc and IIa + IIc	6	17	0	33	0	67[c]

[a]All lesions were chosen suitable for ESD (leading to selection bias, because LST with endoscopic criteria of massively sm-invasive cancer had a priori been excluded). Note the high percentage of HGIN/mucosal cancer in larger LST

[b]Intramucosal HGIN/cancer only, no sm-invasive cancer

[c]4 of 6 cases

and JGES guidelines recommend resection en bloc for LST-NG of size ≥20 mm, LST-GM ≥40 mm, and LST-NGPD [12, 23].

11.4.2 *Distinction of NICE Type 2 (Adenomatous)* Versus *Type 1 (Serrated) Lesions*

Serrated lesions (SL) presumably give rise to 15% of all colorectal carcinomas (CRC) and 25–30% of proximal CRC; they lately have raised endoscopic and histologic attention [24]. The four subtypes of SL exhibit a wide range of CRC potential (see Table 2.6):

- Hyperplastic polyps (HP), nearly none (considered non-neoplastic)
- Serrated sessile adenoma/polyps without dysplasia (SSA/P), moderate CRC potential (13% in 7 years)
- SSA/P with dysplasia (i.e. mixed serrated adenoma, MSA) and traditional serrated adenoma (TSA), high CRC potential (approximately 50% in 5 years) [24].

Serrated adenomas are located predominantly in the rectosigmoid (especially types Ip and Isp, TSA) and in the right colon (especially types 0-II, SSA/P and MSA). On *non-magnifying* NBI, the WASP classification (Workgroup serrAted polypS and Polyposis) accurately (87%) distinguished *type 2 lesions* (brown color, brown vessels, and branched or tubular SP) from *type 1 lesions* (SSA/P, MSA) using two positives of four discriminators (clouded surface [=mucus], vague border,

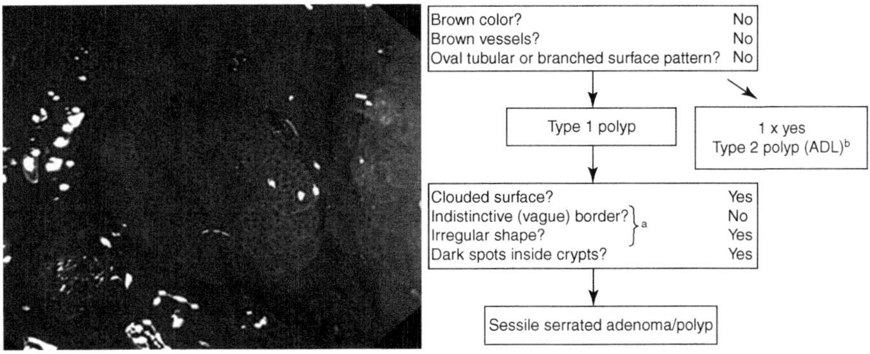

Fig. 11.8 Representative: NBI image of sessile serrated adenoma/polyp (SSA/P) with decision pathway for WASP classification. [a]Indistinct border, irregular shape: Criterion was derived from standard WLI/NBI still images (non-magnified, non-CE), and is not maintained when using magnifying indigo carmine CE or magnifying NBI. [b]ADL—adenomatous/cancerous lesion. (From Ijspeert et al. [26], with permission of John Wiley and Sons Inc)

irregular shape, dark spots inside crypts) (Fig. 11.8) [25, 26]. However, two discriminators, indistinct margins and irregular shape, no longer hold true when using M-NBI or indigo carmine CE. Based on the WASP classification, large European cohorts on screening colonoscopy yielded a prevalence of 30% for HP, 3–8% for SSA/P, less than 1% each for MSA and TSA, and 0.5% for serrated polyposis syndrome (SPS) [27] (*see* Table 2.6). Accurate distinction among NICE type 1 lesions would provide cost-saving policies for HP ("resect and discard" and "resect or leave in") and select serrated neoplasias for endoscopic resection. (*See* Sect. 11.5.3.)

11.5 Differential Diagnosis of Lesions on Magnifying Endoscopy

The basic strategy to analyze VP with M-NBI and then PP with M-CE allows accurate endoscopic differential diagnosis to predict histologic type and tumor category of early neoplasias [19].

Note *Magnified NBI (≥60×)* and often *crystal violet M-CE* is required to accurately (>90%) differentiate with VP (CP) and SP (PP) [5, 16, 19–22]:

- Adenoma *versus* carcinoma
- Intramucosal *versus* submucosal deeply invasive carcinoma
- Hyperplastic lesion *versus* adenoma and serrated neoplasias (The latter distinction is less accurate; *see* Sect. 11.5.3.)

11.5.1 Differential Diagnosis of JNET Type 2 Lesions (Adenoma/Superficial Adenocarcinoma)

Classic adenomas consist of transformed colonocytes with enhanced nucleus/cytoplasm ratio, loss of polar orientation of cell nuclei, enhanced clonal proliferation of colonocytes, and formation of regular pseudoglandular structures *without* goblet cells. By definition, adenomas lack invasive or metastatic potential, and the process of cell-cell adhesion is preserved. Therefore, the lesion forms single-layered, glandular marginal epithelium, seen as *surface pattern* (*SP*) using NBI and CE with magnification (Fig. 11.2). The enhanced proliferation of pseudoglandular structures creates patterns of different surface shapes visualized as *PP* type *III*L or *IV*, rarely *IIIs* or *Virregular* (Fig. 11.2c–f), and regular, dense vessel pattern (VP) *2A, lesion JNET type 2A* (Figs. 11.9 and 11.12b, c). The margin of adenoma is

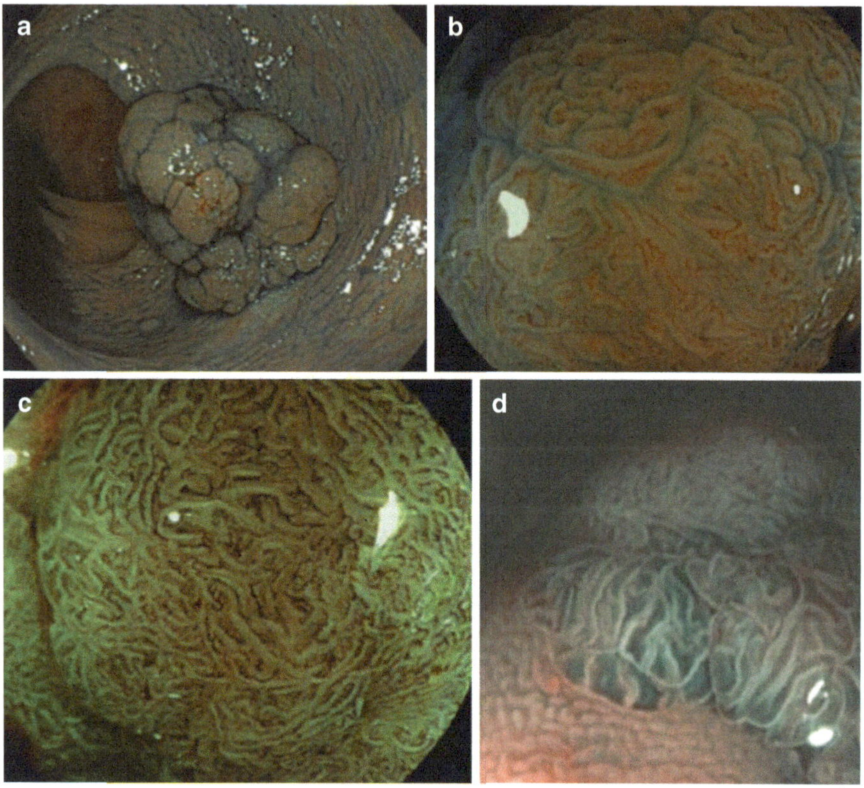

Fig. 11.9 (**a**–**d**) *Protruding neoplasia 0-Isp*, 25 mm in diameter. (**a**) WLI indigo carmine CE. (**b**) With magnification. (**c**) M-NBI (80-fold): JNET type 2A (VP 2A, PP IV). Histology: *tubulovillous adenoma* with focal HGIN. (**d**) *Protruding adenoma 0-Isp*, 15 mm in size, clear margin without demarcation of relief, JNET type 2A with even surface marginal crypt epithelium (PP IIIL, VP 2A); M-NBI 60-fold). EMR *tubular adenoma* with LGIN

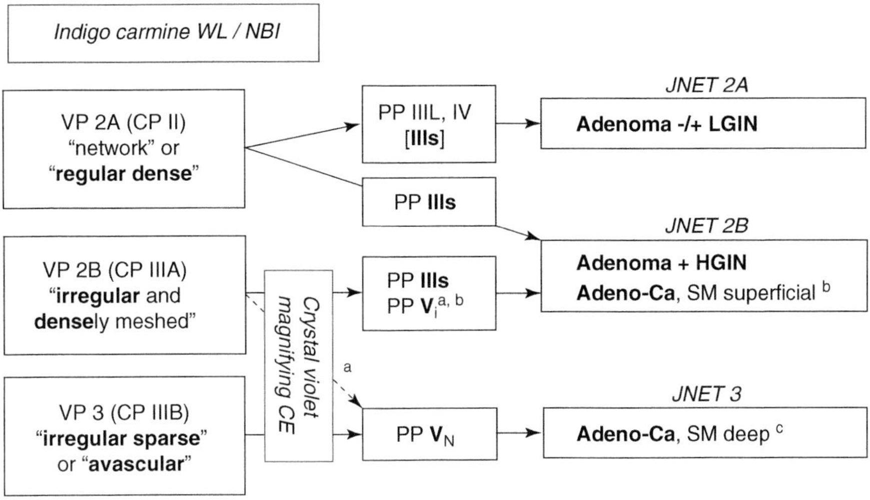

Fig. 11.10 *Analysis of colorectal adenomatous/cancerous lesions* with magnifying NBI/CE, to distinguish malignancy and grade of invasiveness by vessel *VP* and pit pattern *PP* [19], for JNET types 2 and 3. [a] PP type V_I high grade with encroachment of margins signals deep sm invasion. [b] Superficial sm invasion <1000 μm. [c] Deep sm invasion ≥1000 μm

clearly visible on WLI (and M-NBI) by change of SP type, but without encroachment of surface relief (Fig. 11.9d, *compare* Fig. 1.6). The regular epithelial structure of adenomas is well visualized as evenly marginal epithelium (MCE) on M-NBI. The basic diagnostic strategy is very accurate (>90%) [14, 19, 22, 28]; see the algorithm in Fig. 11.10.

Flat HNPCC neoplasias in hereditary nonpolyposis colorectal cancer syndrome (Fig. 11.11a–c) show distinctive 0-IIa/b/c type lesions, mainly *pale* with *clear margins* after indigo carmine enhancement or on magnifying NBI. The overall number of lesions in the colon is *not* significantly increased in HNPCC as compared with sporadic adenoma carriers, but *flat adenomas with pale components* (70–80% mucinous villous) and *CRC* occur at an earlier age (mean 35–40 years) and predominantly (~70%) in the *right hemicolon* [29]. A high proportion (40–80%) contains *HGIN* or *carcinoma*, mainly with mucinous differentiation [29–31]. M-NBI shows VP 2A or 2B and PP IIIL, IV, or V_I/V_N. Indigo carmine-CE is recommended for HNPCC surveillance improving detection rate (0.3 → 0.7 lesions per patient).

Key Points

Adenoma (JNET type 2A) shows typical findings on WLI and indigo carmine:

- Disappearance of submucosal vascular pattern
- Clear lateral margins of the lesion (without encroachment)
- Reddish color, with lobulation on the lesion surface
- Regular pit pattern, tubular (IIIL, sometimes IIIs) or branched (IV)
- Even distension of flat-type adenomas on insufflation/desufflation

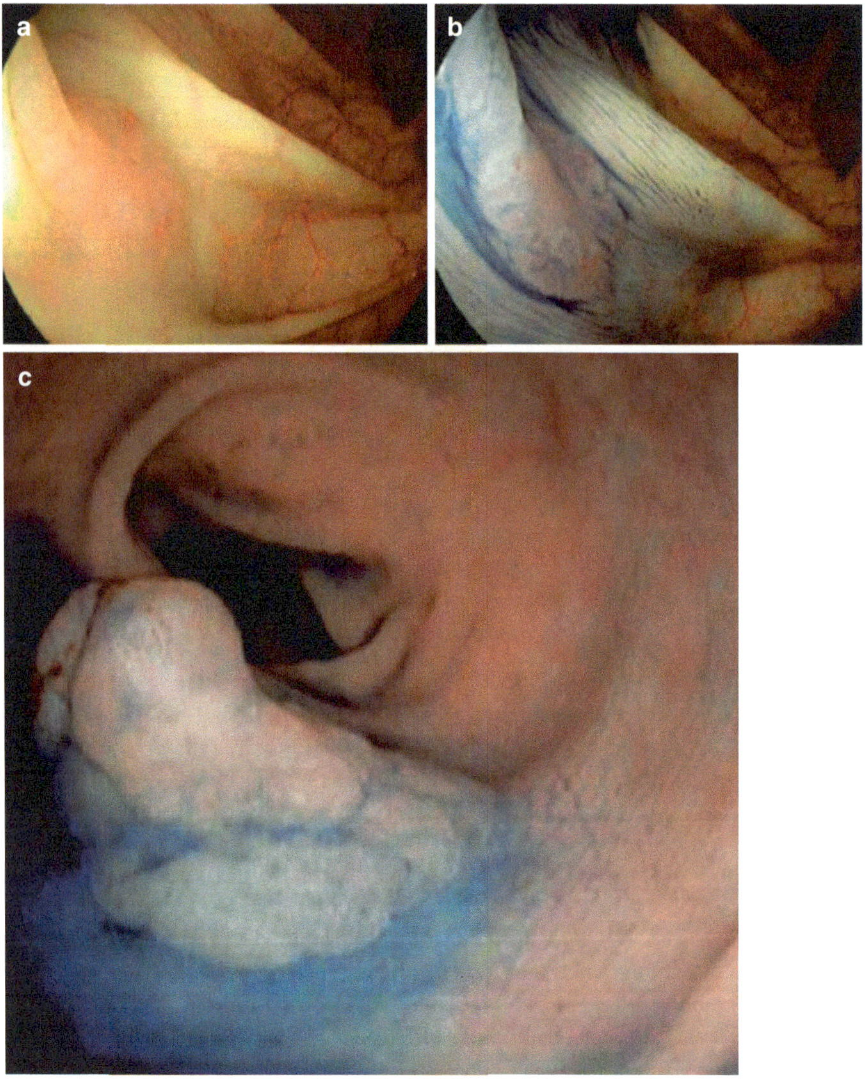

Fig. 11.11 (**a**) LST-NG (0-IIa) isochrome, ascending colon, in a 41-year-old man with HNPCC (*MLH-1* mutation). (**b**) Indigo carmine shows enhanced margins of the neoplasia. (**c**) LST-GM (0-Is + IIa), isochrome, 15 mm, in a 32-year-old woman with HNPCC (*MLH-1* negative), detected at surveillance 24 months after negative colonoscopy, with indigo carmine. (Pan-)chromoendoscopy enhances detection of flat neoplasias in HNPCC. (From Rondagh et al. [29], with permission of Thieme)

Typical structural findings on magnifying NBI:

- Even surface pattern (even white zone = marginal crypt epithelium)
- Regular network vessel pattern (VP 2A)

Differentiated adenocarcinoma (G1, G2) exhibits irregularities in thickness and shape of cancerous marginal crypt cell layers (*irregular SP*) and irregular pseudogland structure (irregular pit pattern *PP type* V_I or V_N on crystal violet M-CE) (Figs. 11.2f–h and 11.7f, Sect. 11.8, case no. 1). Absorptive staining of epithelial cells with *crystal violet* best demonstrates irregular or destroyed pseudoglandular structure (*PP* V_I *or* V_N) (Fig. 11.2f–h). Coherently growing cancer cell clusters exhibit sharp margins with a "*demarcation line*" and *encroachment of surface relief* towards surrounding adenomatous or normal epithelium. Angiogenesis creates an irregular, dense vessel pattern *VP 2B* [16, 17, 19] (Figs. 11.7f and 11.12c).

Undifferentiated carcinoma (G3) is rare (<5%) in the colorectum, and its endoscopic distinction from differentiated cancer is not yet evidence-based.

Key Points
Hallmarks of *superficial differentiated adenocarcinoma* (G1 or G2), *JNET type 2B*:

- Irregular SP (uneven thickness of cancerous epithelium)
- Irregular pit pattern PP III_S or PP V_I
- Irregular vessels VP 2B
- Demarcation of relief (DL and encroachment) at lateral margin towards adenoma/mucosa
- Air-induced deformation (AID) of type 0-II cancer (Fig.11.14a–c).

11.5.2 *Diagnosis of Superficial AC* Versus *Deep sm-Invasive AC (JNET Type 2B* Versus *Type 3)*

The estimated *vertical depth of invasion* guides the decision for or against endoscopic resection of early cancer. Other risk factors for lymph node metastasis, such as lymphovascular invasion and tumor cell budding, are not predictable from endoscopic signs; targeted biopsy is necessary to exclude poorly differentiated CRC G3 (prevalence <5% in CRC).

Protruded-type early colon cancer is highly suspicious for *sm2–3 invasion* in the presence of a small, thick pedicle (*fullness of stalk*), a small nodule on polypoid neoplasia (*Buddha sign*), or an expansive nodule with *loss of lobulation* (Fig. 11.13b). Further evidence is friability, central depression with PP V_N or ulcer-

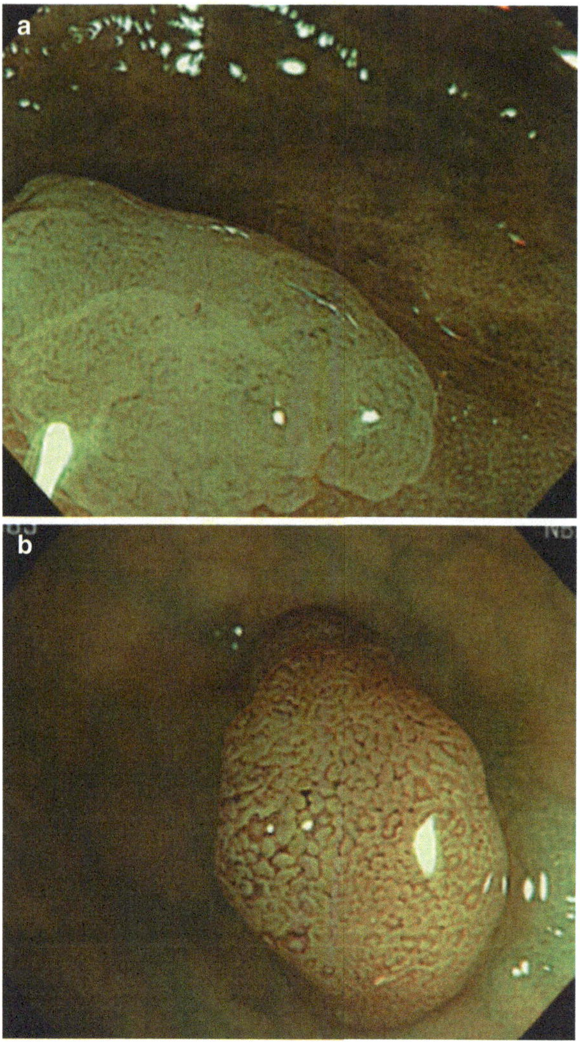

Fig. 11.12 **Vessel pattern (VP) types** (m-NBI, 100×). (**a**) *VP 1* meshed is faintly visible (−) in hyperplastic lesion 0-IIa *JNET type 1* (with PP type II), as compared with VP type 1 (+), visible in adjacent normal mucosa (*right side*). (**b**) *VP 2A*, regularly meshed, in lesion 0-Is *JNET type 2A* is typical for adenoma (probable PP IIIL)

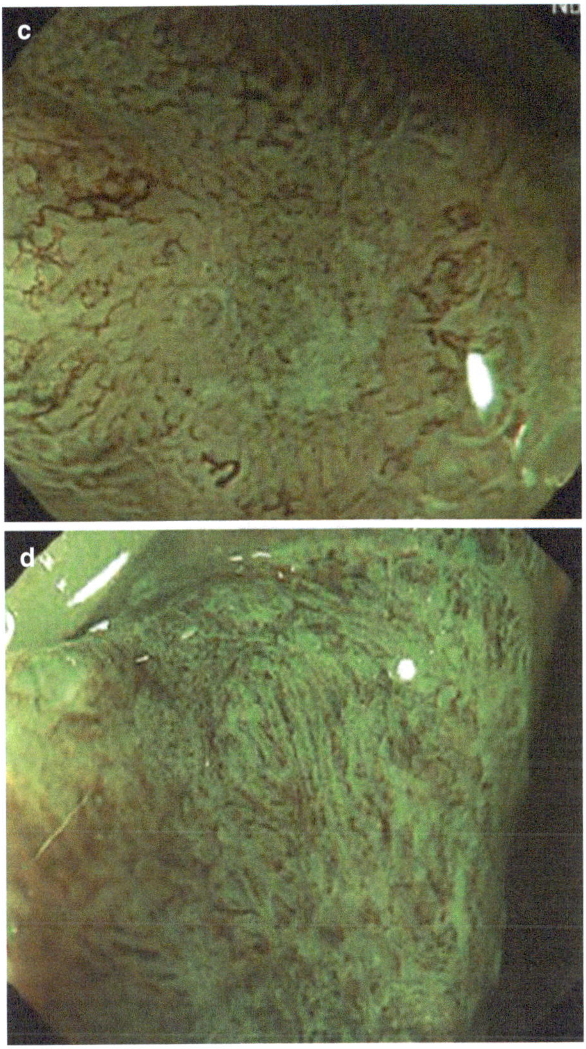

Fig. 11.12 (continued) (**c**) *VP 2B*, irregularly meshed, *dense* vessel pattern, in flat lesion compatible with adenoma and HGIN or intramucosal (or superficially sm-invasive) differentiated cancer. Crystal violet CE is recommended for evaluation of pit pattern, probably lesion JNET type 2B. (**d**) *VP 3*, loosely irregular, and in part *sparse* vessels suggesting sm-invasive early cancer ($\geq$sm2). Crystal violet CE is required to categorize the corresponding pit pattern type V (e.g., high-grade irregular or nonstructured) and diagnose lesion JNET type 3

ation, or fixed deformation of protruding neoplasia upon insufflation/desufflation (Figs. 1.2b, 11.13, and 11.14d–f). *Deep sm-invasive cancer* destroys (at least in part) pseudogland structure and microcapillaries and causes a destructive, amorphous pit pattern (*PP* V_I *high grade*, V_N) and irregular, sparse vessels *VP 3* with varying thick caliber (Figs. 11.2g–h and 11.12d). Typical images are shown in Figs. 11.14e, f and 11.15f.

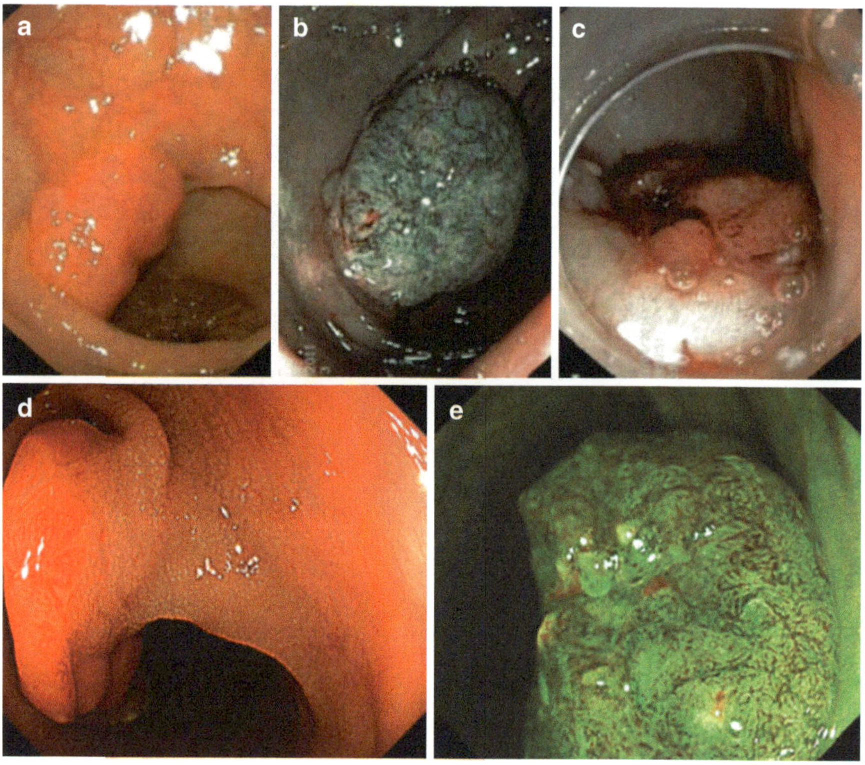

Fig. 11.13 (**a**, **b**) *Nodular neoplasia type 0-Is* with aboral pseudodepression (0-Is + c), friability, and VP 3. (**c**) *Complete non-lifting* on sm injection (3 × 5 mL) in descending colon. Laparoscopic resection disclosed tubulovillous adenoma and *focal adenocarcinoma G2, sm3*. (**d**, **e**) *Polypoid lesion type 0-Ip* in sigmoid colon. (**d**) Short pedestal with "fullness of stalk" (WLI), and (**e**) VP type 3 and PP type Vi high grade (M-NBI). Histology: well-differentiated *adenocarcinoma (G2), sm2*, and lymphovascular invasion (−)

Key Points

Deep submucosal invasion sm ≥ 2 of early CRC 0-IIa may be diagnosed from various findings [5, 16, 20–22, 28, 32, 33]:

- Expansive nodule with *loss of lobulation* in LST-GM
- Central depression or ulcer with PP V_N
- Expansive protrusion or nodule in depression 0-IIc
- *Fixed deformity* of CRC lesion (e.g., constant swollen convergence of folds −/+fusion) (Fig. 11.14d, e).

Typical signs are shown in Figs. 11.13, 11.14, 11.15 and 11.16e, f.

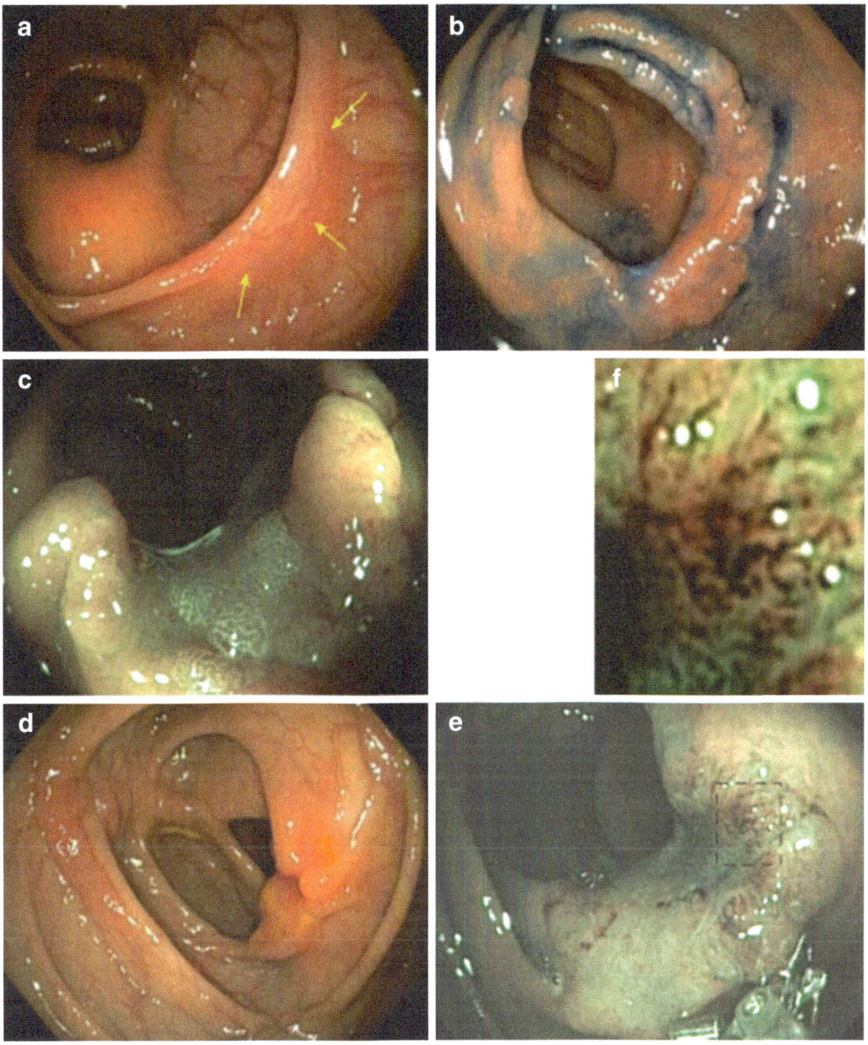

Fig. 11.14 (**a–c**) LST NGPD (0-IIa + c) in ascending colon with *marked air-induced deformation (AID)*: (**a**) Insufflation with adherent mucus; *yellow arrows* mark the margin of the lesion. (**b**) Indigo carmine. (**c**) Desufflation (cleaned). (**d**, **e**) Neoplasia 0-IIc + IIa with *fixed shape* and folds during insufflation/desufflation, transverse colon, WLI. (**f**) VP 3, lesion JNET type 3, NBI 80×. Hemicolectomy: adenocarcinoma G2 (mucoid differentiated), pT1b (sm3), Ly0, V0, N0 (0/9), and sm fibrosis

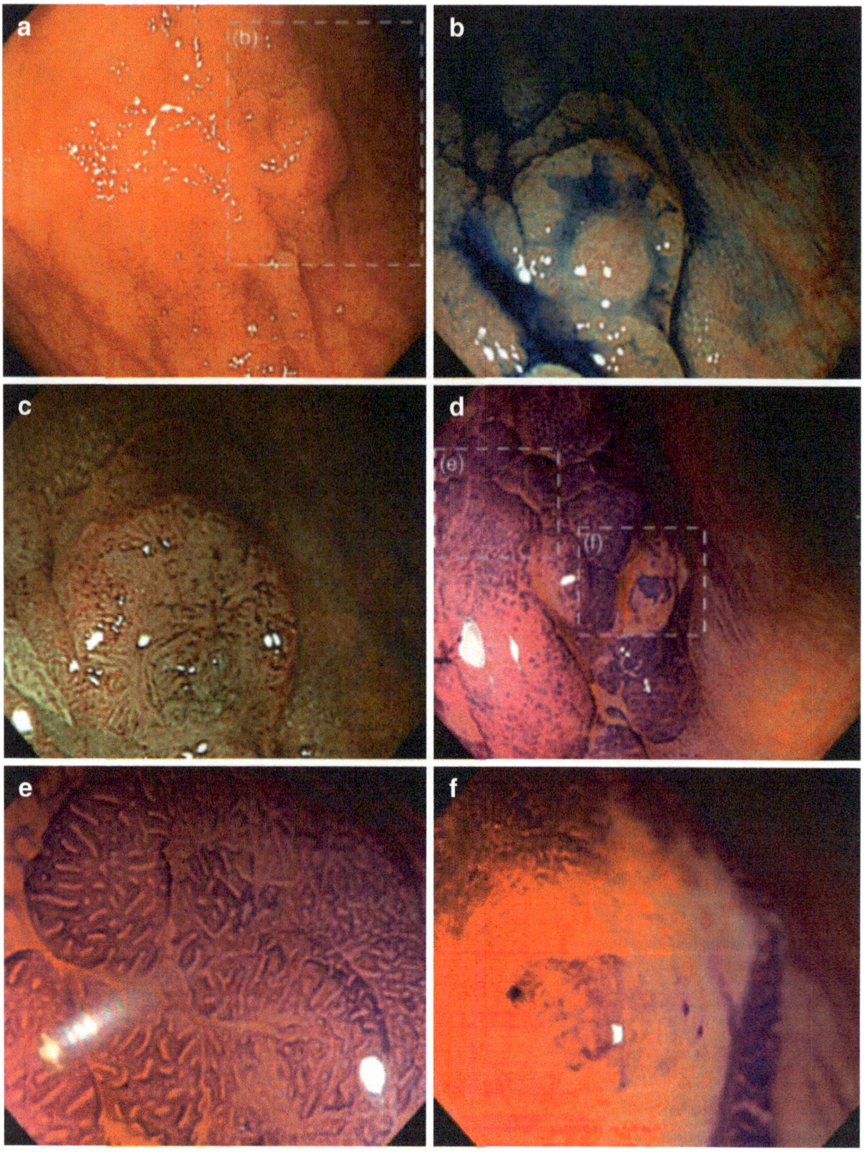

Fig. 11.15 Early CRC 0-IIa + IIc (>sm2 invasive), in sigmoid colon of a 59-year-old man. (**a**) Lesion on WLI. (**b**) Right margin of lesion with protuberance in depression, indigo carmine. (**c**) Protuberance on NBI (V 2B = CP IIIA in center). (**d**) Crystal violet, showing location of (**e**) and (**f**). (**e**) PP IIIL, magnified (80×). (**f**) Tiny area of amorphous PP Vn, magnified (80×). ESD using dual knife → adenocarcinoma G1, psm1 (990 μm), 29 × 20 mm, ly0 v0; curative R0

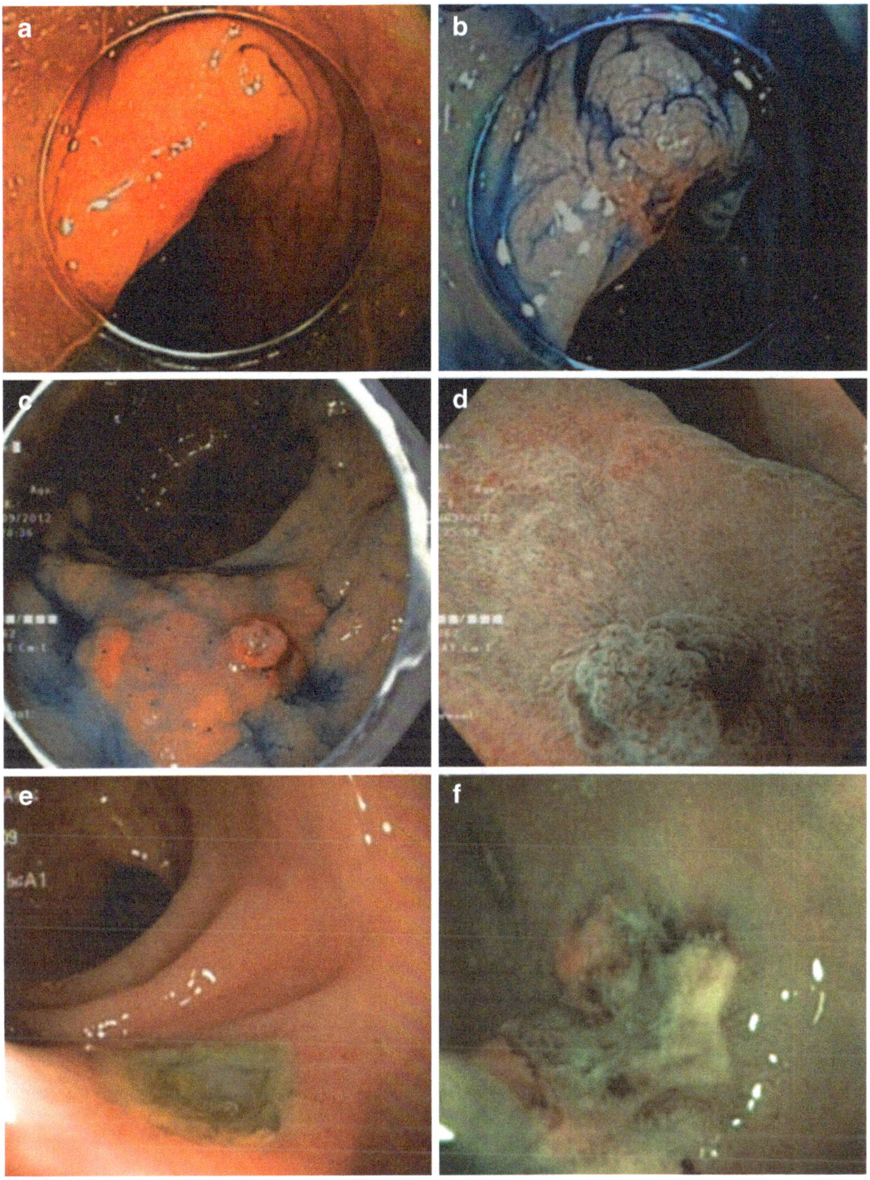

Fig. 11.16 Signs (a–d) suspicious for sm invasion. (**a**, **b**) Early cancer 0-IIa + c, with *constant folds and fusion of folds* (JNET type 2B/3), transverse colon. Laparoscopic hemicolectomy: adenocarcinoma G2, pTis (M), N0 (0/20), ly0, v0; R0. (**c**, **d**) LST-NG (0-IIb, VP 2A, PP IIIs) with polyp (*0-Isp, VP 2B, PP* V_I): lesion JNET type 2B. ESD: adenocarcinoma G2, pTis (M) and tubular adenoma with LGIN and HGIN. (**e**, **f**) *Lesion 0-III*, transverse colon, 18 mm (VP 3, probably PP V_N): lesion JNET type 3. Surgery: *advanced adenocarcinoma* G2, *pT2*

Key Points

Three clues indicate ≥sm2-invasion (JNET type 3) of early CRC [16, 17, 19, 32, 33]:

- *Shape and rigidity* of neoplastic lesion and folds (lack of AID)
- *Highly irregular/amorphous PP* [VI/V_N] and *sparse VP 3*
- *Poor lifting or non-lifting* of neoplasia upon submucosal injection

Predilection sites of sm-invasive carcinomatous foci in LSTs have been analyzed in a series of 511 large, en bloc–resected LSTs of different subtypes [33] (Fig. 11.17). Such predilection sites must be assessed for signs of invasive cancer, such as bleeding sites, sclerous wall change (lack of AID), irregular or sparse VP 2B/VP 3, and amorphous PP V_N. Large nodules (>10 mm) in LST-granular mixed types most likely harbor mucosal or even sm-invasive carcinomatous foci, as do depressed areas in homogenous LST-GH, granular-mixed LST-GM, or non-granular LST-NG. Multiple sm-invasive cancer foci in LST-NG are hardly predictable on endoscopy; the lesion requires resection en bloc.

Key Points

Deep submucosal invasion of early cancer is suspected in the presence of:

- Laterally spreading tumors (LST, Fig. 11.17) with
  - Large nodule >10 mm with PP V_N in LST-GM
  - LST-GM of whole large-nodular type with PP V_I or V_N
  - LST-GM >30 mm size with pit pattern V_I or V_N
  - LST-G with depressed area IIc + IIa and PP V_N
  - LST-NG(PD) >20 mm size with PP V_N
  - Protrusion or ulcer in LST-NG
- Non-lifting upon submucosal injection of any of the above lesions

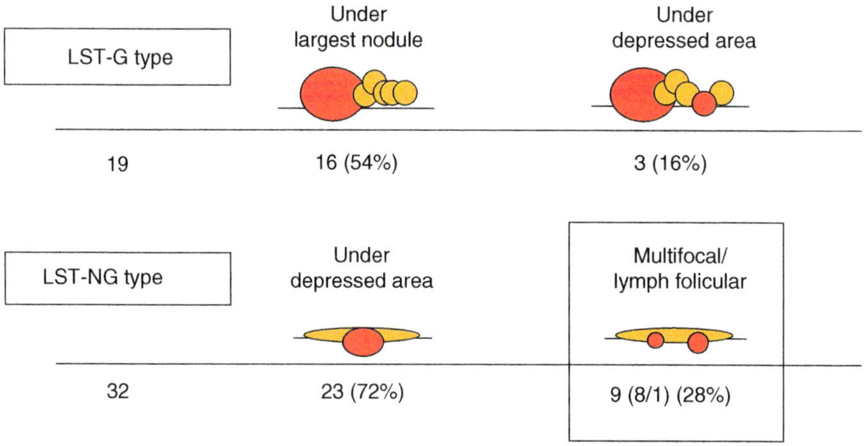

Fig. 11.17 Predilection site (*red nodule*) of *sm-invasive* carcinomatous foci in different types of LST. Parts that are probably non-invasive are shown in *yellow*. (Adapted from Uraoka et al. [33], with permission of John Wiley & Sons Inc)

11.5.3 Tentative Distinction of Serrated Lesions, JNET Type 1

Among JNET type 1 serrated lesions (SL), hyperplastic polyps HP are frequently seen in the rectosigmoid as lesions 0-Is or IIa with indistinct margins, stellate PP II and scanty VP 1 (Fig. 11.4a, b). By contrast, *sessile serrated adenoma/polyp* (SSA/P) differs from HP by distinct margins, and neoplastic variants of hyperplastic pit pattern (PP II-O and III_H) and *varicose microvessels* (VMV) (Fig. 11.18a), whereas *SSA/P with dysplasia* (MSA) in addition shows adenomatous PP IV (Fig. 11.18b, lower right). And *traditional serrated adenoma* (TSA) 0-Ip/s shows stellar PP II combined with adenomatous PP III_L and IV (Fig. 11.18b, upper row). Based on these features, the algorithm in Fig. 11.19 tentatively distinguishes SSA/P (Fig. 11.20a–f) from HP (Fig. 11.21), and from MSA (Fig. 11.22c–f) and TSA (Fig. 11.22a, b). *Focal early serrated adenocarcinoma* (SAC) is identified within a serrated lesion by areals of irregular or amorphous PP Vi or Vn and irregular VP 2B or 3 (Fig. 11.19). However, this analysis has not yet been prospectively validated.

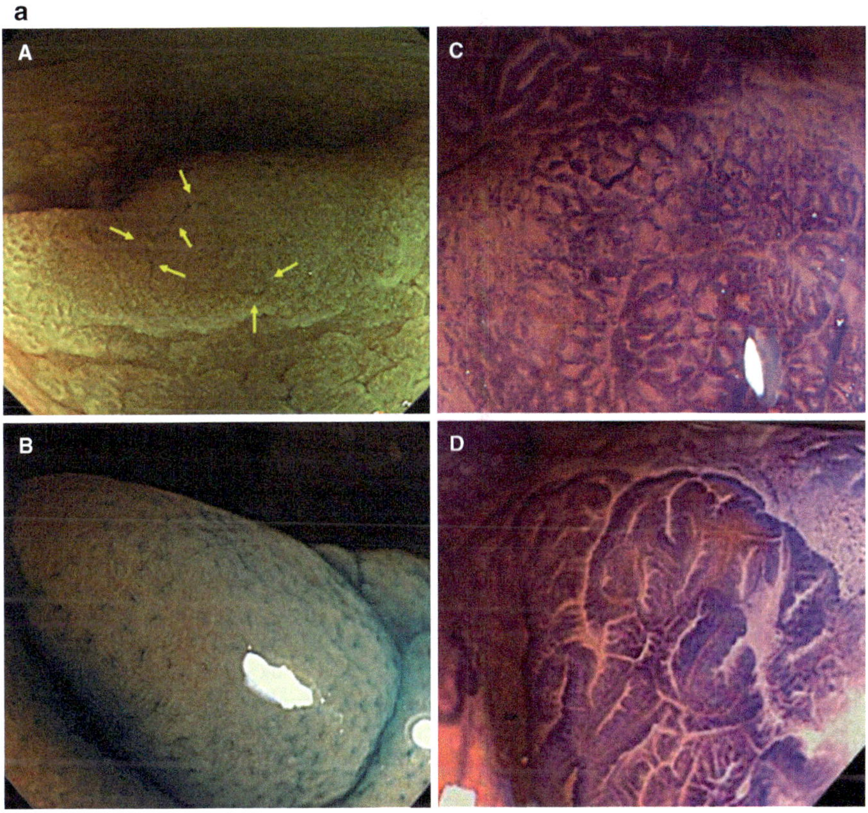

Fig. 11.18 (**a**) ***Surface patterns of serrated neoplasias***. (***A***) Granular surface pattern with 0-II-D appearance and presence of single "*varicose microvessels*" (VMV) (*arrows*) extending beyond periglandular vessels (M-NBI, 40-fold). (***B***) Kudo PP type II (*stellar*) (indigo carmine CE, 60-fold). (***C***) Dilated PP type II-D = II-O. (***D***) Fuji type IIIH pit pattern is wider and more rounded; the dilatation of the crypts produces a "fern-like" appearance. (***C, D***, Crystal violet m-CE, 60-fold.) (From Uraoka et al. [36], with permission of SPRINGER)

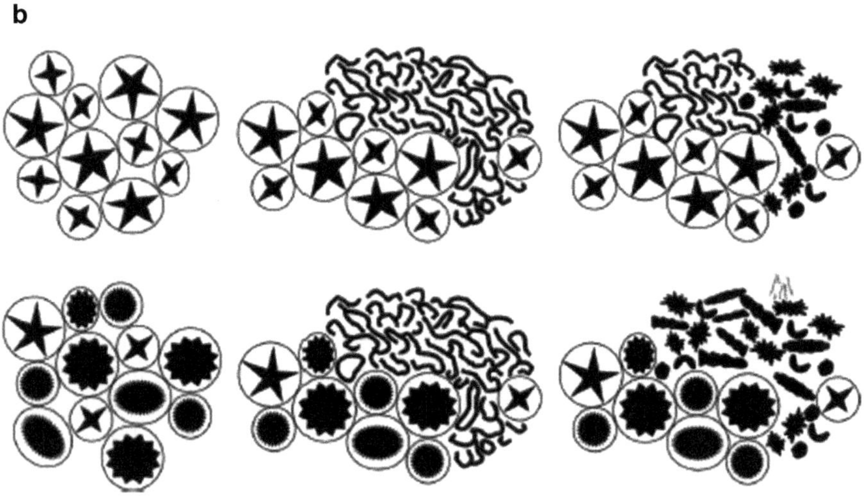

Fig. 11.18 (continued) (**b**) **Traditional serrated adenomas (TSA)** *(upper row)* show stellar PP type II (*left*) alternating or mixed with adenomatous type III (*middle*) or branched type IV (*right*). ***Sessile serrated adenomas (SSA)*** *(lower row)* exhibit wide-open oval or stellar-like crypt orifices, termed PP type II-O ("open") (*lower left*), which may alternate with or progress to a type IV adenomatous surface pattern (*middle*) or type V invasive surface pattern (*right*). (Modified from [34])

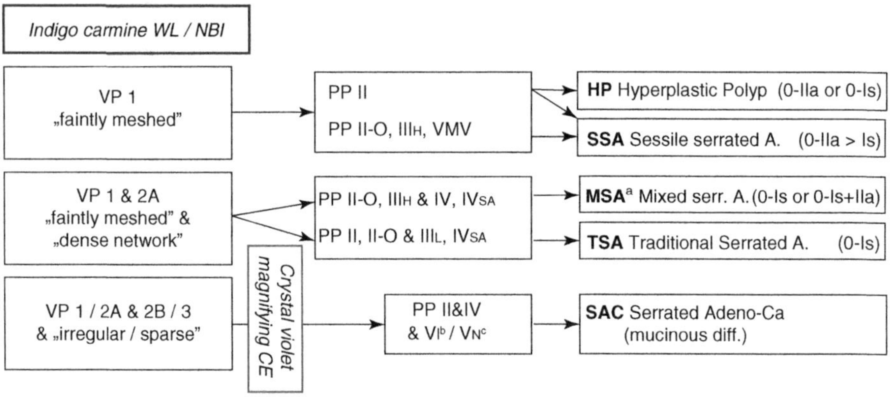

Fig. 11.19 Tentative endoscopic distinction of hyperplastic lesion versus serrated lesions by VP and PP. [a] MSA = SSA/P with dysplasia (according to WHO). [b] Indicating superficial sm invasion <1000 μm. [c] Indicating deep sm invasion ≥1000 μm. PP II-O—II-open (or also: PP III_H—fern-like); PP IV_{SA}—pinecone-like

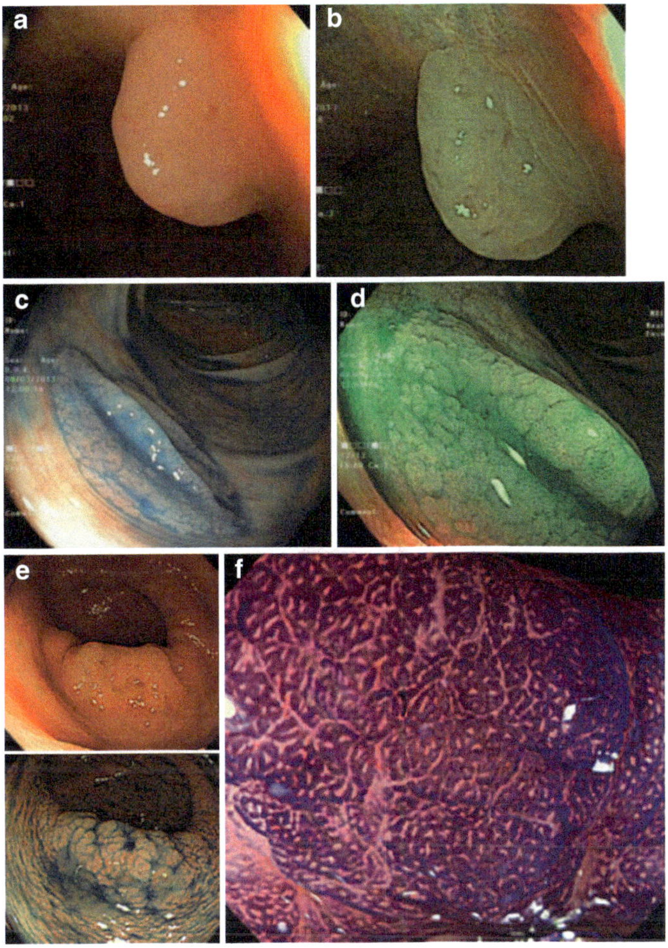

Fig. 11.20 *Sessile serrated adenomas* (confirmed by histology). (**a**, **b**) Pale lesion 0-Is, 15 mm, PP II and VP I(−) ascending colon, WLI and NBI. (**c**, **d**) Pale LST-NG (0-IIa), PP II and II-O, transverse colon, indigo carmine, WLI and NBI. (**e**) Pale LST-GH (0-IIa), ascending colon. WLI (*top*), indigo carmine (*bottom*). (**f**) PP type II-O, crystal violet m-CE (80×)

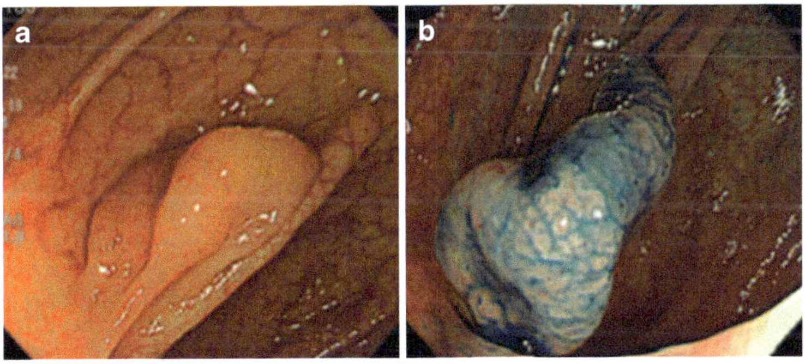

Fig. 11.21 (**a**, **b**) *Hyperplastic polyp 0-Ip*, pale PP II (stellar). WLI and indigo carmine

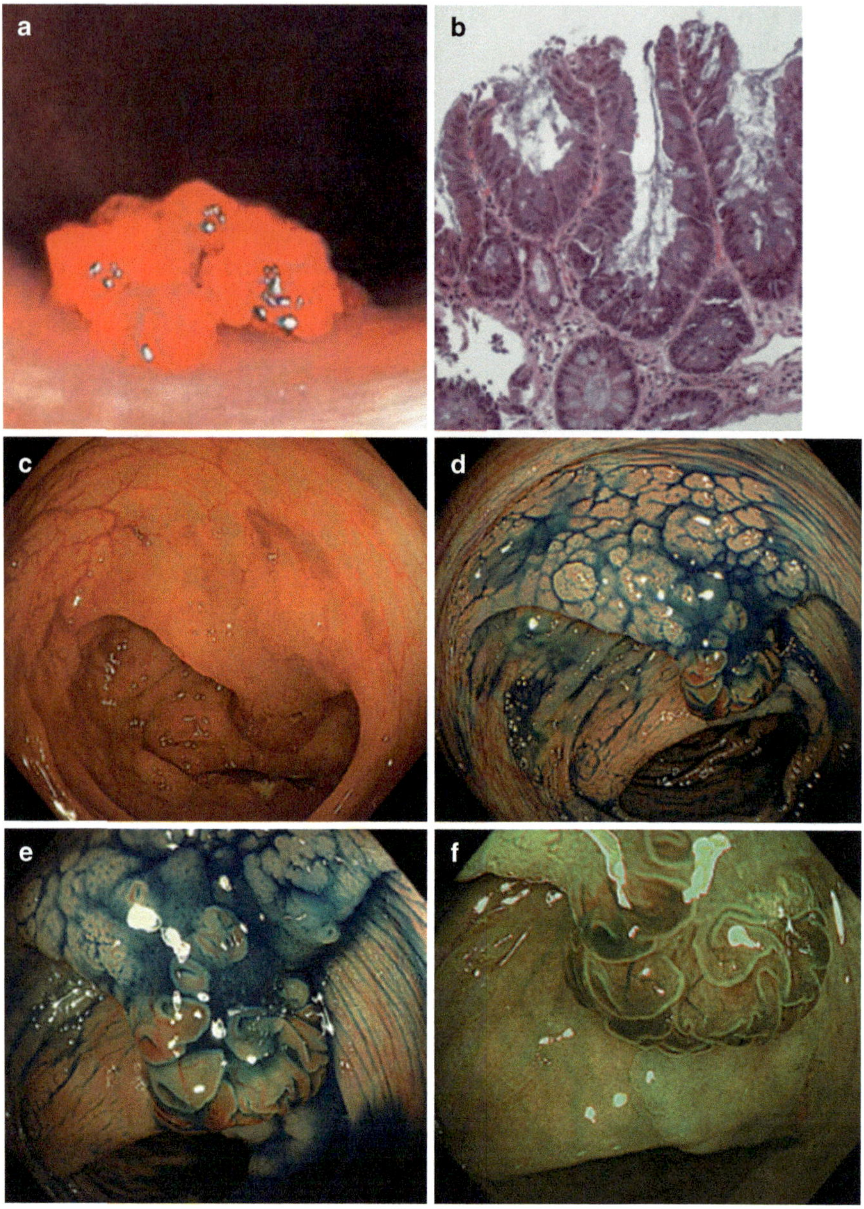

Fig. 11.22 Serrated adenoma (SA) (**a**, **b**, polypoid; **c**–**f**, mixed type). (**a**) Polypoid serrated adenoma (*TSA*) 0-Isp, colon descendens: PP type IV_{SA} (pinecone-like), WLI. (From Morita et al. [35], with permission of Thieme.) (**b**) SA, H&E stain: serrated crypts with goblet cells and mucin and glandular and cellular atypia. (**c–f**) LST-G mixed, isochrome, located in ascending colon. (**c**) WLI. (**d**) Indigo carmine. (**e**) PP IV_{SA} (gyrous, *right*) and II and II-O (*left*); indigo carmine m-CE 80×. (**f**) VP 2A (irregular meshed and dense, *right*) and VP 1 (*left, top): mixed JNET types 2A & 1;* m-NBI 80×. Histology for (**c–f**): mixed-type SA (sessile serrated adenoma/polyp with dysplasia)

Sessile serrated adenomas (*SSA*) (Figs. 11.20a–f and 11.22c–f), without or with dysplasia, present types 0-IIa more often than 0-Is, occur mainly in the right colon, and have high carcinogenic potential with rapid malignant transformation [24, 34–37]. They are often covered with sticky, adherent mucus that requires tenacious flushing with a water jet to clean the mucosal surface; it tends to cover mucosal pathology such as a flat serrated adenoma or even serrated adenocarcinoma, whereas mucus adherent to normal mucosa is easily washed off. On histology, the adenoma contains goblet cells and mucin, often in dilated and serrated crypts (Fig. 11.22b) that are the structural basis for altered pit appearance on imaging. Compared with the normal stellar type II pit pattern, the surface pattern typically shows wider and more rounded pit orifices with serrated margins (Fig. 11.18a(A,C,D) and 11.18b, lower row), named pit pattern *type II-O (open shape)* or *II-D (dilated)* (Fig. 11.19a and 11.20f); these may alternate with adenoma-like pattern *type IV* or pinecone-like *type* IV_{SA} (Fig. 11.22e, f) [34, 35]. SSA/P typically show scant VP 1 with varicose microvessels (VMV) *extending beyond* periglandular vessels (Fig 11.18a(A)). *Mixed-type serrated adenoma, MSA*, is a variant harboring both *flat hyperplastic* parts (stellar PP II) and *sessile adenoma-like* parts (PP II-O, III_H, IV, and IV_{SA}) named *SSA/P with dysplasia* [34, 36, 37] (Fig. 11.22c–f).

Polypoid 0-Ip (traditional) serrated adenomas (TSA), are often reddish due to adenomatous parts with PP type III or IV (Fig. 11.22a, b). TSA show a mixed pattern (Fig. 11.18b, upper row) alternating with areas of stellar pits type II and neoplastic pits *PP type II-O* and *type IV* or variant *PP* IV_{SA} [34–37] (Fig. 11.22a).

Serrated polyposis syndrome (SPS), formerly called hyperplastic polyposis syndrome, is characterized by multiple serrated polyps (typically SSA/P and/or HP) spread throughout the colon. This rare syndrome is associated with multiple SSAs, HPs, conventional adenomas, and increased risk for colon cancer (serrated adenocarcinoma); it requires surveillance and removal of all hyperplastic or serrated lesions [24, 27, 38] (Fig. 11.23a–d). By contrast, true *hyperplastic polyposis* may be seen in *rectal prolapse syndrome* (*RPS*) as a consequence of chronic mechanical stress causing mucosal and fibromuscular hyperplasia of the distal rectal submucosa and mucosa (Fig. 11.23e–g). This condition is treatable with laparoscopic rectopexia.

Fig. 11.23 (**a–d**) *Serrated polyposis syndrome (SPS)* with multiple serrated adenomas, and 20-mm traditional serrated adenoma (pinecone-like aspect) in ascending colon (>30 hyperplastic/serrated polyps in colorectum). (**a**, **b**) *TSA and SSA in SPS*, WLI and indigo carmine CE. (**c**, **d**) Serrated adenocarcinoma (*SAC*) in SPS patient. WLI and indigo carmine. (From Miwata et al. [38], with permission of John Wiley & Sons). (**e–g**) *Hyperplastic polyposis with rectal prolapse syndrome*. (**e**, **f**) Mucous and fibrin pseudomembranes on hyperplastic polyps (WLI). (**g**) Note entirely normal PP I and II, VP 1 (meshed) (NBI 60×)

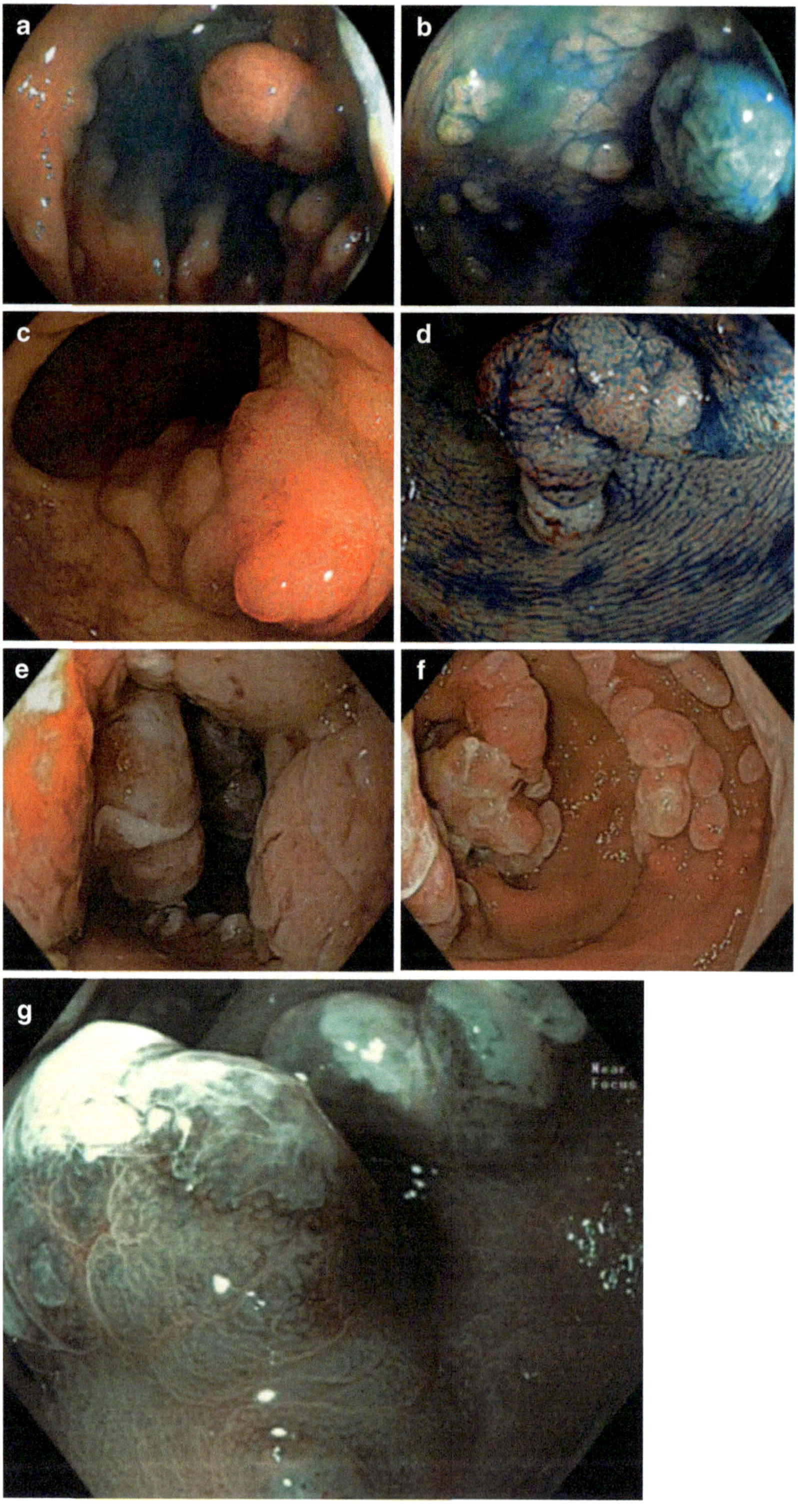
a
b
c
d
e
f
g
Near
Focus

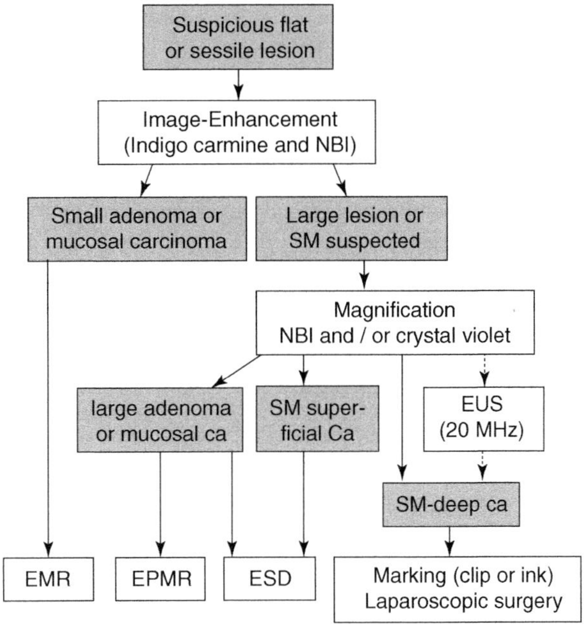

Fig. 11.24 Recommended colonoscopic approach for suspicious flat or sessile lesions. Endoscopic mucosal resection with snaring (*EMR*) removes small mucosal neoplasias en bloc, and large noninvasive adenoma (−/+HGIN) in piecemeal fashion (*EPMR*). NBI with at least 50-fold magnification should be available for analysis. We recommend crystal violet stain to assess for a pit pattern (PP V) characteristic of sm invasion. High-resolution endoscopic ultrasound (Hr-EUS, 20 MHz) is helpful when available, but is not standard

11.6 Endoscopic Resection of Mucosal Neoplasias

Endoscopic analysis on WLI, M-CE, and M-NBI of macroscopic lesion type, pit pattern, and vessel pattern according to the JNET classification is superior to high-resolution endoscopic ultrasound (Hr-EUS) (*see* Chap. 5) for the diagnosis of *superficial versus deep sm-invasive* cancer. The decision on the presence of superficial or deep sm invasion is challenging but is key for resective strategy (Fig. 11.24).

All colonic polyps (0-I lesions), including diminutive polyps, are indications for *endoscopic resection*. Removal of hyperplastic polyps smaller than 5 mm (especially multiple hyperplastic polyps in the rectum) is not generally necessary [23, 39].

Note: All hyperplastic lesions proximal to the sigmoid colon and hyperplastic lesions in the rectosigmoid larger than 5 mm in size, as well as all serrated adenomas/polyps, must be completely removed [23, 39, 40].

11.6.1 Snaring Resection Techniques

Snare polypectomy (without sm injection under the polyp) is the preferred ablation procedure for semipedunculated, pedunculated, or sessile polyps (adenomas −/+ focal mucosal carcinomas). *Endoscopic mucosa resection (EMR)* with sm injection under the lesion removes slightly larger sessile or flat neoplasias (diameter 10–20 mm) en bloc with free margins. EMR of flat lesions using the cold snaring technique (en bloc and EPMR) yields superior specimens for histology and probably a lower recurrence rate [40].

EMR has limitations such as piecemeal resection for flat lesions larger than 20 mm, resection of lesions involving the dentate line or the ileocecal valve, and resection of lesions with a non-lifting sign. Piecemeal resection results in less accurate histological assessment and often leads to local recurrence. Nevertheless, LSTs suspicious for malignant foci and neoplasias 0-IIc require endoscopic or surgical resection en bloc [23, 39].

Note *Indications for EMR* [23, 39]:

- Adenomas type 0-IIa/IIb (PP type IIIL, IV, [IIIs]), diameter ≤20 mm
- Neoplasias type 0-IIc (PP IIIs) of size ≤15 mm with lifting sign upon sm injection
- LST of homogenous granular type (LST-GH) without signs of submucosal invasion (piecemeal EPMR)

Limitations of large-sized EMR [23, 39, 41–43]:

- Lesions exceeding 2 cm diameter are not resectable en bloc
- Submucosal fibrosis (e.g., in chronic inflammatory disease or often in LST-NG)
- Technical limitations for snaring (e.g., mucosal folds, colonic angulation, small rectal carcinoid tumors)
- High rate of local recurrence (up to 30%) after EPMR of large lesions (HGIN or T1a cancer, diameter >3 cm) [42].

Complications of EMR [39–42]:

- Perforation (risk 4–5%, higher in cases with technical limitations)
- *Post-polypectomy coagulation syndrome* (risk 0.5–1.2%; high risk of delayed perforation and severe peritonitis)
- *Recurrent or late bleeding* (risk ~5%) at the EMR site

11.6.2 Endoscopic Submucosal Dissection (ESD)

Colonic endoscopic submucosal dissection (ESD) is more difficult but is standard in experienced centers [7, 43–45]. In Japan, ESD is standard for early malignant or difficult-to-snare flat neoplastic lesions (complex lesions) (Table 11.4). The basic principles for en bloc resection of flat neoplasias have been accepted in the British Guideline: En bloc resection is mandatory for neoplasias suspicious for malignant foci or for complex flat lesions with high risk of incomplete or complicated endoscopic snaring. These patients should be referred to specialized interdisciplinary centers [39]. Many Western guidelines still accept EPMR for such lesions, however. Depending on national guidelines, LST-GM may also be resected in piecemeal fashion, with the larger nodule resected first [33]. The outcome of ESD is discussed in Chap. 3.

Note Mucosal or submucosal (sm1)-invasive cancer (G1 or G2, Ly0 V0, without tumor cell budding) seldom recurs (<2%) when it is resected en bloc with free margins (R0). The risk of lymph node metastasis is near zero if the depth of submucosal invasion is <1000 μm [23, 46].

Table 11.4 Indications of ESD for Colorectal Tumors[a] (JGES Guideline 2015 [23])

Lesions for which endoscopic en bloc resection is required:
1. Lesions for which en bloc resection with snare EMR is difficult to apply
LST-NG, particularly LST-NGPD
Lesions showing a V_I type pit pattern
Carcinoma with shallow T1 (SM) invasion
Large depressed-type tumors (0-IIc)
Large protruded-type lesions (0-Is/Isp) suspected to be carcinoma[b]
2. Mucosal tumors with submucosal fibrosis [c]
3. Sporadic localized tumors in conditions of chronic inflammation such as ulcerative colitis
4. Local residual or recurrent early carcinomas after endoscopic resection

[a]Partially modified from the draft proposed by the Colorectal ESD Standardization Implementation Working Group
[b]Including LST-G, nodular-mixed type
[c]As a result of a previous biopsy or prolapse caused by peristalsis of the intestine

Surgery is indicated *after ESD* for any of the following conditions:

- Vertical (deep) margin that is tumor-positive (R1)
- Deep submucosal invasion (>1000 μm below MM)
- Lympho−/ vascular tumor infiltration is positive (Ly 1 or V 1)
- Cancer grading is poorly differentiated or undifferentiated (G3, G4)
- Tumor budding Bd 2 or Bd 3 at the deepest front of invasion (differentiated AC)

Indication for *a priori surgical resection:*

- Signs of deep submucosal invasion of proven carcinoma [23, 47]

11.7 Lesions of the Anal Canal

The *surgical anal canal* extends for 4–5 cm from the rostral end of the inner sphincter (oral end of the contracted anal canal) down to the anal verge, which corresponds to the end of the outer anal sphincter. The inner 3 cm with anal papillae all around (median 8 [6–11]) and crypts are covered with columnar epithelium, and the anoderm (1.5–2 cm transition zone aboral to the dentate line) has stratified squamous epithelium down to the end of the intersphincteric groove, where, on the anal verge (~1 cm), the keratinized anal skin starts. Somatic sensation (pudendus nerve branches) starts at the dentate line.

Using standard endoscopes (with M-WLI and M-NBI), most of the anal canal and anoderm (distended by insufflation) is well visualized on retroflex view from the rectum. On NBI, the dentate line is displayed as a sharp border between brownish columnar rectum epithelium and greenish-white squamous epithelial anoderm (Figs. 11.26d and 11.33a).

Anal lesions, in the anoderm, show some similarities to squamous epithelial lesions in the esophagus. Condylomata acuminata (wart-like lesions type 0-Is/p or II-a) are caused by human papillomavirus (HPV) infection and show many elongated regular-caliber capillaries in squamous epithelium (similar to esophageal papillomas) on M-WLI and M-NBI. Most neoplastic anal lesions (dysplasia and early squamous cell cancer) are triggered by infection with HPV subtypes, especially in high-risk individuals with anal intercourse or extensive condylomata acuminata [48]. *Anal neoplasias* display irregular alterations in capillary and surface architecture similar to squamous epithelial neoplasias in esophagus. *High-grade anal dysplasias* (*AIN III*) are Lugol-voiding [49] (*see* Case 10 and Fig. 11.33 in Sect. 11.8). Retroflex inspection of the anal canal and anoderm with high-definition magnifying WLI/NBI endoscope allows excellent diagnostic imaging. We recommend an interdisciplinary diagnostic and therapeutic work-up of such lesions, involving dermatology, anorectal surgery, and gastroenterology [49].

11.8 Cases: Adenomas, Dysplasia, and Early Colorectal Cancer

Case 1: Small Lesion 0-Is + 0-IIc Located at the Sigmoid Colon

A small lesion 0-IIc with central bulging (0-Is), 8 mm in diameter, was detected on

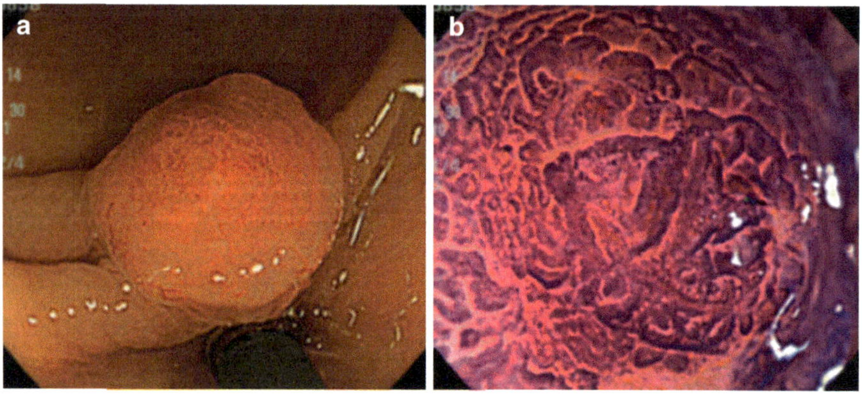

Fig. 11.25 (**a–d**) *Lesion 0-Is + IIc* (d 4 cm, *bulging in IIc*) on haustral fold in sigmoid colon. (**a**) WLI. (**b**) Crystal violet CE (WLI, 80×), PP type V_I *high grade*

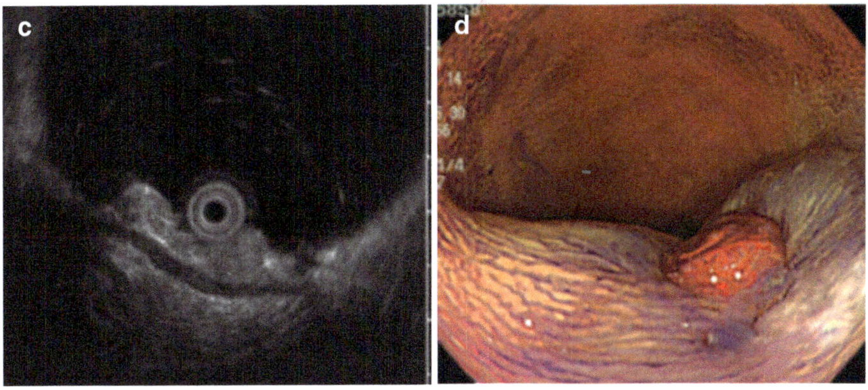

Fig. 11.25 (continued) (c) Radial Hr-EUS shows a 4-mm-wide *break in sm echo layer*. (d) Complete *non-lifting sign* after sm injection of 3 × 2 mL fluid. *Diagnosis*: Deeply sm-invasive early CRC. *Surgery*: well-differentiated AC, pT1b, *deeply sm invasive* (2000 μm), ly 1 v 0

a haustral fold in sigmoid colon. Magnifying view (80×) with crystal violet staining revealed a highly irregular-type Vi pit pattern, and Hr-EUS (20 MHz) disclosed a 4-mm-wide break in the sm echo band. Both findings supported deeply sm-invasive cancer, a diagnosis further strengthened by complete non-lifting sign upon sm injection. The patient underwent curative laparoscopic resection: adenoca (tub2), pT1bsm (2000 μm), ly1, v0, pPM0, pDM0, pRM0, and 0-Is + IIc (Fig. 11.25).

Note All four signs of sm invasiveness (macroscopic/PP/EUS/non-lifting), when combined, allow highly accurate diagnosis.

Case 2: Large Rectal LST-G Mixed Type Invading Anal Canal

Rectal LST-G mixed type (0-IIa + Is) consisting of homogenous granular parts and one triangular-shaped sessile lesion (4 × 3 cm, 1 cm elevated) was diagnosed in a woman in her mid-40s. CE showed PP type IIIL and IV (Fig. 11.26) and on the sessile part some PP type IIIs but no ulcerations or friability. Surgical full-wall resection would certainly have interfered with anal function and fecal continence. Therefore, the patient favored diagnostic ESD en bloc. Circular dissection of the anal margin and anal channel in prograde fashion, followed by stepwise partial circumferential incision and submucosal dissection in retroflex fashion, allowed en bloc resection of the entire lesion including the sm vascular plexus.

Note ESD en bloc of advanced adenoma or mucosal cancer of the anorectum can provide cure and preserve normal anorectal function.

Fig. 11.26 (a–d) Large LST-G mixed type (0-IIa + Is), extending about 9 cm from squamocolumnar junction (= dentate line, shown on top of panel d) (c, d; 70% circumferential) at the posterior wall over the Houston fold (a, b) into the rectum (WLI, indigo carmine CE). (e) Specimen was resected by dual knife with safety margin and (f) intact sm vascular stratum (sml-2); submucosal view of specimen → *histopathology*: *focal differentiated adenocarcinoma, depth M*, in tubulovillous adenoma 130 × 103 mm, ly0, v0, pLM0, pVM0; curative resection R0. (g, h) Follow-up after 6 months showed a scar after ESD with regenerative mucosa and no narrowing of the anal channel

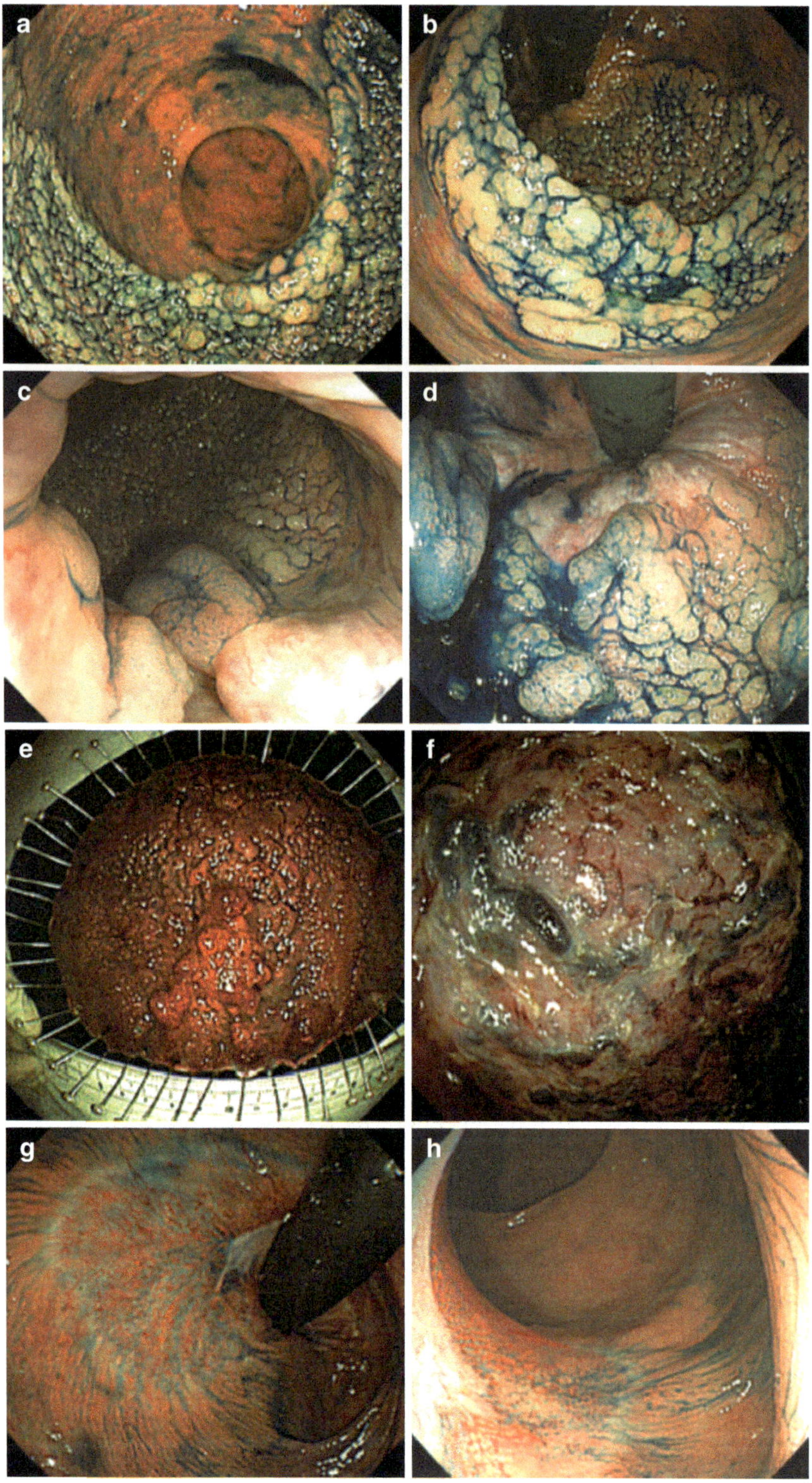
a
b
c
d
e
f
g
h

Case 3: Small Lesion 0-IIa + c at the Sigmoid Colon

Screening colonoscopy in a 77-year-old woman showed a small (d 1 cm) lesion type 0-IIa + c with PP type IIIs (on biopsy HGIN) at the inner curve of the rectosigmoid flexure (Fig. 11.27). Hybrid-ESD with snaring of final sm bridge resected the lesion en bloc, without thermal damage to resection bed or to the specimen, which revealed tubular adenoma with HGIN, resected R0.

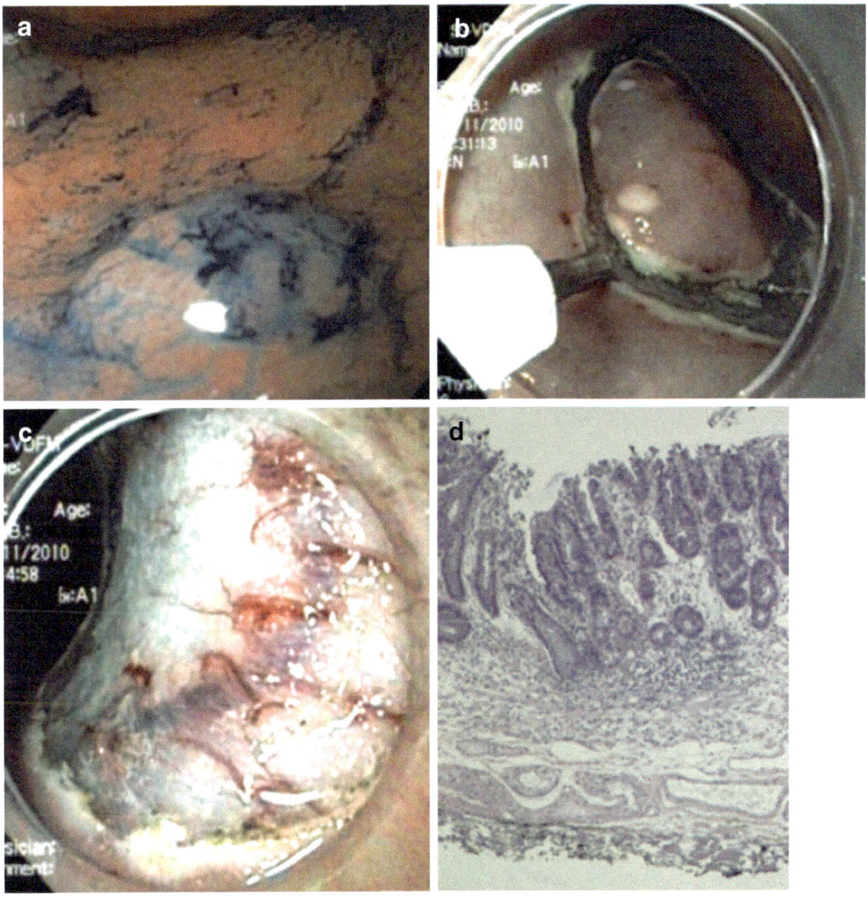

Fig. 11.27 (**a**) Small lesion type 0-IIa + c with PP IIIs on M-CE (40×) using indigo carmine. Previous targeted biopsy: HGIN. (**b**) Simplified ESD with final snaring. (**c**) Bare resection bed. (**d**) Cross section of the specimen, showing tubular adenoma with focal HGIN and no thermal damage at the deep margin

Note Simplified hybrid-ESD (with low-power snaring) has advantages:

- Shorter procedure time (during the ESD learning curve)
- High-quality ESD specimen for histology, without thermal artifacts

Case 4: LST-G Whole Nodular Type (0-Is + Isp), Sigmoid Colon

A polypoid lesion, LST-GN-whole nodular, in sigmoid colon showed signs of deep sm invasion (Fig. 11.28), a contraindication for snaring polypectomy.

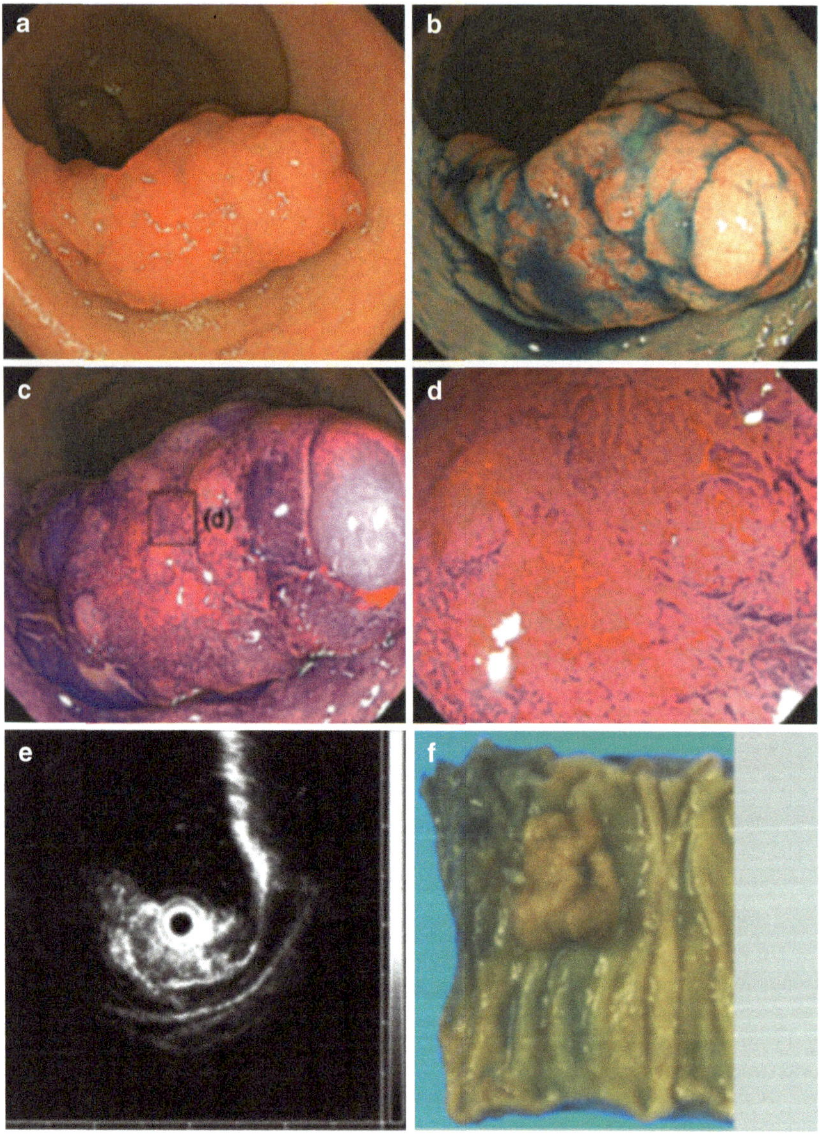

Fig. 11.28 LST-GN whole nodular type (0-Is + Isp), 20 mm in diameter. (**a**) WLI. (**b**) Indigo carmine. (**c**) Crystal violet CE, which disclosed (**d**) focal areas with *PP type* V_I *high grade*. (**e**) Hr-EUS (20 MHz) showed a *break of sm echo band* beneath the lesion. (**f**) Specimen of laparoscopic resection: adenocarcinoma G1, pT1b*sm2, ly1, v1*, pN0

Note Accurate endoscopic analysis of neoplastic polyps prevents polypectomy (R2 resection) on deeply sm-invasive cancer type 0-Is/p.

Case 5: Relatively Large Cecal Lesion LST-G Whole Nodular (0-Is)
On complete colonoscopy performed for a positive fecal occult blood test, a lesion 0-Is, whole nodular, 5 × 3 cm in size, was found located on the last lateral haustral fold of the cecum. Detailed endoscopic analysis was performed and ESD was conducted for diagnostic and possibly curative intention (Fig. 11.29).

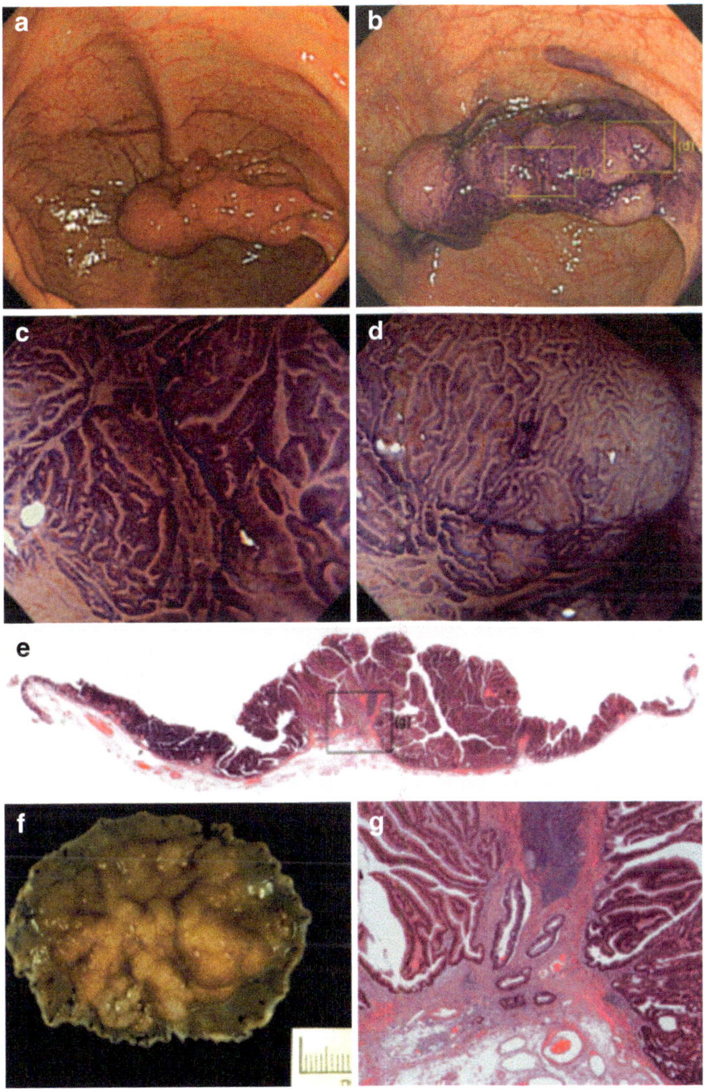

Fig. 11.29 (**a**) A lesion 0-Is, whole nodular, 5 × 3 cm in size, on the last lateral haustral fold of the cecum. (**b**) On crystal violet CE, the lesion showed PP type IIIL and IV and irregular PP V in small depressed areas (*insert* **c, d**), which revealed on M-CE (80×) (**c**) PP type Vi low grade and (**d**) PP type Vi high grade. (**f**) ESD en bloc performed for diagnostic purpose yielded a single specimen of the entire lesion with safety margins. (**e**) Sequential transverse sections showed lateral and vertical margins negative. (**g**) *Histology*: adenocarcinoma, tub1, size 50 × 35 mm (specimen 55 × 40 mm), sm1 (500 μm), ly0, *v1*. Laparoscopic hemicolectomy with lymph node dissection was recommended

Case 6: LST-NG Located at the Sigmoid Colon

Screening colonoscopy showed a LST-NG, (d 4 cm) with slight pseudodepression extending over a haustral fold (Fig. 11.30). Analysis suggested *intramucosal cancer*. ESD en bloc was performed.

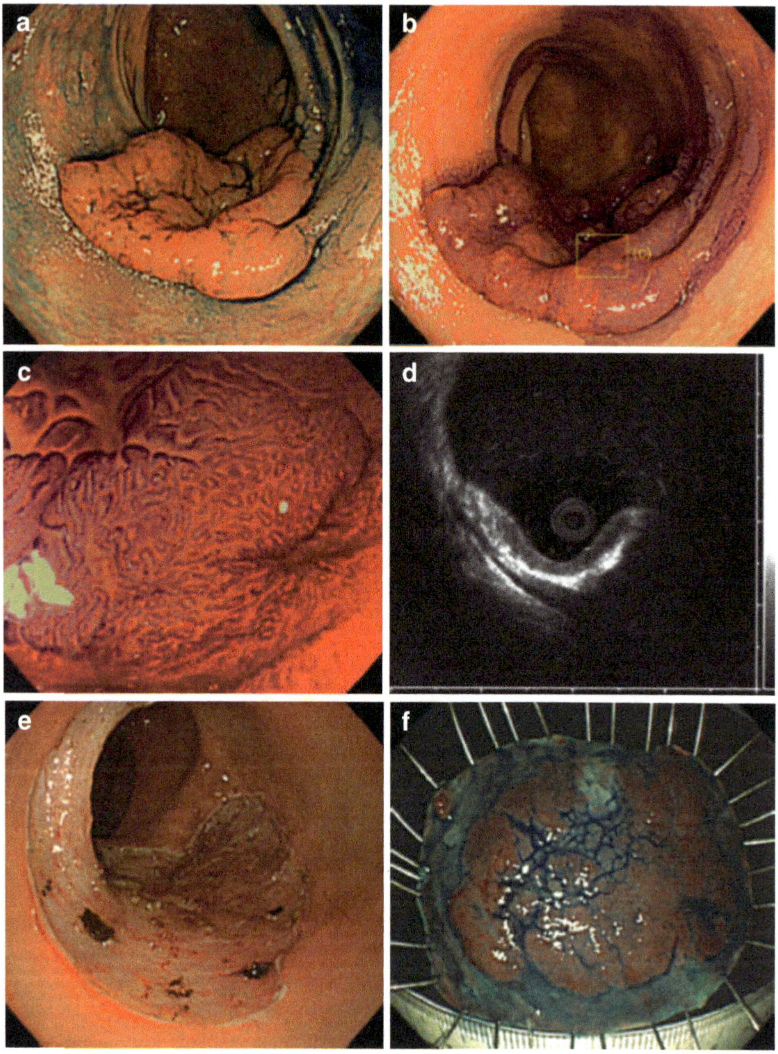

Fig. 11.30 (**a–f**) *LST-NGPD* (d 4 cm) in sigmoid colon. (**a**) Indigo carmine CE. (**b**) Crystal violet CE. (**c**) M-CE (80×) with crystal violet stain: PP type V_I *low grade*. (**d**) Radial Hr-EUS shows *intact sm echo layer* (white echo band). (**e**) Resection bed. (**f**) ESD specimen (indigo carmine). Histology: adenocarcinoma, pT1b *sm1* (990 μm), tub1, ly0, v0, HM0, VM0

Note Attempt ESD for cure on LST-NGPD, unless signs of *deep* sm invasion.

Case 7: LST-NG (Sized ~5 cm) Located at the Transverse Colon

In this 76-year-old man on anticoagulant therapy, colonoscopy for anemia showed mucosal irregularity at transverse colon (Fig. 11.31).

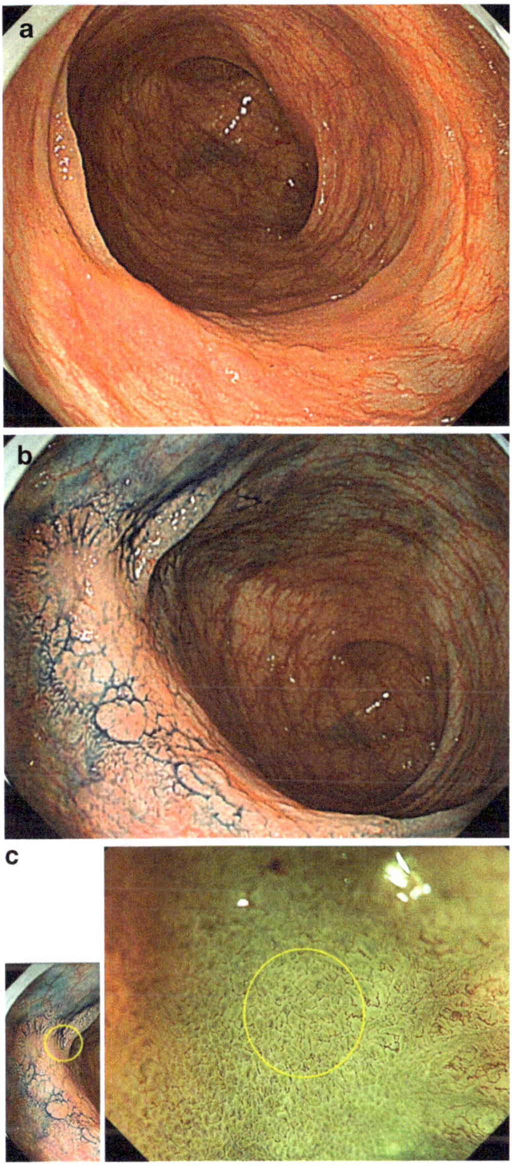

Fig. 11.31 (**a**) Reddish surface irregularity with loss of sm vascular pattern (*bottom*). (**b**) Indigo carmine spraying revealed a flat lesion 0-IIb, further analyzed by magnifying imaging (80×) using (**c**) NBI (VP 2B)

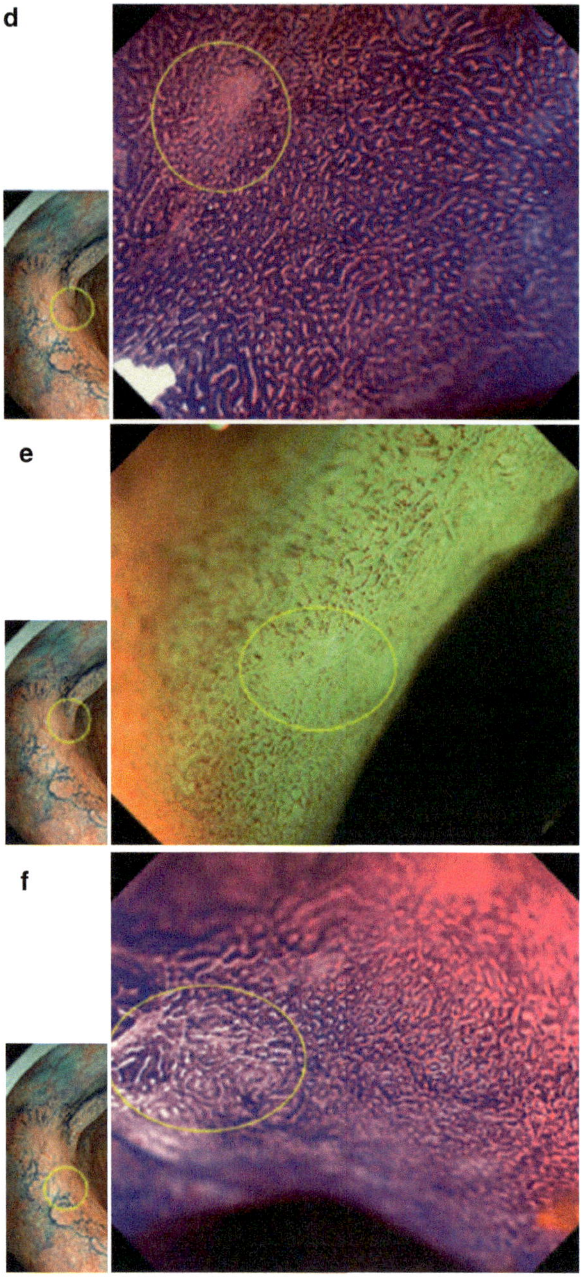

Fig. 11.31 (continued) (**d**) crystal violet (PP Vi low grade). One tiny spot showed (**e**) VP 3 on m-NBI and (**f**) PP V_I high grade on crystal violet m-CE. *Clinical diagnosis*: LST-NG JNET type 2B and focal type 3 suspicious for sm-invasive, differentiated adenocarcinoma, diameter nearly 5 cm. ESD was recommended (for diagnostic purpose)

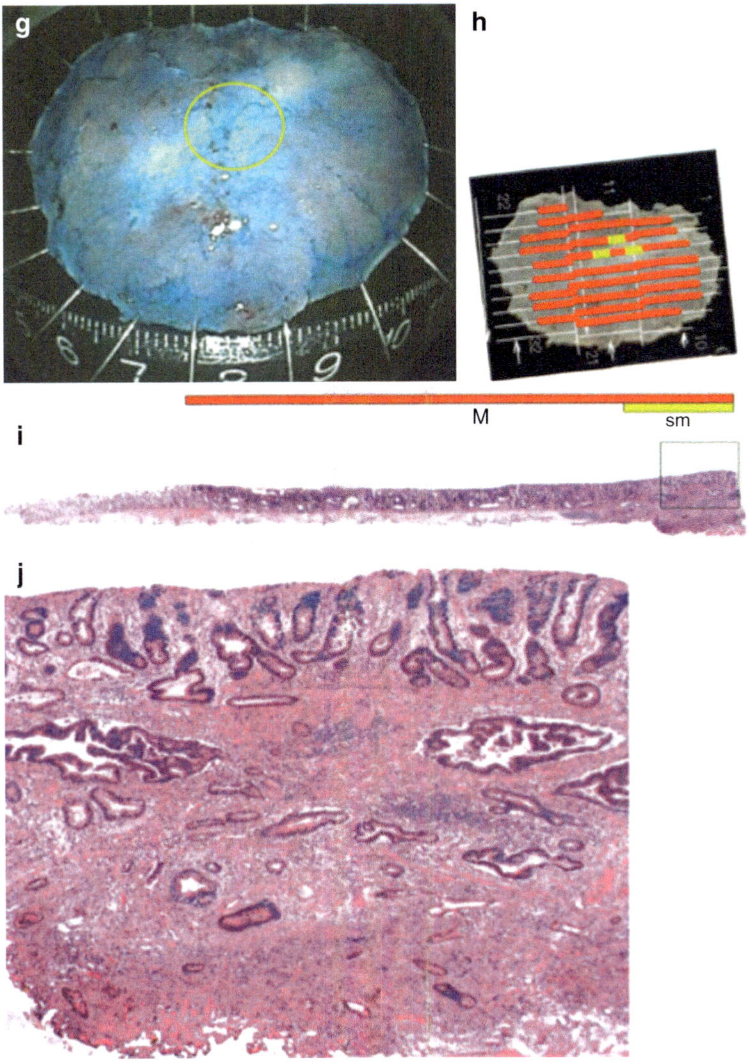

Fig. 11.31 (continued) (**g**) The specimen with safety margin was pinned and documented (*suspicious area marked*). (**h**) Specimen sections mapped for intramucosal (*red*) and sm-invasive (*yellow*) cancer. (**i**) Section (H&E stain) with maximum sm invasion (**j**). (**j**) H&E stain 100-fold. *Histopathology*: adenocarcinoma, tub1 > tub2, 48 × 37 mm, p*sm* > *3000 μm*, ly0, v0, HM0, *VM1*. Hemicolectomy with lymph node dissection was recommended

Note:

- ESD can provide precise histological information, especially when the pathologist is informed about suspicious areas.
- Histology may change the clinical strategy for cancer therapy.

Case 8: Rectal LST-G (Size ~5 cm)

Total colonoscopy was performed for a positive fecal occult blood test in this 48-year-old woman. A large rectal lesion (~5 cm) was pointed out (Fig. 11.32).

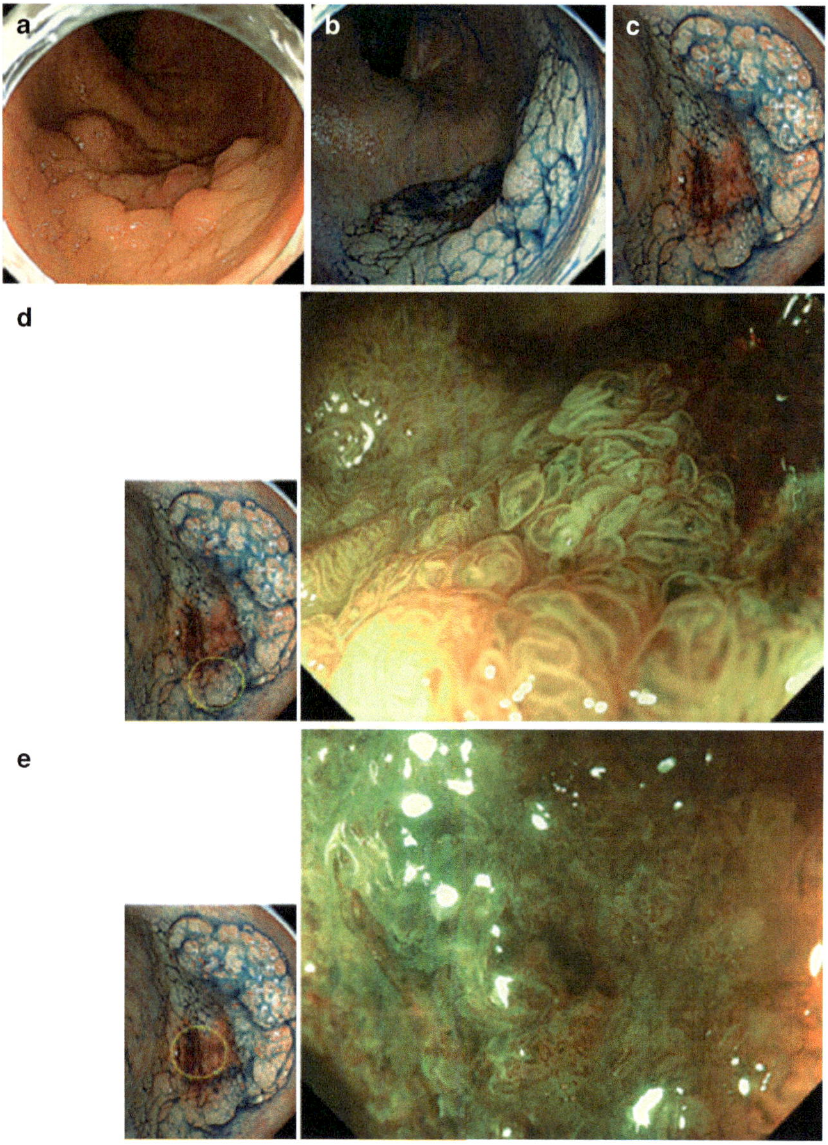

Fig. 11.32 (**a**) Rectal *LST-G (0-IIa + c)*, d ~5 cm, on WLI and (**b**, **c**) indigo carmine CE. (**d**) Vessels VP 2A (in 0-IIa margin, *left*) and (**e**) VP 2B (in 0-IIc lesion, *left*): Lesion JNET type 2B, on m-NBI (80×)

Note Preoperative endoscopic diagnosis is not always perfect.
Consider diagnostic ESD before recommending major surgery (especially anorectal surgery)

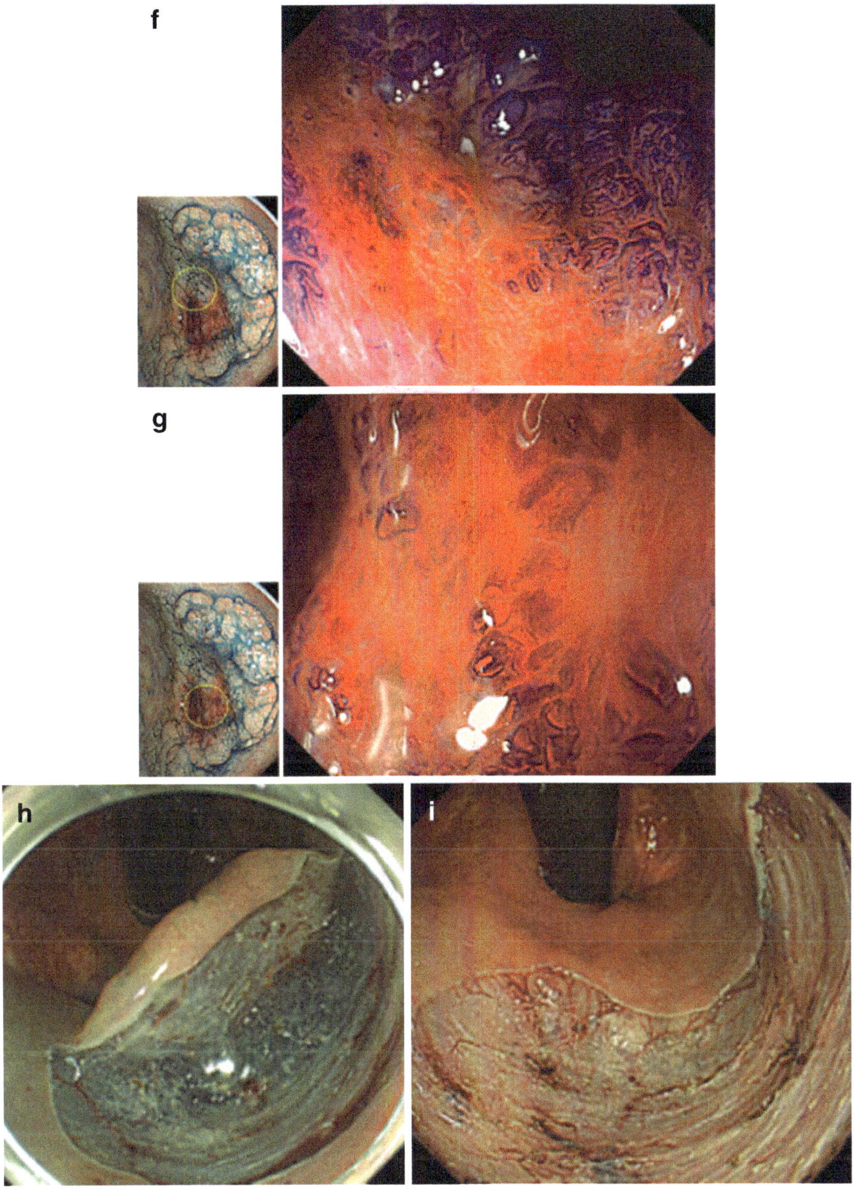

Fig. 11.32 (continued) Crystal violet stain (with little sticky mucus) shows (**f**) PP type IIIL in 0-IIa and (**g**) PP type Vn in 0-IIc part. *Clinical diagnosis*: *LST-G with deeply sm-invasive cancer (focal JNET type 3)*, sized 5 cm. (**h**, **i**) ESD was attempted for diagnostic purpose

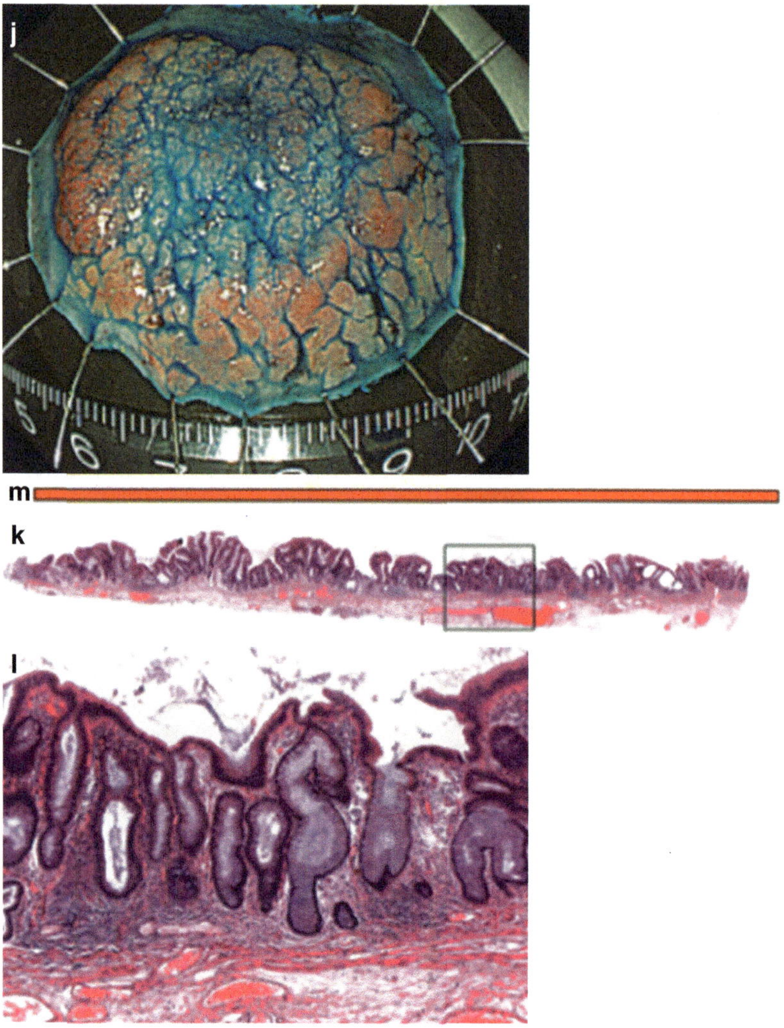

Fig. 11.32 (continued) (**j**) ESD specimen (indigo carmine): the surface structure of the neoplasia was slightly irregular after clearance of mucus. *Histology*: (**k**) Noninvasive (*m, red line = entirely mucosal*) tubulovillous adenoma (H&E stain, box **l**) with (**l**) focal high-grade dysplasia (H&E stain, 100-fold)

Case 9: Anal Squamous Cell Lesion 0-IIb-G (Size ~10 mm)

A 39-year-old woman had experienced painful anal itching and occasional minor contact bleeding for 2 months. Ano-/rectoscopy with magnifying (60-fold) colonoscope displayed in retroflex view a reddish, velvety lesion 0-IIb (10 × 10 mm) in the anoderm between the dentate line and anal verge at the left lateral side. Diagnostic biopsy was performed, and later curative ESD (Fig. 11.33).

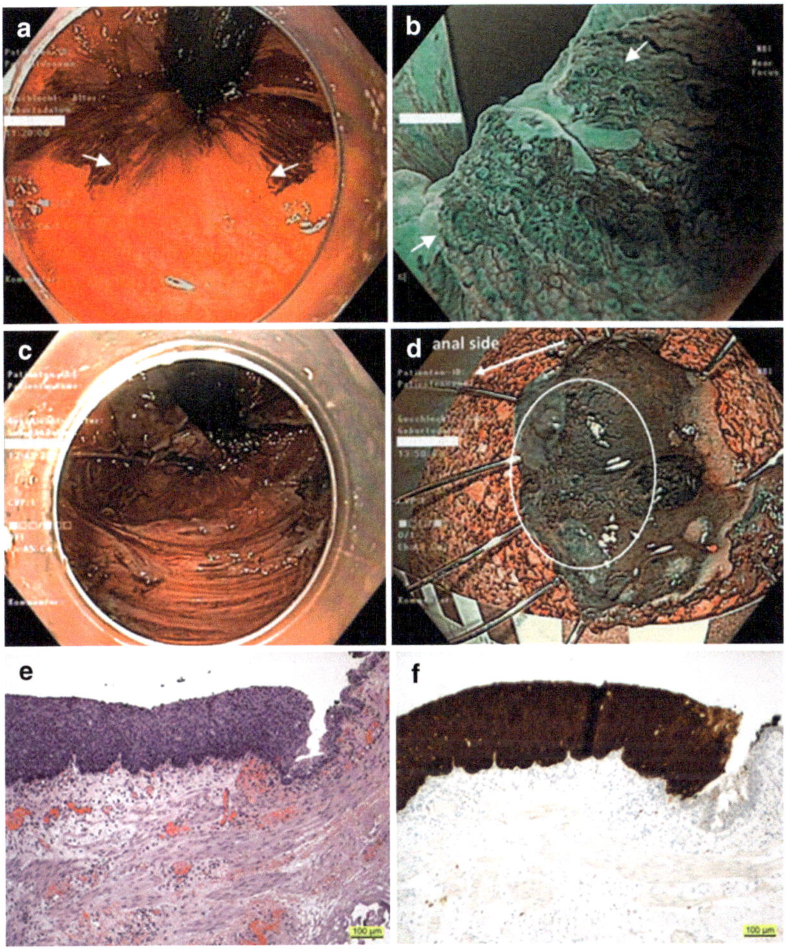

Fig. 11.33 (**a**) Lugol-voiding reddish lesion 0-IIb with clear margin (*arrows*) to Lugol-staining anoderm that also contrasts to columnar mucosa (squamocolumnar junction = dentate line), seen on WLI. (**b**) M-NBI (60×) showed a brownish-greenish discolored area (dense irregular MV) with irregular surface relief, loss of permeation of sm veins, and clear margins to non-keratinized anoderm, suspect for anodermal neoplasia. *Biopsy:* High-grade dysplasia (HGD), positive for HPV-16. (**c**) Resection bed after ESD en bloc. (**d**) ESD specimen (2.5 × 1.7 cm, with complete markings of safety margin). (**e**) Histology (H&E stain, 100×): *High-grade intraepithelial dysplasia,* free resection margins (*AIN III, R0*). (**f**) Immunohistochemistry (IHC) strongly positive for p16 protein (confirming AIN III). Not shown: In-situ hybridization ++ for high-risk HPV-16 in AIN (negative in anoderm). Follow-up after 9 months: Complete remission of the HPV-16–induced AIN (Modified from Wagner et al. [49] with permission of Thieme)

Note ESD can be considered for cure of intraepithelial neoplasias in anoderm, preferably in cooperation with dermatologist and proctologic surgeon.

Acknowledgments We gratefully acknowledge the contribution of some cases by Dr. Tsuneo Oyama of Nagano, Japan, and the contribution of histology by Dr. Daniel Neureiter and Dr. Tobias Kiesslich, Salzburg, Austria.

References

1. O'Brien MJ, et al. Flat adenomas in the National Polyp Study: Is there increased risk for high-grade dysplasia initially or during surveillance? Clin Gastroenterol Hepatol. 2004;2:905–11.
2. The Paris endoscopic classification of superficial neoplastic lesions: esophagus, stomach, and colon: November 30 to December 1, 2002. Gastrointest Endosc. 2003;58:S3–43.
3. Endoscopic Classification Review Group. Update on the Paris classification of superficial neoplastic lesions in the digestive tract. Endoscopy. 2005;37:570–8.
4. George SM, et al. Classification of advanced colorectal carcinomas by tumor edge morphology: evidence for different pathogenesis and significance of polypoid and nonpolypoid tumors. Cancer. 2000;89:1901–9.
5. Kudo S, et al. Nonpolypoid neoplastic lesions of the colorectal mucosa. Gastrointest Endosc. 2008;68:S3–47.
6. Rembacken BJ, et al. Flat and depressed colonic neoplasms: a prospective study of 1000 colonoscopies in the UK. Lancet. 2000;355:1211–4.
7. Fuccio L, et al. Clinical outcomes after endoscopic submucosal dissection for colorectal neoplasia: a systematic review and meta-analysis. Gastrointest Endosc. 2017;86:74–86.
8. Kaminski MF, et al. Performance measures for lower gastrointestinal endoscopy: a European Society of Gastrointestinal Endoscopy (ESGE) quality improvement initiative. United European Gastroenterol J. 2017;5:309–34.
9. Rotondano G, et al. The Cooperative Italian FLIN Study Group: prevalence and clinicopathological features of colorectal laterally spreading tumors. Endoscopy. 2011;43:856–61.
10. Soetikno RM, et al. Prevalence of nonpolypoid (flat and depressed) colorectal neoplasms in asymptomatic and symptomatic adults. JAMA. 2008;299:1027–35.
11. Bogie RM, et al. Endoscopic subtypes of colorectal laterally spreading tumors (LSTs) and the risk of submucosal invasion: a meta-analysis. Endoscopy. 2018;50:263–82.
12. Matsuda T, et al. Our perspective on endoscopic resection for colorectal neoplasms. Gastroenterol Clin Biol. 2010;34:367–70.
13. Niimi K, et al. Long-term outcomes of endoscopic submucosal dissection for colorectal epithelial neoplasms. Endoscopy. 2010;42:723–9.
14. Kudo S, et al. Pit pattern in colorectal neoplasia: endoscopic magnifying view. Endoscopy. 2001;33:367–73.
15. Sano Y, et al. Magnifying observation of microvascular architecture of colorectal lesions using a narrow-band imaging system. Dig Endosc. 2006;18:s44–51.
16. Hayashi N, et al. Endoscopic prediction of deep submucosal invasive carcinoma: validation of the Narrow-Band Imaging International Colorectal Endoscopic (NICE) classification. Gastrointest Endosc. 2013;78:625–32.
17. Sano Y, et al. Narrow-band imaging (NBI) magnifying endoscopic classification of colorectal tumors proposed by the Japan NBI Expert Team. Dig Endosc. 2016;28:526–33.
18. Komeda Y, et al. Magnifying narrow band imaging (NBI) for the diagnosis of localized colorectal lesions using the Japan NBI Expert Team (JNET) Classification. Oncology. 2017;93(Suppl 1):49–54.
19. Wada Y, et al. Diagnostic accuracy of pit pattern and vascular pattern analyses in colorectal lesions. Dig Endosc. 2010;22:192–9.
20. Matsuda T, et al. Efficacy of the invasive/non-invasive pattern by magnifying chromoendoscopy to estimate the depth of invasion of early colorectal neoplasms. Am J Gastroenterol. 2008;103:2700–6.
21. Backes Y, et al. Narrow band imaging, magnifying chromoendoscopy, and gross morphological features for the optical diagnosis of T1 colorectal cancer and deep submucosal invasion: a systematic review and meta-analysis. Am J Gastroenterol. 2017;112:54–64.
22. Zhang QW, et al. Narrow-band imaging in the diagnosis of deep submucosal colorectal cancers: a systematic review and meta-analysis. Endoscopy. 2017;49:564–80.
23. Tanaka S, et al. JGES guidelines for colorectal endoscopic submucosal dissection/endoscopic mucosal resection. Dig Endosc. 2015;27:417–34.
24. East JE, et al. Serrated lesions in colorectal cancer screening: detection, resection, pathology and surveillance. Gut. 2015;64:991–1000.

25. Hazewinkel Y, et al. Endoscopic features of sessile serrated adenomas: validation by international experts using high-resolution white-light endoscopy and narrow-band imaging. Gastrointest Endosc. 2013;77:916–24.
26. Ijspeert JE, et al. Development and validation of the WASP classification system for optical diagnosis of adenomas, hyperplastic polyps and sessile serrated adenomas/polyps. Gut. 2016;65:963–70.
27. Ijspeert JE, et al. Detection rate of serrated polyps and serrated polyposis syndrome in colorectal cancer screening cohorts: a European overview. Gut. 2017;66:1225–32.
28. Kanao H, et al. Narrow-band imaging magnification predicts the histology and invasion depth of colorectal tumors. Gastrointest Endosc. 2009;69:631–6.
29. Rondagh EJ, et al. Nonpolypoid colorectal neoplasms: a challenge in endoscopic surveillance of patients with Lynch syndrome. Endoscopy. 2013;45:257–64.
30. De Jong AE, et al. The role of mismatch repair gene defects in the development of adenomas in patients with HNPCC. Gastroenterology. 2004;126:42–8.
31. Vasen HF, et al. Familial colorectal cancer risk: ESMO clinical recommendations. Ann Oncol. 2009;20(Suppl 4):51–3.
32. Kato H, et al. Lifting of lesions during endoscopic mucosal resection (EMR) of early colorectal cancer: implications for the assessment of resectability. Endoscopy. 2001;33:568–73.
33. Uraoka T, et al. Endoscopic indications for endoscopic mucosal resection of laterally spreading tumours in the colorectum. Gut. 2006;55:1592–7.
34. Kimura T, et al. A novel pit pattern identifies the precursor of colorectal cancer derived from sessile serrated adenoma. Am J Gastroenterol. 2012;107:460–9.
35. Morita T, et al. Evaluation of endoscopic and histopathological features of serrated adenoma of the colon. Endoscopy. 2001;33:761–5.
36. Uraoka T, et al. Prospective evaluation of endoscopic criteria characteristic of sessile serrated adenomas/polyps. J Gastroenterol. 2015;50:555–63.
37. Yano Y, et al. Clinicopathological and molecular features of colorectal serrated neoplasias with different mucosal crypt patterns. Am J Gastroenterol. 2011;106:1351–8.
38. Miwata T, et al. Clinicopathologic features of hyperplastic/serrated polyposis syndrome in Japan. J Gastroenterol Hepatol. 2013;28:1693–8.
39. Rutter MD, et al. British Society of Gastroenterology/Association of Coloproctologists of Great Britain and Ireland guidelines for the management of large non-pedunculated colorectal polyps. Gut. 2015;64:1847–73.
40. Ferlitsch M, et al. Colorectal polypectomy and endoscopic mucosal resection (EMR): European Society of Gastrointestinal Endoscopy (ESGE) Clinical Guideline. Endoscopy. 2017;49:270–97.
41. Cao Y, et al. Meta-analysis of endoscopic submucosal dissection versus endoscopic mucosal resection for tumors of the gastrointestinal tract. Endoscopy. 2009;41:751–7.
42. Hochdorffer R, et al. Endoscopic resection of "giant" colorectal lesions: long-term outcome and safety. Z Gastroenterol. 2010;48:741–7.
43. Saito Y, et al. Clinical outcome of endoscopic submucosal dissection versus endoscopic mucosal resection of large colorectal tumors as determined by curative resection. Surg Endosc. 2010;24:343–52.
44. Saito Y, et al. A prospective, multicenter study of 1111 colorectal endoscopic submucosal dissections (with video). Gastrointest Endosc. 2010;72:1217–25.
45. Yahagi N, et al. Endoscopic submucosal dissection for the reliable en bloc resection of colorectal mucosal tumors. Dig Endosc. 2004;16:s89–92.
46. Kitajima K, et al. Correlations between lymph node metastasis and depth of submucosal invasion in colorectal carcinoma: J Gastroenterol. 2004;39:534–43.
47. Watanabe T, et al. Japanese Society for Cancer of the Colon and Rectum (JSCCR) guidelines 2016 for the treatment of colorectal cancer. Int J Clin Oncol. 2018;23:1–34.
48. Long KC, et al. Screening, surveillance, and treatment of anal intraepithelial neoplasia. Clin Colon Rectal Surg. 2016;29:57–64.
49. Wagner A, et al. Endoscopic submucosal dissection (ESD) for anal high-grade intraepithelial dysplasia: a case report. Z Gastroenterol. 2018;56:495–8.

Chapter 12
Chronic Inflammatory Bowel Disease in Remission: Mucosal Neoplasias

Naohisa Yahagi, Tadateru Maehata, and Atsushi Nakayama

The cumulative risk of colorectal cancer (CRC) in patients with ulcerative colitis (UC) amounts to 2% at 10 years, 9% at 20 years, and 18% at 30 years after onset of symptoms [1]. The risk of CRC is increased about 2.5-fold for Crohn's disease (CD) [2] and 5.6-fold for Crohn's colitis [3] and is equivalent in long-standing UC and Crohn's colitis [4].

In spite of the known increased risk of CRC and in spite of endoscopic surveillance, overall 5-year survival for CRC associated with inflammatory bowel disease (IBD) may not be better than for sporadic CRC. In a study of 28 patients with CD-associated CRC and 52 with UC-associated CRC, the overall 5-year survival rates were only 46% for CD- and 50% for UC-associated CRC; the median duration of IBD was 15 years for CD and 18 years for UC. Dysplasia was associated with CRC in 73% of CD and 79% of UC [4]. Hence, the detection rate of dysplastic lesions must rise in surveillance colonoscopy for IBD. We must intensify detection and analysis of neoplasias in IBD surveillance using HD endoscopy with magnification (>50-fold) and chromoendoscopy (indigo carmine) or (to a lesser extent) virtual chromoendoscopy (NBI). (Compare Chap. 1.)

12.1 Factors Increasing Risk of Colonic Neoplasias in IBD

The relative risk of CRC is significantly elevated after 8–10 years of colitis in IBD, which is the time point when surveillance should start in both UC and Crohn's colitis, whereas in left-sided UC, surveillance may start at 15-year disease duration [1,

N. Yahagi (✉) · T. Maehata · A. Nakayama
Division of Research and Development for Minimally Invasive Treatment, Cancer Center, Keio University School of Medicine, Shinjuku-ku, Tokyo, Japan
e-mail: yahagi-tky@umin.ac.jp

F. Berr et al. (eds.), *Atlas of Early Neoplasias of the Gastrointestinal Tract*,
https://doi.org/10.1007/978-3-030-01114-7_12

2, 5, 6]. A more recent study stressed that 9–15% of cancers occur earlier and would be missed with this recommendation [7], in spite of evidence gathered from retrospective analyses [2, 5, 6].

Young onset of IBD even raises the risk of CRC [5, 8]. The risk of CRC is increased twofold in UC patients with first- or second-degree relatives with CRC [8], and fourfold with long-standing primary sclerosing cholangitis (PSC) [8, 9] (Table 12.1). Patients with IBD and PSC should undergo annual colonoscopy beginning at the time of diagnosis of PSC and continuing indefinitely, even after liver transplantation [9, 10].

12.2 Colonoscopic Surveillance for CRC Risk in Long-Standing IBD

12.2.1 Surveillance Protocol

Surveillance colonoscopy (using white-light imaging, WLI) is best performed in stable remission of colitis (Truelove activity index ≤2) [11] and combined with chromoendoscopy (CE) using indigo carmine (or methylene blue) for targeted

Table 12.1 Risk Factors for Development of Colorectal Cancer (CRC) in IBD

Risk factor	Absolute risk	RR[a]	References
Disease duration	At 10 years: 2–3%	2.4	[1, 5]
	At 20 years: 8%	2.8	
	At 30 years: 18%		
Extent:			
Ulcerative pancolitis		14.8	[3]
Left-sided ulcerative colitis (UC)		2.8	
Ulcerative proctitis		1.7	
Presence of primary sclerosing cholangitis (PSC)[b]	At 10 years: 9%	4.8	
	At 20 years: 31%		[9, 10]
	At 25 years: 50%		
CRC in first-degree relative (FDR)			
>50-year-old FDR		2.5	
<50-year-old FDR		9.2	[9, 10]
Disease onset at			
Age < 15 years	40%		[8]
Age 15–39 years	25%		

Modified from Farraye et al. [4]

[a]Relative risk ratio

[b]The risk of CRC is increased in PSC even without UC [9, 10]

biopsy strategy [4]. After 8 years of UC, screening and further surveillance colonoscopy is recommended, with targeted biopsies of suspicious lesions or quadrant biopsies every 10 cm from suspicious sections of the involved colon (e.g., with pseudopolyposis or postinflammatory narrowing). Analogous recommendations pertain to Crohn's colitis when at least 30% of the colon is involved [4, 12, 13]. The typical result is a minimum of 28–32 biopsy samples. However, a recent randomized multi-center prospective study showed equality of targeted biopsy for detecting neoplastic lesions compared with random biopsy [14]. The procedure report in UC or Crohn's colitis should number the locations of all biopsies sampled from flat mucosa, from any superficial lesion 0-II (image documented), or any suspicious polypoid lesion sampled or removed.

12.2.2 Chromoendoscopy and Magnifying Narrow-Band Imaging (NBI)

In well-cleaned, mucus-depleted large bowel, image-enhanced endoscopy (IEE) using panchromoendoscopy with indigo carmine (or methylene blue) should be employed to take targeted biopsies. Panchromoendoscopy and targeted biopsies resulted in a higher yield of dysplasia than systematic four-quadrant biopsies in non–dye-sprayed colon [14–16]. Chromoendoscopy and virtual chromoendoscopy using NBI do not differ significantly for detection of colitis-associated neoplasia. Given the shorter procedural time and easier applicability, NBI may replace classic chromoendoscopy in the future [17].

Note Recommendations of surveillance for IBD-associated CRC [12, 18]:

- Start at 8 years after onset of symptoms in pancolitis.
- Examine when colonic disease is in remission.
- IEE-colonoscopy every 1–2 years after onset of surveillance, or every 2–3 years after two negative examinations (no dysplasia/CRC).
- Use high-definition (HD) endoscopy with >50× magnifying NBI and indigo carmine CE for analysis of lesions and mucosal patterns.
- Take representative targeted biopsy specimens from each anatomic section (or two protocol biopsies every 10 cm) of the involved colon.
- With PSC, colonoscopic surveillance starts at diagnosis and requires annual surveillance colonoscopy.

An exemption is *ulcerative proctitis/proctosigmoiditis*, which does not carry increased risk and may be managed with average-risk recommendations.

12.3 Diagnosis of Visible Dysplasia on Surveillance Colonoscopy

12.3.1 Lesions in IBD

To detect areas suspicious for neoplastic lesions in regenerative chronic inflammatory mucosa, you must focus on subtle alterations in microsurface structure and vascular pattern, as well as on visible surface alterations likely to harbor premalignant or malignant tissue [6, 14, 19, 20]. Nevertheless, previous intensity of inflammatory activity correlates positively with an increased risk of high-grade intraepithelial neoplasia (HGIN) or cancer. By analogy, the presence of postinflammatory pseudopolyps approximately doubles the risk of HGIN or cancer in UC [4, 6]. Long-standing UC with stricture or foreshortened colon has a high probability of even advanced cancer [19].

Previously, the term "dysplasia-associated lesion or mass" (DALM) was commonly used for endoscopically unresectable, raised dysplastic lesions (0-IIa or 0-Is) with *concomitant dysplasia* of the surrounding flat mucosa. Also, "adenoma-like lesion or mass" (ALM) was commonly used for endoscopically resectable protruded lesions with a distinct margin and smooth surface. Endoscopic diagnosis of those lesions was subjective, however, and it sometimes became difficult to distinguish between them [21]. Therefore, new criteria, visible polypoid dysplasia (lesion height ≥ 2.5 mm) and non-polypoid dysplasia (lesion height < 2.5 mm) was proposed by SCENIC (Surveillance for Colorectal Endoscopic Neoplasia Detection and Management in Inflammatory Bowel Disease Patients: International Consensus Recommendations) [12, 20] and the European Crohn's and Colitis Organisation (ECCO) guideline [13].

Note Be observant for the *principal premalignant/malignant lesions in IBD*:

- *Sporadic adenoma/dysplasia* (outside IBD-involved colon)
- Visible Polypoid dysplasia (lesion height ≥ 2.5 mm, 0-Is, Isp, Ip)
- Visible Non-polypoid dysplasia (lesion height < 2.5 mm, 0-IIa, IIb, IIc)
- Sites for risk of *Invisible Dysplasia*: (→ random biopsies) in: Pseudopolyposis, postinflammatory narrowing, surroundings of visible lesions

Sugimoto et al. were the first to apply the Paris classification, as proposed by SCENIC, to a well-documented series of visible high-grade dysplasia (HGD) ($n = 39$) in a cohort of 62 patients diagnosed with HGD or CRC in chronic UC [22]. HGD lesions typically were reddish (80%) or discolored (20%) *versus* background mucosa in remission; mostly elevated, flat, or sessile; and mainly (80%) located in the rectosigmoid (Table 12.2). Typically, most sessile/elevated lesions spread out in a flat area (Is+IIb/IIa + IIb) but were not classified as mixed types. The two depressed lesions were next to an ulcer. All flat (IIb) and depressed (IIc) HGD showed up in red, sessile (0-Is) and elevated lesions (0-IIa) in red (66% each) or as discolored

Table 12.2 Morphologic Types of Visible High-Grade Dysplasia in Chronic UC [22]

Paris type	0-Ip	0-Is	0-IIa	0-IIb	0-IIc
Percent (n = 39)	0	15%	49%	31%	5%

(a third each). All were diagnosed with targeted biopsy. Borders were indistinct in 57% of HGD lesions on CE, but were distinct in all (100%) on M-NBI [22]. A recent classification (FACILE) for optical diagnosis of visible dysplasia achieved moderate 76% accuracy by experts based on evaluation of 4 criteria on still images in non-magnifying CE [23]. But prospective clinical data on prevalence of macroscopic types of HGD or early CRC in IBD colitis are not yet available.

Note The flat II-b component, when the demarcation line is identified on M-NBI, must be classified, since mixed lesions (0-Is+IIb; 0-IIa + IIb) are a good indication for endoscopic resection, whereas invisible dysplasia near such lesions suggests colectomy because of high and non-manageable cancer risk.

Endoscopic diagnosis of surface (S) and vascular (V) structure of IBD-associated lesions is usually very difficult even for experts. Morphology of the lesions in IBD patients is altered by long-standing inflammation, and regeneration of the tissue comes in a variety of forms. At present, there is no consensus regarding pit pattern diagnosis or NBI magnification findings in IBD patients. It is sometimes difficult to distinguish between sporadic dysplasia and UC-associated dysplasia by gross appearance, surface structure, and vascular pattern of the lesions. A *p53 immunohistochemical (IHC) staining* is mandatory to distinguish between them, after complete removal of the lesion (Figs. 12.1 and 12.2). However, chromoendoscopy with magnification and NBI with magnification (M-NBI) are very useful to identify abnormal surface structure and vascular pattern of the lesions in IBD patients, although interpretation of those findings has not yet been established (Figs. 12.3 and 12.4).

Sometimes, invisible dysplasias or flat dysplasias (similar to lesions type 0-IIb or IIc) are detected by chance during surveillance colonoscopy. In cases of HGD, cancer may already be present in 42–67% of patients [18, 24]. By contrast, low-grade dysplasia (LGD) may carry only a 3% initial risk of concomitant CRC, with a 10% subsequent rate of progression to CRC within 10 years [25].

12.3.2 Prevalent Versus Incident Low-Grade Dysplasia

A review of 10 prospective studies reported that when LGD was detected at *initial* surveillance colonoscopy (*prevalent LGD*), HGD or CRC developed in 29% (16 of 55 patients) at some time during further follow-up, and CRC developed in 13% (7 patients) [26]. But when LGD was found during *further surveillance* (*incident LGD*), only 16% (33 of 204 patients) progressed to HGD or CRC, with 8% (17 patients) progressing to CRC [5]. When no dysplasia was found on initial colonoscopy, the rate of progression to CRC ranges from 1% to 3% per year [4, 27].

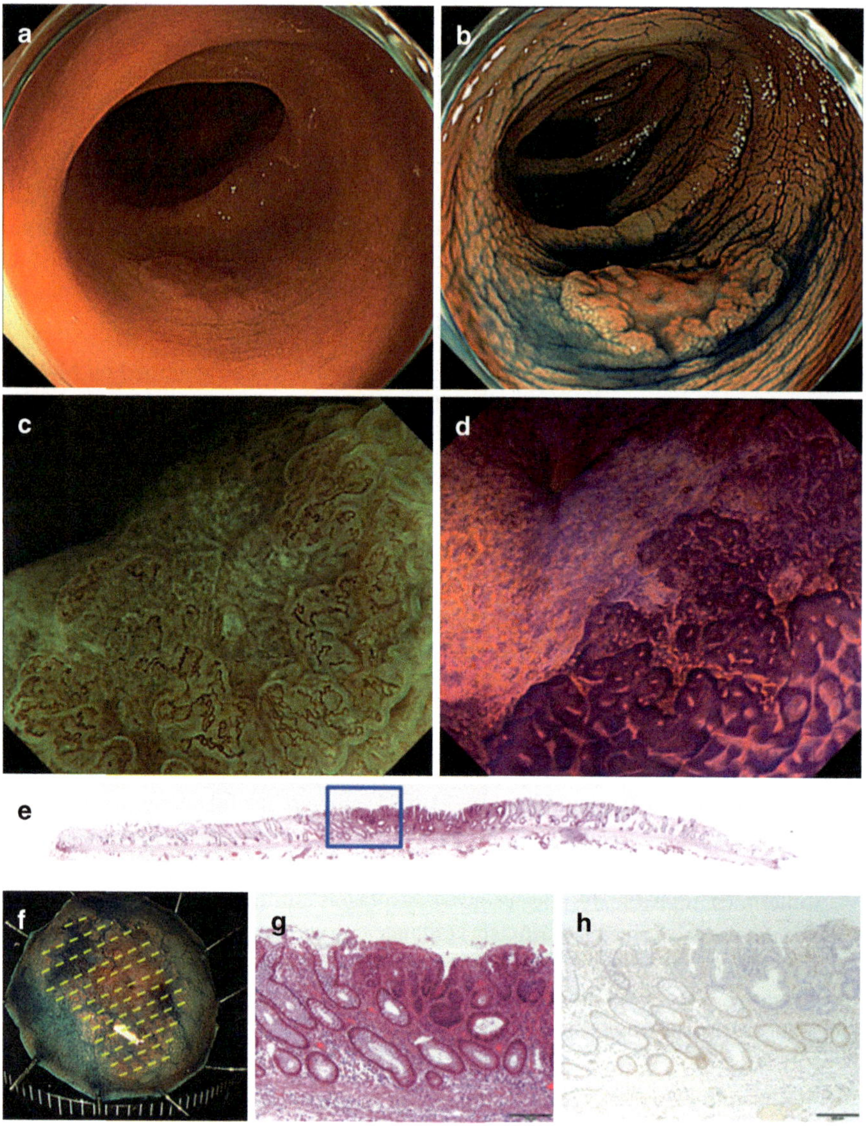

Fig. 12.1 A case of *sporadic mucosal cancer*. (**a**) A laterally spreading tumor (LST)-NG (PD) around 25 mm located at the sigmoid colon was found by WLI in a 63-year-old man with long-lasting ulcerative colitis (UC), which was in remission. (**b**) Demarcation line and surface structure become much clear with indigo carmine dye spraying. (**c**) Irregular and uneven microvessels, as well as irregular surface structure, were observed with NBI magnification. (**d**) Dense, uneven small pits at the peripheral part of the lesion and loose, unclear small pits at the central part were observed by crystal violet staining and magnification. (**f**) Margin-free resection was achieved by endoscopic submucosal dissection (ESD). (**e, g**) Histopathological result was Is+IIc, 28 × 18 mm, tubular adenocarcinoma (tub1) with tubular adenoma, pM, int, INFα, ly0, v0, pHM0, pVM0. (**h**) *p53* immuno-histochemical staining was negative, so this lesion was judged to be a *sporadic mucosal cancer*

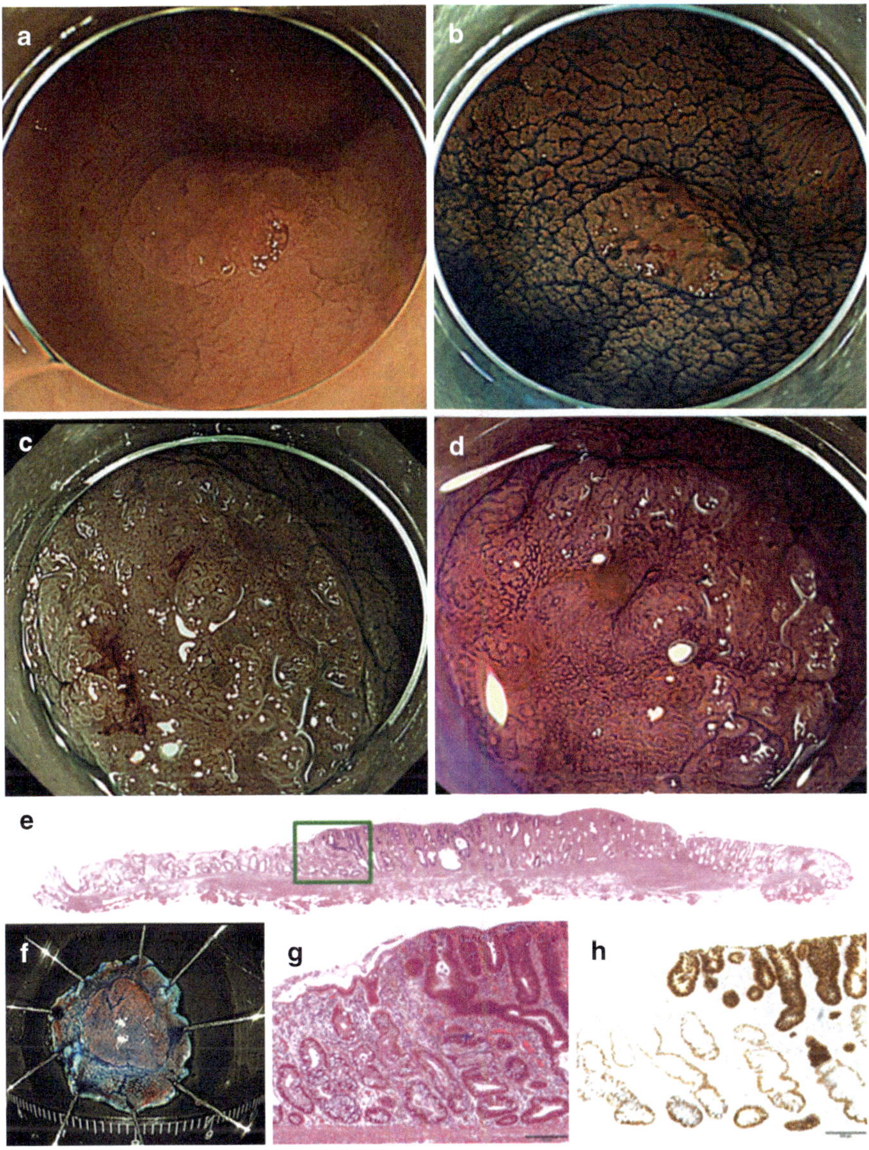

Fig. 12.2 A case of *UC-associated mucosal cancer*. (**a**) A slightly reddish IIa lesion about 10 mm in size was found at the upper rectum by WLI in a 65-year-old man with 15 years history of UC, in remission. (**b**) Demarcation line and surface structure become much clear with indigo carmine dye spraying. (**c**) Slightly irregular microvessels and irregular surface structure were observed with NBI magnification. (**d**) Dense, uneven small pits were observed at the central part of the lesion by crystal violet staining and magnification. (**f**) Margin-free resection was achieved by ESD. (**e, g**) Histopathological result was IIa, 9×9 mm, tubular adenocarcinoma (tub1), pM, int, INFα, ly0, v0, pHM0, pVM0. (**h**) Overexpression of p53 protein was observed by immuno-histochemical staining, so this lesion was judged to be *UC-associated mucosal cancer*

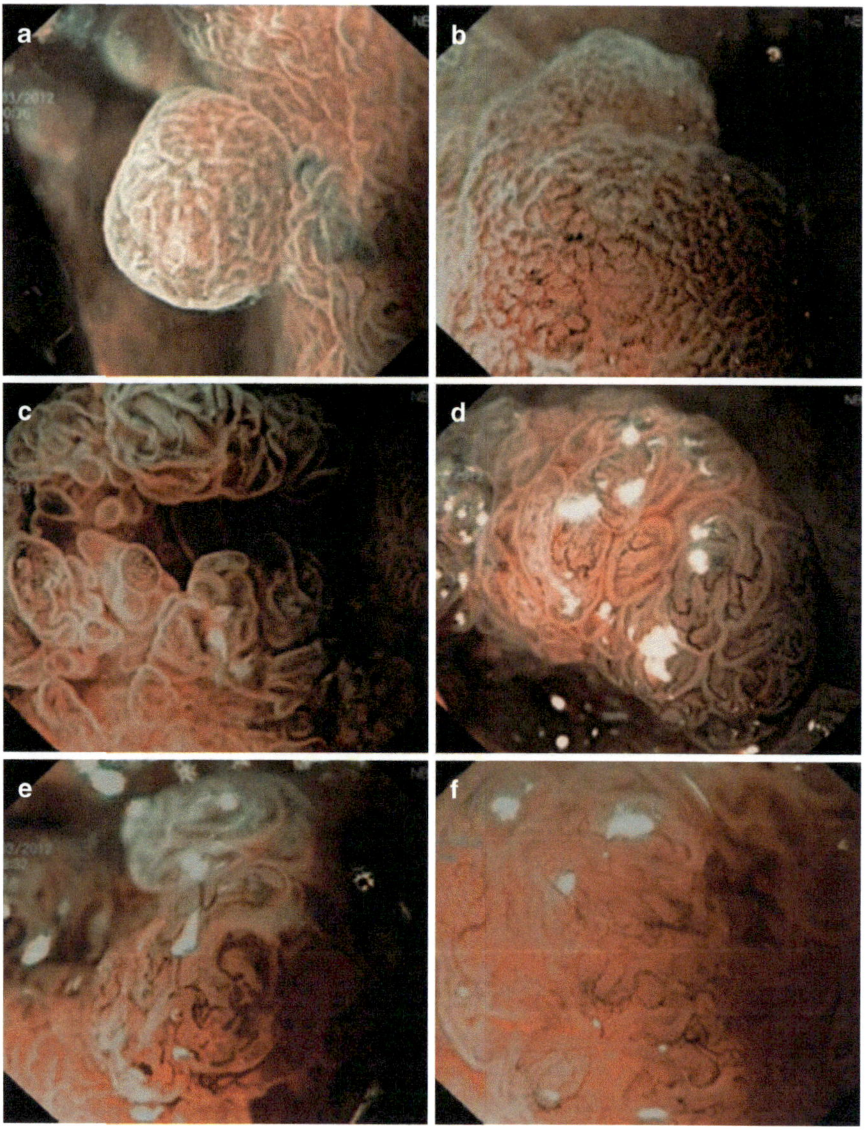

Fig. 12.3 0-Is lesions in long-standing ulcerative regenerative pancolitis with pseudopolyps (**a**, **b**) as well as raised dysplasia (**c**–**f**, M-NBI, 100×). (**a**, **b**) Regularly arranged, meshed capillary and surface structure, regenerative pseudopolyp. (**c**) Dense capillary network and slightly irregular surface structure in rectal LST-GM (0-IIa + Is): Tubulovillous adenoma. (**d**) Irregular meshed capillary and enlarged irregular surface structure in sigmoid 0-Is lesion. *Histology*: Tubulovillous low-grade intraepithelial neoplasia (LGIN). (**e**, **f**) Highly irregular capillary and surface structure in rectal 0-Is lesion. *Histology*: HGIN (differentiated mucosal cancer T0 m1)

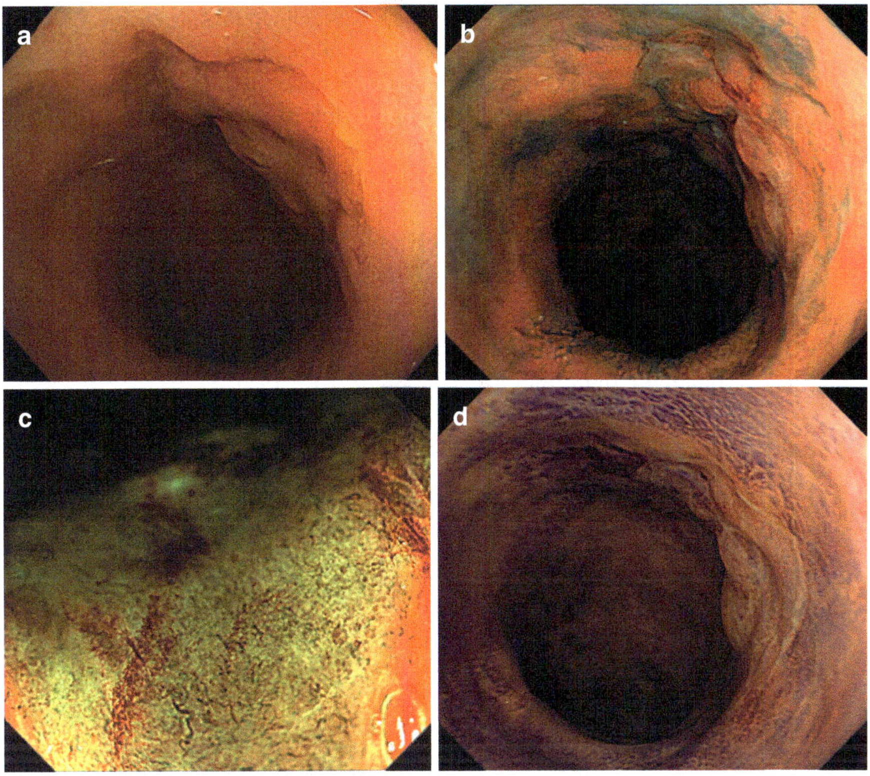

Fig. 12.4 A case of *flat dysplasia* (0-IIc like advanced cancer). (**a**) An irregular depressed lesion about 2 cm in size is seen in the descending colon of a 63-year-old man with 16 years history of ulcerative pancolitis. (**b**) Rigid colonic wall and tense nodules. (**c**) Non-structured surface and sparse vascular network was observed with NBI magnification. (**d**) Stainability of crystal violet was poor within the depressed area. Because the biopsy revealed adenocarcinoma, the patient underwent total colectomy. This lesion had already became advanced cancer although the lesion size was just 2 cm. *Final histopathological diagnosis*: Tubular adenocarcinoma (tub2 + por2), 0-IIa + IIc, 20 mm, pT2(MP), sci, INFc, ly0,v0,pPM0, pDM0, pRM0

12.3.3 Focality of Dysplasia

The overall 5-year progression rate of flat prevalent LGD to either HGD or CRC was 53%. The rate was nearly identical among 39 patients with unifocal LGD and 7 patients with multifocal LGD [4, 28].

12.4 Management of Neoplastic Lesions in IBD Patients

Sporadic adenomas in *uninvolved* parts of the colon in UC (or Crohn's colitis) carry a low risk (<5%) of associated dysplasia or CRC, as do protruding lesions in *non-dysplastic* mucosa of IBD-involved colon [26]. Those are very good indications for endoscopic resection. The clinical course of UC-associated lesions can be followed with a strict surveillance program after complete endoscopic resection of dysplastic lesions [27]. Therefore, it is recommended to conduct endoscopic resection for both polypoid dysplastic lesions and non-polypoid dysplastic lesions without invisible dysplasia around the lesion or distant area, if technically possible [12, 13]. Endoscopic submucosal dissection (ESD) by expert endoscopists is feasible for neoplasia in UC patients and may avoid unnecessary surgery [29]. However, patients with endoscopically unresectable non-polypoid dysplasia should undergo a total colectomy, as a meta-analysis involving 477 patients indicated that even low-grade flat dysplasia (LGD) had a risk of 22% for synchronous cancer and a 5-year progression rate of 36% to advanced neoplasia (HGD or CRC) [4].

Note According to SCENIC and ECCO guidelines [4, 12, 13]:

- *Endoscopic resection* (en bloc) is indicated for:
  - Sporadic lesions
  - Polypoid dysplasia and non-polypoid dysplasia without invisible dysplasia around the lesion or in a distant area
- *Total colectomy* is indicated for IBD with:
  - Endoscopically unresectable non-polypoid dysplasia
  - Invisible HGD detected by random biopsy

12.5 Cases: Neoplastic Lesions in IBD

Case 1: Flat adenoma in Chronic Ulcerative Colitis
In a patient with long-lasting UC, surveillance colonoscopy showed discolored, slightly irregular mucosa in the sigmoid colon on a background of UC in remission (Fig. 12.5). Irregular surface structure with less vascular network was observed by NBI magnification. Uneven, irregular pits were observed by crystal violet staining magnification. The lesion was resected en bloc by ESD; histology revealed tubular adenoma, resected R0, 46 × 33 mm.

Note Endoscopic diagnosis of flat neoplasia and lateral margins is sometimes difficult, but chromoendoscopy and magnification are helpful in recognizing irregular mucosal structure and demarcation line.

Case 2: Flat Carcinoma in Long-Standing Ulcerative Colitis
A small nodule and slight reddish area was recognized during surveillance colonoscopy in a 63-year-old man with 18 years' history of ulcerative pancolitis in remission (Fig. 12.6). A very flat lesion became obvious after chromoendoscopy with indigo carmine, and a highly dilated neoplastic vessel was observed by NBI magnification. The nodular area showed almost non-structure pit after crystal violet staining, and biopsy revealed well-differentiated adenocarcinoma. The patient underwent total colectomy.

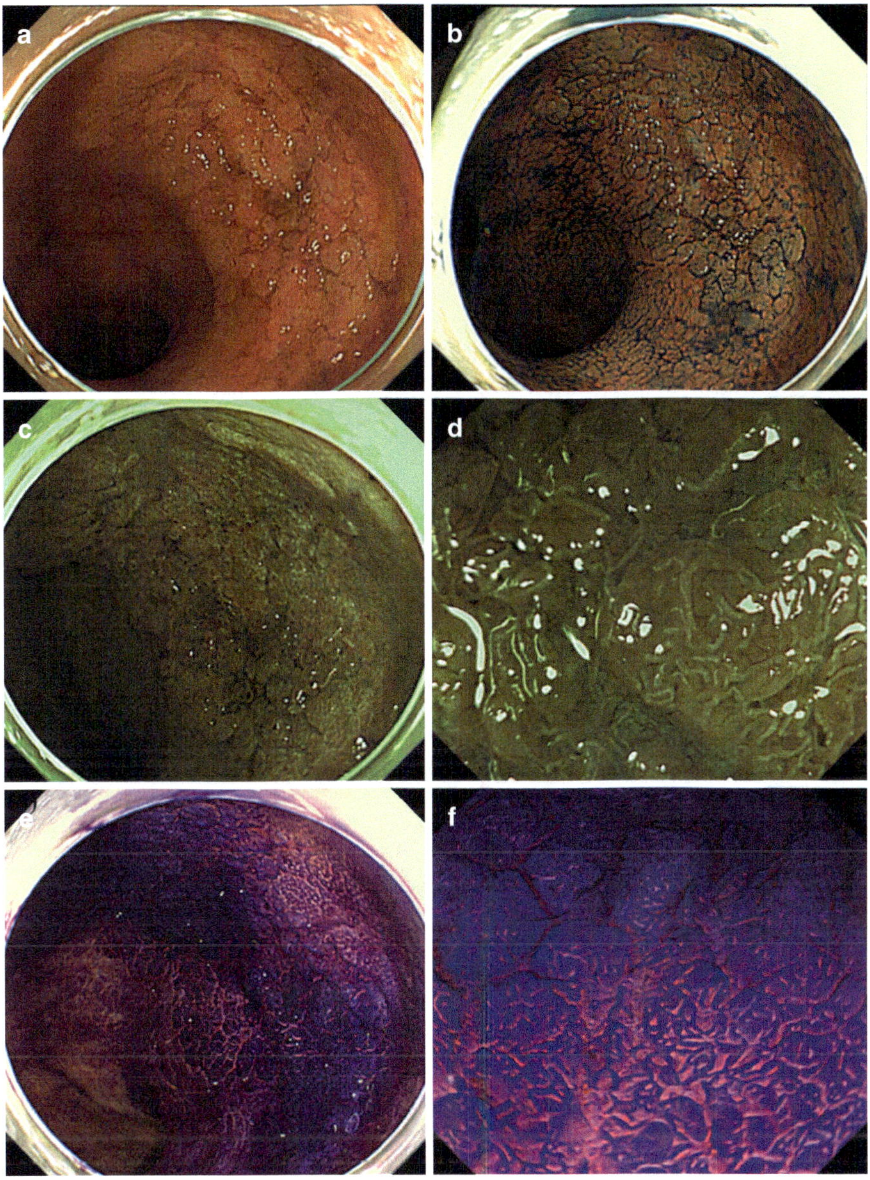

Fig. 12.5 UC Case 1: (**a**) Slightly irregular, discolored mucosa was observed in a patient with long-standing UC in remission. (**b**) Irregular mucosal surface and tumor border became much clearer with indigo carmine dye spraying. (**c**) The tumor border was clearly seen with NBI. (**d**) Irregular surface structure with less vascular network was observed by NBI magnification. (**e**) Crystal violet staining. (**f**) Uneven, irregular pits were observed by crystal violet staining magnification. The lesion was resected by ESD, and histology revealed tubular adenoma, 46 × 33 mm

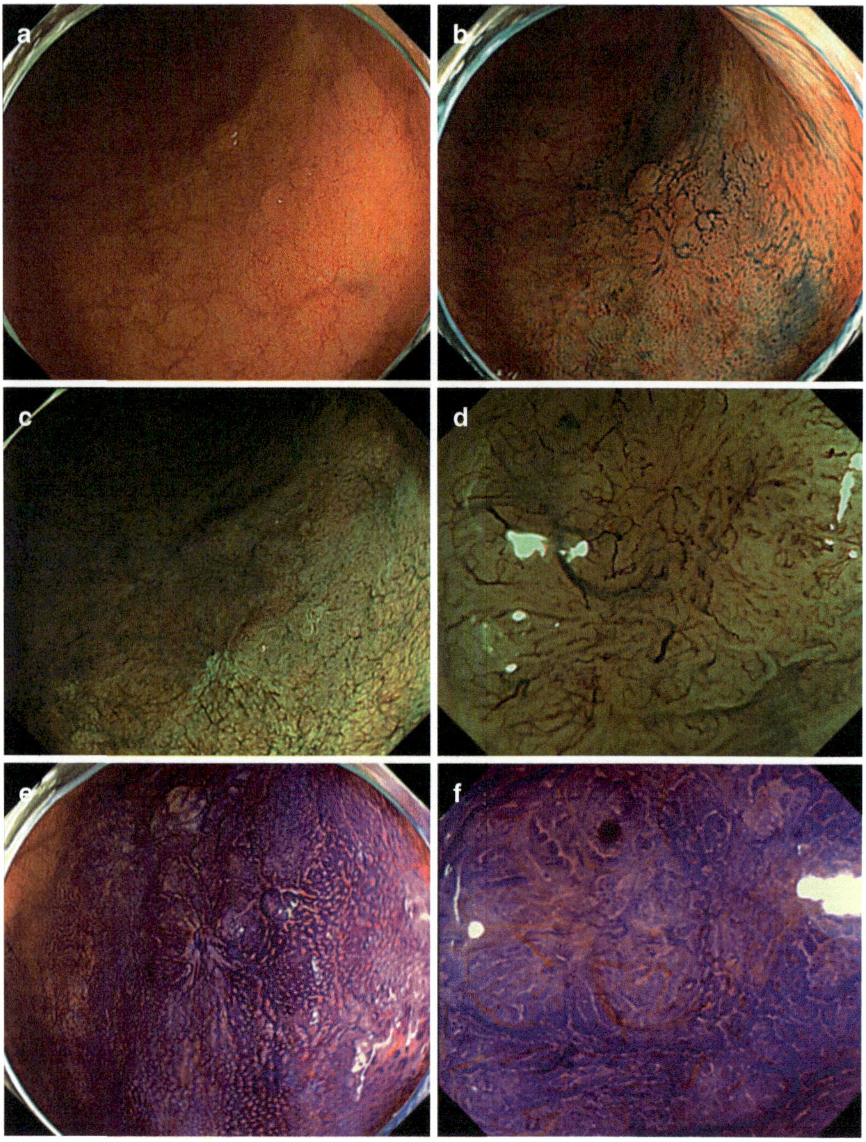

Fig. 12.6 UC Case 2: (**a**) A small nodule and slight reddish area were recognized during surveillance colonoscopy. (**b**) An irregular mucosal surface and very flat lesion became obvious after indigo carmine dye spraying. (**c, d**) A highly dilated neoplastic vessel, suggesting invasive cancer, was observed with NBI magnification. (**e, f**) An almost non-structure pit pattern, also suggesting invasive cancer, was observed at the nodular area with crystal violet staining magnification. The biopsy specimen revealed well-differentiated adenocarcinoma, and the patient underwent total colectomy. The final histopathological result was a well-differentiated tubular adenocarcinoma (tub1), pSM (200 μm), 11 × 5 mm, int, INFb, ly(+),v(−)

Note Be observant for subtle differences in mucosal color or pattern of flat neoplasia when performing surveillance colonoscopy in patients with ulcerative colitis in remission.

Case 3: Raised Dysplasia

A 51-year-old otherwise healthy man was referred for endoscopic resection of a rectal LST-granular-mixed (LST-GM) of 4 cm estimated diameter, with focal HGD. He had chronic ulcerative pancolitis for 18 years and had been in remission for 3 years. The rectal LST was much larger than expected (diameter 7 cm), and he had a variety of suspicious discolored lesions. Therefore, he was reevaluated with a magnifying (100-fold) endoscope up to the hepatic flexure, looking for additional dysplastic lesions. He presented a variety of raised lesions with irregular surface structure and vascular pattern; challenging endoscopic differential diagnoses of regenerative versus neoplastic lesions were clarified by targeted biopsies (Fig. 12.7).

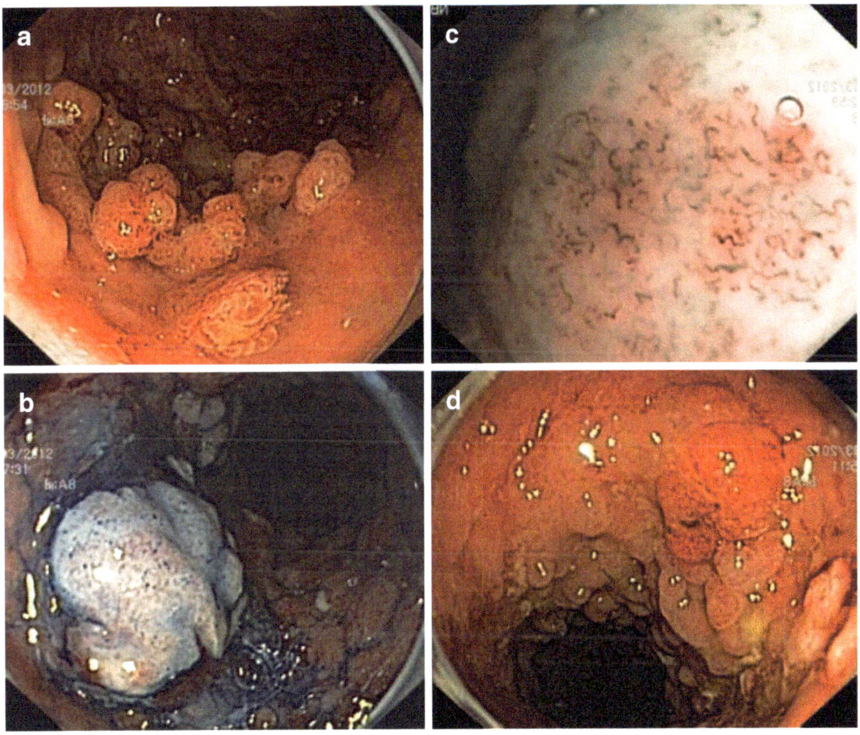

Fig. 12.7 UC Case 3: (**a**) Rectal LST-mixed (75 × 35 mm; 0–7.5 cm p.a) in chronic pancolitis in remission. *Histology*: polypoid dysplasia with focal HGIN (in two areas). Raised lesion with LGIN + focal HGIN. (**b**) Sessile whitish lesion (0-Is, 15 mm) in descending colon (60 cm p.a.), chronic ulcerative pancolitis. (**c**) Absent, but very smooth surface, tortuous vascular pattern (NBI 80×; same lesion as in **b**). *Histology*: nonneoplastic fibrotic mucosa and submucosa with mucinophages: *Fibrotic pseudopolyp*. (**d**) *Protruding reddish lesion* (0-IIa + Is, 20 mm) in descending colon (60 cm p.a.). Same lesion 0-Is as in Fig. 12.3e, f (NBI 80×). *Targeted biopsy*: polypoid dysplasia with focal HGIN

Diagnosis: Multiple raised dysplasias (three distantly separated lesions with HGIN) in chronic ulcerative pancolitis. The patient was referred for sphincter-preserving total colectomy with ileoanal pouch.

Note On such a background of extensive regenerative mucosa and multiple endoscopic lesions in long-standing (mildly active) IBD-associated colitis:

- Endoscopic diagnosis of neoplasias and malignancy is extremely difficult, even for expert endoscopists.
- Risk of advanced-stage CRC is very high when endoscopic resection of lesions and follow-up would be attempted.
- Colectomy with ileal pouch is preferable.

Acknowledgments The contribution of a case by Dr. Gerhard Kleber of Aalen, Germany, and the evaluation of histology by Dr. Daniel Neureiter of Salzburg, Austria, are gratefully acknowledged.

References

1. Eaden JA, et al. The risk of colorectal cancer in ulcerative colitis: a meta-analysis. Gut. 2001;48:526–35.
2. Jess T, et al. Increased risk of intestinal cancer in Crohn's disease: a meta-analysis of population-based cohort studies. Am J Gastroenterol. 2005;100:2724–9.
3. Ekbom A, et al. Increased risk of large-bowel cancer in Crohn's disease with colonic involvement. Lancet. 1990;336:357–9.
4. Farraye FA, et al. AGA technical review on the diagnosis and management of colorectal neoplasia in inflammatory bowel disease. Gastroenterology. 2010;138:746–74.
5. Bernstein CN, et al. Cancer risk in patients with inflammatory bowel disease: a population-based study. Cancer. 2001;91:854–62.
6. Rutter MD, et al. Thirty-year analysis of a colonoscopic surveillance program for neoplasia in ulcerative colitis. Gastroenterology. 2006;130:1030–8.
7. Lutgens MW, et al. High frequency of early colorectal cancer in inflammatory bowel disease. Gut. 2008;57:1246–51.
8. Beaugerie L, et al. Cancers complicating inflammatory bowel disease. N Engl J Med. 2015;372:1441–52.
9. Soetikno RM, et al. Increased risk of colorectal neoplasia in patients with primary sclerosing cholangitis and ulcerative colitis: a meta-analysis. Gastrointest Endosc. 2002;56:48–54.
10. Broome U, et al. Primary sclerosing cholangitis and ulcerative colitis: evidence for increased neoplastic potential. Hepatology. 1995;22:1404–8.
11. Lichtiger S, et al. Cyclosporine in severe ulcerative colitis refractory to steroid therapy. N Engl J Med. 1994;330:1841–5.
12. Laine L, et al. SCENIC international consensus statement on surveillance and management of dysplasia in inflammatory bowel disease. Gastrointest Endosc. 2015;81:489–501.
13. Magro F, et al. Third European evidence-based consensus on diagnosis and management of ulcerative colitis. Part 1: definitions, diagnosis, extra-intestinal manifestations, pregnancy, cancer surveillance, surgery, and ileo-anal pouch disorders. J Crohns Colitis. 2017;11:649–70.
14. Watanabe T, et al. Comparison of targeted vs random biopsies for surveillance of ulcerative colitis-associated colorectal cancer. Gastroenterology. 2016;151:1122–30.

15. Kiesslich R, et al. Methylene blue-aided chromoendoscopy for the detection of intraepithelial neoplasia and colon cancer in ulcerative colitis. Gastroenterology. 2003;124:880–8.
16. Marion JF, et al. Chromoendoscopy-targeted biopsies are superior to standard colonoscopic surveillance for detecting dysplasia in inflammatory bowel disease patients: a prospective endoscopic trial. Am J Gastroenterol. 2008;103:2342–9.
17. Bisschops R, et al. Chromoendoscopy versus narrow band imaging in UC: a prospective randomised controlled trial. Gut. 2018;67:1087–94.
18. Farraye FA, et al. AGA medical position statement on the diagnosis and management of colorectal neoplasia in inflammatory bowel disease. Gastroenterology. 2010;138:738–45.
19. Gumaste V, et al. Benign and malignant colorectal strictures in ulcerative colitis. Gut. 1992;33:938–41.
20. Soetikno R, et al. Paradigm shift in the surveillance and management of dysplasia in inflammatory bowel disease (West). Dig Endosc. 2016;28:266–73.
21. Chiu K, et al. DALM, rest in peace: a pathologist's perspective on dysplasia in inflammatory bowel disease in the post-DALM era. Mod Pathol. 2018;31:1180–90.
22. Sugimoto S, et al. Endoscopic morphologic features of ulcerative colitis-associated dysplasia classified according to the SCENIC consensus statement. Gastrointest Endosc. 2017;85:639–46.
23. Iacucci M, et al. A multimodal (FACILE) classification for optical diagnosis of inflammatory bowel disease associated neoplasia. Endosc 2019;51:133–41.
24. Rubio CA, et al. Villous and serrated adenomatous growth bordering carcinomas in inflammatory bowel disease. Anticancer Res. 2000;20:4761–4.
25. Lim CH, et al. Ten year follow up of ulcerative colitis patients with and without low grade dysplasia. Gut. 2003;52:1127–32.
26. Odze RD. Adenomas and adenoma-like DALMs in chronic ulcerative colitis: a clinical, pathological, and molecular review. Am J Gastroenterol. 1999;94:1746–50.
27. Odze RD, et al. Long-term follow-up after polypectomy treatment for adenoma-like dysplastic lesions in ulcerative colitis. Clin Gastroenterol Hepatol. 2004;2:534–41.
28. Ullman TA, et al. The fate of low grade dysplasia in ulcerative colitis. Am J Gastroenterol. 2002;97:922–7.
29. Kinoshita S, et al. The role of colorectal endoscopic submucosal dissection in patients with ulcerative colitis. Gastrointest Endosc. 2018;87:1079–84.

Appendix: Terminology

Observation Methods

1. White light endoscopy (WLI)
2. Chromoendoscopy (CE)
   - Lugol's staining (squamous epithelial esophagus)
   - Indigo carmine (stomach, small intestine, colon)
   - Crystal violet (colon, irregular or amorphous pit pattern)
3. Narrow band imaging (NBI): specify as below
   - Non-magnifying NBI
   - Magnifying NBI (M-NBI)
4. Magnifying (magnification) endoscopy (M-E)

Endoscopic Appearance

1. **Macroscopic appearance**

   (a) superficial lesions, type 0
   - polypoid and protruding 0-I
     - pedunculated, 0-Ip
     - sessile, 0-Is
   - flat (non-polypoid and non-excavated) 0-II
     - slightly elevated (elevated), 0-IIa
     - completely flat (flat), 0-IIb
     - slightly depressed (depressed), 0-IIc
   - excavated
     - ulcerated type, 0-III
     - excavated and depressed types, 0-IIc + III, 0-III + IIc

F. Berr et al. (eds.), *Atlas of Early Neoplasias of the Gastrointestinal Tract*,
https://doi.org/10.1007/978-3-030-01114-7

Advanced carcinoma in Upper GI Tract (GIT):
(b) polypoid carcinomas, type 1
(c) ulcerated carc. sharply demarcated, raised margins, type 2
(d) ulcerated, infiltrating carc. without definite limits, type 3
(e) non-ulcerated, diffusely infiltrating carcinomas, type 4

Macroscopic appearance (adenoma, carcinoma) in Lower GIT
Laterally spreading type lesions (LST, d > 10 mm), subtypes:

- Granular, – homogenous (LST-GH) i.e. 0-IIa
  - mixed nodular (LST-GM), i.e. 0-IIa + Is
  - whole nodular (LST-GN), i.e. 0-Is
- Non-Granular LST (LST-NG)
  - non-granular flat (LST-NGF)
  - pseudodepressed (LST-NGPD)

2. **Chromoendoscopy**
   - Lugol-unstained area (squamous epithelial esophagus)
   - multiple Lugol-voiding lesions
3. **NBI**
   - brownish area
4. **Magnifying endoscopy (M-E), magnifying NBI (M-NBI)**

   (a) **demarcation line**
   (b) **microvascular pattern/architecture (MVP)**
   - regular, irregular, absent
   - <u>squamous epithelium</u>
     - intrapapillary capillary loop (IPCL)
       dilatation
       tortuosity
       caliber change
       variety in shape
     - submucosal dendritic (branched) veins
   - <u>columnar epithelium</u>
     - collecting venule (CV), submucosal
     - subepithelial capillary network (SECN)
     - irregular microvessel pattern (IMVP)
       fine network pattern
       non-network pattern (corkscrew pattern)

   (c) **mucosal (micro-)surface pattern / structure**

   - regular, irregular, absent
   - columnar epithelium
     - crypt opening, pit
     - pit patterns (colorectum)
     - tubular pattern (tubular, villous or ridge type)

- marginal crypt epithelium, white zone (WZ)
- irregular microsurface pattern (IMSP)
- absent microsurface pattern (AMSP)
- white opaque substance (WOS)
- light blue crest (LBC, typical of intestinal metaplasia)

Subepithelial Lesions

- High-resolution endoscopic ultrasound (hr-EUS, 12–30 MHz), echo layers:
  - ep, epithelial echo of mucosa (1st layer, hyperechoic)
  - lpm, lamina propria of mucosae (2nd layer, hypoechoic)
  - sm, submucosa (3rd layer, hyperechoic, sometimes with upfront echo of mm, muscularis mucosae
  - pm, proper muscle (4th layer, hypoechoic)
  - ad/ss, adventitia/subserosa
  - correlated with anatomic / histopathologic wall layers
- Layer of origin
  - ep, lpm: adenoma/dysplasia and HGIN/cancer
  - lpm: MALT lymphoma, NET
  - mm: (rarely) GIST, leiomyoma
  - sm: GCT, (NET), lipoma, lymphoma, fibroma, lymphangioma, others
  - pm: GIST, leiomyoma

Index

A
Aberrant pancreas, 86
Abrikosoff tumors, 67
Acetic acid chromoendoscopy, 152
Acute perforations, 56
Adenocarcinoma (AC) of the esophagus, 108, 109
Adenoma-like lesion or mass (ALM), 296
Adenomas
  anal squamous cell lesion 0-IIb-G, 287, 289
  large rectal LST-G mixed type invading anal channel, 278, 280
  LST-G whole nodular type (0-Is + Isp), 278, 279
  LST-NG, 275, 277, 281, 283–285
  rectal LST-G, 286–288
  relatively large cecal lesion LST-G whole nodular, 281, 282
  small lesion 0-IIa + c, 276, 278
  small lesion 0-Is + 0-IIc, 275, 276
Adenomatous/hyperplastic mucosal lesions, 32
Altered pit pattern, 203
Altered villi, 203
Ampullary adenomas, 225, 226
Anal canal, lesions of, 274, 275
Anal lesions, 275
Anal neoplasias, 275
Anechoic, 80
Angiodysplasia, 186
Antibiotic prophylaxis, 114
Atrophic gastritis, 17, 208
Avascular area (AVA), 126, 128

B
Barrett's adenocarcinoma, 38, 40
Barrett's esophagus (BE), 22, 149
  diagnosis and examination of, 150, 151
  dysplasia and early cancer
    early Barrett neoplasia type 0-Is, 160
    mucosal adenocarcinoma, underwater and acetic acid delineation of, 166, 167
    with mucosal cancer, 167, 169
    multifocal Paris 0-Is lesions, 165
    0-Ip/s + IIa, 163, 164
    with Paris 0-Is submucosal lesion, 166, 168
    and submucosal lesion, 165, 166
    type 0-IIa, 162
  early neoplasias, endoscopic resection of, 158–160
  procedure, detection and analysis of, 152–154
  sm-invasive cancer, endoscopic diagnosis of, 155–158
Barrett's mucosa, 22
Bleeding, risk, 57
Blue Light Imaging (BLI), 4
Budding sign, 82

C
Cancerous villi, 196
Candida, 130, 131
Capillary patterns (CP), 14
Chromoendoscopy (CE), 122, 195
  IBD, 295
  mucosal neoplastic lesions, 4, 6

F. Berr et al. (eds.), *Atlas of Early Neoplasias of the Gastrointestinal Tract*,
https://doi.org/10.1007/978-3-030-01114-7

Chromosomal instability, 35
Chronic ulcerative colitis, 302, 303
Classic polypoid adenoma–carcinoma pathway, 31
Classic tubular adenoma, 15
Cold polypectomy, 231
Cold snare polypectomy (CSP), 235
Colonic mucosa, 13
Colonic neoplasias, 7, 13, 15
Colonic neoplastic lesions, characteristics of, 30, 33
  classic polypoid adenoma–carcinoma pathway, 31
  flat/depressed colonic adenoma–carcinoma pathway, 31
  HNPCC, 34
  serrated adenoma–carcinoma pathway, 31, 34
Colonic pit pattern, 244
Colonic wall, 80
Colonoscopy, 102, 111
Colorectal cancer (CRC), 103–105
Colorectal lesions, 247–253
Colorectal mucosa, 243, 244, 246
Colorectum
  adenomas, dysplasia and early colorectal cancer
    anal squamous cell lesion 0-IIb-G, 287, 289
    large rectal LST-G mixed type invading anal channel, 278, 280
    LST-G whole nodular type (0-Is + Isp), 278, 279
    LST-NG, 275, 277, 281, 283–285
    rectal LST-G, 286–288
    relatively large cecal lesion LST-G whole nodular, 281, 282
    small lesion 0-IIa + c, 276, 278
    small lesion 0-Is + 0-IIc, 275, 276
  anal canal, lesions of, 274, 275
  colorectal lesions
    NICE types, 247–251
    macroscopic type and appearance of, NICE type 2, 252, 253
  colorectal mucosa and neoplasias, structure of, 243, 244, 246
  curative endoscopic resection in, 30
  macroscopic types, prevalence and carcinoma risk of, 242
  magnifying endoscopy, differential diagnosis of lesions, 253
    JNET type 2 lesions, differential diagnosis of, 254–259
    superficial AC *vs.* deep sm-invasive AC, diagnosis of, 257, 259–264
    tentative distinction of serrated lesions, JNET type 1, 265–270
  mucosal neoplasias, endoscopic resection of, 271
    ESD, 273, 274
    snaring resection techniques, 272, 273
Columnar epithelial mucosa, 13
Columnar epithelium-lined esophagus, *see* Barrett's esophagus
Columnar intraepithelial neoplasia (CIN), 38
Columnar mucosa-lined esophagus, microarchitecture of, 21, 22
Concomitant dysplasia, 296
Condylomata acuminata, 275
Crohn's colitis, 295
Curative endoscopic resection, in esophagus, stomach, and colorectum, 30
Cylinder epithelial dysplasia, 38, 40

D

Deeper muscularis mucosae (DMM), 159
Deeply sm-invasive carcinoma, 206, 207
Deep sm-invasion, 156
Deep sm-invasive AC, diagnosis of, 257, 259
Delayed perforation, 56
Depressed lesions, differential diagnosis of, 185–193, 248
Differentiated adenocarcinoma, 179, 257
Diffuse/signet-ring type gastric cancer, 36
Duodenal adenocarcinoma, 235, 237
Duodenal adenomatosis, 230
Duodenal neoplasias, 230–235
Duodenal NET, 72
Duodenum, 114
  adenoma and adenocarcinoma in, 229, 230
  ampullary adenomas, 225, 226
  duodenal neoplasias, endoscopic resection of, 230–235
  endoscopic analysis of, 226, 227
  incidence and risk of malignant transformation, 223–225
  non-ampullary duodenal adenomas
    duodenal adenocarcinoma with submucosal invasion, 235, 237
    low-grade duodenal adenoma, 234–236

Duplication cyst, 84–86
Dysplasia, 34
  anal squamous cell lesion 0-IIb-G, 287, 289
  Barrett's lesion type 0-IIa, 162
  Barrett's esophagus and submucosal lesion, 165, 166
  circular Barrett's carcinoma 0-Ip/s + IIa, 163, 164
  early Barrett neoplasia type 0-Is, 160
  large rectal LST-G mixed type invading anal channel, 278, 280
  LST-G whole nodular type (0-Is + Isp), 278, 279
  LST-NG, 275, 277, 281, 283–285
  mucosal adenocarcinoma, underwater and acetic acid delineation of, 166, 167
  with mucosal cancer, 167, 169
  multifocal Paris 0-Is lesions, 165
  with Paris 0-Is submucosal lesion, 166, 168
  rectal LST-G, 286–288
  relatively large cecal lesion LST-G whole nodular, 281, 282
  small lesion 0-IIa + c, 276, 278
  small lesion 0-Is + 0-IIc, 275, 276
Dysplasia-associated lesion or mass (DALM), 296

E
Early gastric cancer (EGC)
  gastroscopy for detection, 176
    early gastric neoplasia, endoscopic structure of, 179, 180
    gastric mucosa, 176–179
  stomach
    endoscopic resection of, 207
    mucosal early gastric cancer, invasion depth, 194, 195
    shape of lesion, invasion depth, 180–193
    shape of mucosal folds, invasion depth, 180–193
Early gastric neoplasias (EGN), 207, 208
Echogenicity, 80
EFTRD, 48, 49
Electrocoagulation syndrome, 56
Electrosnaring, 48
Endoscopic en-bloc resection, 49, 51–53
Endoscopic mucosal resection (EMR), 41, 42, 48, 137, 272
Endoscopic resection techniques, 71
Endoscopic submucosal dissection (ESD), 41, 42, 47, 49, 53, 55, 273, 274, 302
  complications, 56, 57
  minor invasive endoscopic surgery, 57, 58
  outcome of, 55, 56
Endoscopy
  gastric cancer, 106, 107
    adenocarcinoma of esophagus/gastroesophageal junction, 108, 109
    SCC, 107
  screening and surveillance, rationale for, 102
    colonoscopy, for CRC prevention, 102
    colorectal cancer, individuals with increased risk for, 103–105
  standards for screening and surveillance, 109, 110
    colonoscopy, 111
    periprocedural precautions, 114, 115
    upper gastrointestinal endoscopy, 112, 113
Esophageal columnar epithelium, surface pattern, 170
Esophageal neoplastic lesions, characteristics of, 38
  Barrett's adenocarcinoma, 38
  squamous epithelial cell dysplasia–cancer pathway, 40, 41
Esophageal squamous cell cancer, 107
Esophageal wall, 81
Esophagitic lesions, 128
Esophagus, curative endoscopic resection in, 30
Expanded snaring techniques, 48

F
Familial adenomatous polyposis (FAP)
  duodenal adenomatosis in, 230
  resection of adenomas, 234, 235
Familial diffuse gastric cancer (FDGC), 35
Familial intestinal gastric cancer (FIGC), 35
FAP duodenal adenomatosis, 224
Five-layered echo-structure, 80
Flat adenoma, 302, 303
Flat carcinoma, 302, 304
Flat/depressed colonic adenoma–carcinoma pathway, 31
Flat dysplasia, 301
Flat HNPCC neoplasias, 255
Flat lesions, 7, 248

G

Gastric adenocarcinoma
    analysis of, 195–206
        histological type, prediction of, 196–206
        pit patterns, 197–206
        surface pattern and vascular pattern, 201
        vascular patterns, 197–206
        villous pattern, 196–206
    characteristics of, 35
        diffuse/signet-ring type gastric cancer, 36
        gastric phenotype carcinoma, 36
        HDGC, 38
        intestinal-type gastric adenocarcinoma, 36
Gastric cancer, 102, 106–109
Gastric GIST, 73, 76
Gastric metaplasia, 226
Gastric mucosa, 176–179
Gastric neoplastic lesions
    atrophic gastritis with tiny reddish area type 0-IIb, 208, 214–218
    pale lesion type 0-IIc, 208, 209
    reddish lesion type 0-IIa+b, 208, 210
    reddish lesion type 0-IIa+c, 208, 211–213
    small lesion 0-IIa, 213, 219
    suspect lesion 0-IIa+c, 213, 221
Gastric NET, 70
Gastric phenotype carcinoma, 36
Gastric wall, 80, 81
Gastroesophageal junction (GEJ), 108, 109, 141–143
Gastrointestinal (GI) tract, 80, 81, 101
    indications for endoscopic en-bloc resection in, 51, 53
    minimally invasive resection techniques, 71
        endoscopic resection techniques, 71
        LECS, 71
    subepithelial gastrointestinal tumors
        duodenal NET with fibrosis, 72, 75
        duodenum, NET in, 73
        gastric GIST, 73, 76
        SM layer, esophageal SET of, 72
        symptomatic esophageal SET, 72, 74
Gastrointestinal stromal tumor (GIST), 66, 87
Genomically stable tumor, 35
GI tract, morphologic carcinogenesis
    colonic neoplastic lesions, characteristics of, 30, 33
        classic polypoid adenoma–carcinoma pathway, 31
        flat/depressed colonic adenoma–carcinoma pathway, 31
        HNPCC, 34
        IBD, inflammation–dysplasia–cancer pathway, 34
        serrated adenoma–carcinoma pathway, 31, 34
    EMR/ESD, 41, 42
    endoscopic features, 25
    esophageal neoplastic lesions, characteristics of, 38
        Barrett's adenocarcinoma, 38
        squamous epithelial cell dysplasia–cancer pathway, 40, 41
    gastric adenocarcinomas, characteristics of, 35
        diffuse/signet-ring type gastric cancer, 36
        gastric phenotype carcinoma, 36
        HDGC, 38
        intestinal-type gastric adenocarcinoma, 36
    Paris Classification
        malignant mucosal neoplasms, classification of, 26, 27
        malignant potential, 27–29
    Western and Japanese classifications, 25
Glycogenic acanthosis, 130
Granular cell tumors (GCT), 67, 87

H

Hamartomatous polyps, 225
Hereditary diffuse-type gastric cancer (HDGC), 38
High-definition (HD) endoscopy, 4
High-grade anal dysplasias, 275
High-grade intraepithelial neoplasia (HGIN), 26, 121, 206, 207
High-resolution endoscopic ultrasound (hr-EUS), 79
    early neoplasia 0-IIc, 92, 97
    gastric lesion 0-IIc, 92
    gastrointestinal tract, endosonographic anatomy of, 80, 81
    neoplasia type 0-IIc, 92, 95
    performance of, 80
    small rectal lesion 0-Is, 90
    superficial epithelial neoplasias, staging, 82
        differential diagnosis of, 84
        limitations, 83, 84
        N staging, 83
        SEL, differential diagnosis of, 84, 86

SM/PM layer, tumors originating from, 87, 88, 90
tumor category, 82
Homogeneous protuberant lesions, 187–188
Human papillomavirus (HPV) infection, 275
Hybrid ESD, 53
Hyperechoic, 80
layer, 80
structure, 86
Hyperplastic (non-neoplastic) polyps (HP), 247
Hyperplastic polyposis (HPS), 269, 270
Hypoechoic, 80
arch, 82
fan, 82
layer, 80
lesion, 82
Hypopharynx
minute esophageal red spot, 140, 141
reddish lesion 0-IIb in, 144–146
SCC, endoscopic surveillance for, 121, 122

I

Image-enhanced endoscopy (IEE)
analysis, 12
mucosal neoplastic lesions, 10, 11
Incident low-grade dysplasia, 297
Inflammation–dysplasia–carcinoma pathway, 30
Inflammatory bowel disease (IBD)
colonic neoplasias, factors increasing risk, 293, 294
CRC risk, colonoscopic surveillance for
chromoendoscopy and magnifying NBI, 295
surveillance protocol, 294, 295
inflammation–dysplasia–cancer pathway, 34
neoplastic lesions
chronic ulcerative colitis, flat adenoma in, 302, 303
long-standing ulcerative colitis, flat carcinoma in, 302, 304
management of, 301, 302
raised dysplasia, 305, 306
surveillance colonoscopy for
dysplasia, focality of, 301
prevalent *vs.* incident low-grade dysplasia, 297
visible dysplasia , diagnosis of, 296–301
Inflammatory lesions, 128
Inflammatory polyps, 133
Inflammatory pseudopolyps, 247
Intestinal-type gastric adenocarcinoma, 36
Intraepithelial neoplasia (IEN), 38
Intramucosal cancer, 190
Intrapapillary capillary loops (IPCL), 12
Inverted diverticulum, 247
Invisible dysplasia, 35
Irregular microvessels, 201
Irregular narrowing of sm-echo, 82

J

Japan Esophageal Society (JES), 126
Japan NBI Expert Team (JNET), 14, 18

L

Lamina propria mucosa (LPM), 4, 5, 38
Laparoscopic-endoscopic cooperative surgery (LECS), 50, 72
Laparoscopic resection (LR), 47
Laterally spreading-type (LST) neoplasia, 7
Leiomyoma (LM), 67, 87
Light blue crests (LBC), 177
Lipoma, 86
Long-standing ulcerative colitis, flat carcinoma in, 302, 304
Low-grade dysplasia (LGD), 297
Lugol-unstained areas, 124
Lymphomas, 65, 86
Lypmphangioma, 84

M

Magnifying narrow-band imaging (M-NBI), 226
Malignant mucosal neoplasms, classification of, 26, 27
Massive submucosal invasion, 190
Microsatellite instability (MSI), 105
Microvascular patterns, 126, 128, 129
Minor invasive endoscopic surgery, 57, 58
Mixed-type serrated adenoma (MSA), 268
Modified Spigelman score, 224
Mucosa-associated lymphoid tissue (MALT) lymphoma, 65
Mucosal adenocarcinoma, underwater and acetic acid delineation of, 166, 167

Mucosal neoplasias
chronic inflammatory bowel disease (*see* Inflammatory bowel disease (IBD))
colorectum (*see* Colorectum)
duodenum and small bowel (*see* Small bowel adenomas)
endoscopic resection of, 271
ESD, 273, 274
snaring resection techniques, 272, 273
endoscopic submucosal dissection, 53, 55
complications, 56, 57
minor invasive endoscopic surgery, 57, 58
outcome of, 55, 56
GI tract, indications for endoscopic en-bloc resection in, 51, 53
squamous cell-lined esophagus and hypopharynx (*see* Squamous cell-lined esophagus)
stomach (*see* Stomach)
superficial epithelial neoplasias
endoscopic en-bloc resection techniques, 49, 50
laparoscopic resection techniques, 50, 51
polypectomy, EMR, and EFTRD, 48, 49
Mucosal neoplastic lesions
characteristics of, 6–9
IEE, analysis, 10–12, 14
colonic neoplasias, microarchitecture of, 13, 15
columnar mucosa-lined esophagus, microarchitecture of, 21, 22
gastric mucosa and neoplasia, microarchitecture of, 16, 18
magnifying endoscopy, 8, 10
squamous mucosa and neoplasias, capillary structure of, 12
standard endoscopy and chromoendoscopy techniques, 4
WLI and chromoendoscopy CE, 5, 6
Mucosal smooth muscle (MM) layer, 38
Multi Light™ system, 9

N
Narrow-band imaging (NBI), 4, 10, 295
Narrow-Band Imaging International Colorectal Endoscopic (NICE) classification, 14, 18
Neoplasias, 12, 128
Neoplastic lesions, 122, 133
Neoplastic non-ampullary mucosal lesions, differential diagnosis, 226, 228, 229
Neoplastic pits, 198
Neoplastic villi, 197–206
Neuroendocrine tumors (NET), 68–70, 88
Non-ampullary duodenal adenomas
duodenal adenocarcinoma with submucosal invasion, 235, 237
low-grade duodenal adenoma, 234–236
Non-exposed endoscopic wall inversion surgery (NEWS), 50, 51
Nonneoplastic lesions, 128
Non-neoplastic non-ampullary mucosal lesions, differential diagnosis, 226–229
Non-neoplastic polyps, 179
Nottingham classification, 156

O
Optical biopsy, 136

P
Panchromoendoscopy, 295
Pancreatobiliary reflux, 131
Partial circumferential incision (PCI) method, 53, 54
Periprocedural precautions, 114, 115
Permeation, 133
Pharyngeal squamous cell cancer, 107
Pigmented melanosis, 129
Pink color sign, 124
Pit-like structure, 201
Pit patterns, 14, 197–206
Pocket creating method (PCM), 53
Polyp–cancer sequence, 30
Polypectomy, 48
Polypoid lesions, 64
Poorly differentiated adenocarcinoma (*PDAC*), 20, 201
Poorly differentiated/undifferentiated early cancers, 29
Prevalent low-grade dysplasia, 297
Primary sclerosing cholangitis (PSC), 294
Proctosigmoiditis, 295
Protruded-type early colon cancer, 257
Protruded-type polyps, 241
Protruding lesions, 226
Protruding neoplasia, 254
Protuberant lesions, differential diagnosis of, 181–184
Pyloric type gastric adenomas, 183–184

R
Rare malignant neoplasias, 90
Rectal prolapse syndrome (RPS), 269
Reddish flat lesions, 128
Reddish protruding lesions, 133

S

Sentinel node navigation surgery (SNNS), 50
Serrated adenocarcinoma (SAC), 265
Serrated adenoma (SA), 31, 33, 252, 267
Serrated lesions (SL), 265
Serrated polyposis syndrome (SPS), 268, 270
Sessile/elevated SET, 64
Sessile hyperplastic polyp, 248
Sessile serrated adenomas (SSA), 265, 266, 268–269
Severe stenosis, 57
Shape pattern, 82
Small bowel adenomas
  ampullary adenomas, 225, 226
  endoscopic analysis of, 226, 227
  incidence and risk of malignant transformation, 223–225
  non-ampullary duodenal adenomas
    duodenal adenocarcinoma with submucosal invasion, 235, 237
    low-grade duodenal adenoma, 234–236
  non-neoplastic *vs.* neoplastic non-ampullary mucosal lesions, differential diagnosis, 226, 228, 229
Small early gastric cancer, 17
Snare polypectomy, 272
Soft tissue sarcoma, 66
Solid gastrointestinal SET
  gastric NET, 70
  GCT, 67, 68
  GIST, 66, 67
  leiomyoma, 67
  NET, 68, 70
  solid SET, 65
Solitary rectal ulcer, 249
Sporadic adenomas, 301
Sporadic mucosal cancer, 298
Sporadic non-ampullary duodenal adenomas, 223
Squamous cell cancer (SCC), esophageal and pharyngeal, 107
Squamous cell-lined esophagus
  endoscopic diagnosis of, 128, 131, 134–135, 138
  endoscopic resection, 137–140
  gastroesophageal junction, flat reddish area oral to, 141–143
  microvascular patterns, 126, 128, 129
  minute esophageal red spot, 140, 141
  SCC, endoscopic surveillance for, 121, 122
  WLI observation, endoscopic signs of neoplastic lesions, 122–124
Squamous epithelial cell dysplasia, 40, 41
Squamous mucosa, capillary structure of, 12
Stomach, 113
  curative endoscopic resection in, 30
  EGC, gastroscopy for detection, 176
    early gastric neoplasia, endoscopic structure of, 179, 180
    gastric mucosa, 176–179
  EGC on WLI
    mucosal early gastric cancer, invasion depth, 194, 195
    shape of lesion, invasion depth, 180–193
    shape of mucosal folds, invasion depth, 180–193
  EGN, endoscopic resection of, 207, 208
  gastric adenocarcinoma
    histological type, prediction of, 196–206
    pit patterns, 197–206
    surface pattern and vascular pattern, 201
    vascular patterns, 197–206
    villous pattern, 196–206
  gastric cancer, individuals with increased risk for, 175
  gastric neoplastic lesions
    atrophic gastritis with tiny reddish area type 0-IIb, 208, 214–218
    pale lesion type 0-IIc, 208, 209
    reddish lesion type 0-IIa+b, 208, 210
    reddish lesion type 0-IIa+c, 208, 211–213
    small lesion 0-IIa, 213, 219
    suspect lesion 0-IIa+c, 213, 221
  HGIN/superficially sm-invasive *vs.* deeply sm-invasive carcinoma, 206, 207
  observation with conventional WLI endoscopy, 180
    depressed lesions, differential diagnosis of, 185–193
    protuberant lesions, differential diagnosis of, 181–184
Subepithelial gastrointestinal tumors
  differential diagnosis of, 64, 65
  GI tract
    duodenal NET with fibrosis, 72, 75
    duodenum, NET in, 73
    endoscopic resection techniques, 71
    gastric GIST, 73, 76
    LECS, 71
    SM layer, esophageal SET of, 72
    symptomatic esophageal SET, 72, 74
  solid gastrointestinal SET
    gastric NET, 70
    GCT, 67, 68
    GIST, 66, 67
    leiomyoma, 67
    NET, 68, 70
    solid SET, 65
Subepithelial lesions (SEL), 63, 79
Submucosal fibrosis, 231
Submucosal invasion, 190

Submucosal lesion, 165, 166
Submucosal protuberant lesions, 195
Submucosal tunneling endoscopic resection (STER), 71, 74
Superficial AC, 257, 259
Superficial differentiated adenocarcinoma, 257
Superficial epithelial neoplasias
  endoscopic en-bloc resection techniques, 49, 50
  hr-EUS, 82
    differential diagnosis of, 84
    limitations, 83, 84
    N staging, 83
    SEL, differential diagnosis of, 84, 86
    SM/PM layer, tumors originating from, 87, 88, 90
    tumor category, staging of, 82
  laparoscopic resection techniques, 50, 51
  polypectomy, EMR, and EFTRD, 48, 49
Superficially sm-invasive carcinoma, 206, 207
Superficial muscle layer (SMM), 38
Superficial protruding lesions, 7
Superficial sm invasion, 156
Surface enhanced endoscopy, 196–206
Surface pattern, 170, 201
Systematic screening protocol for the stomach (SSS), 114

T
Tangential approach, 53
Tenting sign, 86
Traditional serrated adenomas (TSA), 268–269
Tumor budding, 28
Tunnelling technique, 53

U
UC-associated mucosal cancer, 299
Ulcerative colitis (UC), 298
Ulcerative proctitis, 295
Uncertain surface pattern, 204
Underwater EMR (UEMR), 231, 232
Undifferentiated adenocarcinoma, 195
Undifferentiated carcinoma, 257
Undifferentiated gastric cancers (PDAC), 180
Upper gastrointestinal endoscopy, 112, 113
Uppermost intact, 82

V
Vascular pattern (VP), 18, 197–206
Vascular tumors, 84
Vessel pattern (VP), 258–259
Villous pattern, 196–206
Villous structure, 201
Visible dysplasia, 35

W
Well differentiated adenocarcinoma (WDAC), 195
Well-differentiated mucosal cancer, 27
White light imaging (WLI), 5, 6

9783030011130

9783030011130